Lorraine,

One of the most rewarding things I have experienced working in VA telehealth is meeting and working with people I greatly admire & respect.

Passion, energy & integrity.

May we always travel the same!

Love & friendship,
Rita

Dear Lorraine -

While I never meant to harm our friendship, I know how much you mean to me in terms of our friendship! I know that it would be very important to have your professional advice to help me grow and flourish in my work & love. I will always cherish our friendship & will be very grateful to...

Home Telehealth: Connecting Care Within the Community

Edited by Richard Wootton, Susan L Dimmick and Joseph C Kvedar

Home Telehealth: Connecting Care Within the Community

Edited by

Richard Wootton

*Centre for Online Health, University of Queensland,
Royal Children's Hospital, Brisbane, Queensland, Australia*

Susan L Dimmick

*Office of Community Affairs, University of Tennessee Health
Science Center, Memphis, Tennessee, US*

Joseph C Kvedar

*Partners Telemedicine and Department of Dermatology,
Harvard Medical School, Boston, Massachusetts, US*

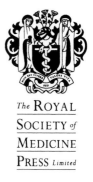

The ROYAL
SOCIETY *of*
MEDICINE
PRESS *Limited*

© 2006 Royal Society of Medicine Press Ltd

Published by the Royal Society of Medicine Press Ltd
1 Wimpole Street, London W1G 0AE, UK
Tel: +44 (0)20 7290 2921
Fax: +44 (0)20 7290 2929
Email: publishing@rsm.ac.uk
Website: www.rsmpress.co.uk

British Library Cataloguing in Publication Data
A catalogue record for this book is available from the British Library

ISBN 1-85315-657-4

Distribution in Europe and Rest of World:

Marston Book Services Ltd
PO Box 269
Abingdon
Oxon OX14 4YN, UK
Tel: +44 (0)1235 465500
Fax: +44 (0)1235 465555
Email: direct.order@marston.co.uk

Distribution in the USA and Canada:

Royal Society of Medicine Press Ltd
c/o BookMasters Inc
30 Amberwood Parkway
Ashland, OH 44805, USA
Tel: +1 800 247 6553/+1 800 266 5564
Fax: +1 419 281 6883
Email: order@bookmasters.com

Distribution in Australia and New Zealand:

Elsevier Australia
30-52 Smidmore Street
Marrikville NSW 2204, Australia
Tel: +61 2 9517 8999
Fax: +61 2 9517 2249
Email: service@elsevier.com.au

Typeset by Phoenix Photosetting, Chatham, Kent
Printed in the Netherlands by Alfabase, Alphen aan den Rijn

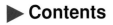# Contents

▶ List of contributors

Allyson M. Beach Oxford HealthCare, Springfield, MO, US

Mark Bensink Centre for Online Health, University of Queensland, Royal Children's Hospital, Brisbane, Queensland, Australia

Alicia Bergman Purdue University, West Lafayette, IN, US

David A. Bradley University of Abertay Dundee, Dundee, UK

Simon Brownsell Department of Medical Physics and Clinical Engineering, Barnsley Hospital NHS Foundation Trust, Barnsley, UK

Sam G. Burgiss University of Tennessee, Knoxville, TN, US

César Cáceres Bioengineering and Telemedicine Unit, Universidad Politécnica de Madrid, Madrid, Spain

Neale R. Chumbler Veterans Administration HSR&D Rehabilitation Outcomes Research Center, University of Florida, Gainesville, FL, US

Nhedti Colquitt Partners HealthCare and the Center for the Integration of Medicine and Innovative Technology, Boston, MA, US

Francisco Del Pozo Bioengineering and Telemedicine Unit, Universidad Politécnica de Madrid, Madrid, Spain

George Demiris University of Missouri-Columbia, Columbia, MO, US

Susan L. Dimmick Office of Community Affairs, University of Tennessee Health Science Center, Memphis, TN, US; ORAU/ORISE, US

Kathy Duckett Partners Home Care, Waltham, MA, US

Dottie Fazenbaker Home Nursing Agency, Altoona, PA, US

Penny Ford Carleton Partners HealthCare and the Center for the Integration of Medicine and Innovative Technology, Boston, MA, US

Felipe García Infectious Diseases Unit, Clinic Hospital, Barcelona, Spain

Amerigo Giordano Fondazione Salvatore Maugeri IRCCS Cardiology Division, Gussago/Lumezzane (BS), Italy

Enrique J. Gomez Bioengineering and Telemedicine Unit, Universidad Politécnica de Madrid, Madrid, Spain

David Hailey Centre for Online Health, University of Queensland, Royal Children's Hospital, Brisbane, Queensland, Australia

Val J. Halamandaris National Association for Homecare, Washington, DC, US

Mark S. Hawley Department of Medical Physics and Clinical Engineering, Barnsley Hospital NHS Foundation Trust, Barnsley, UK

Marilynne A. Hebert Health Telematics Unit, Faculty of Medicine, University of Calgary, Alberta, Canada

M. Elena Hernando Bioengineering and Telemedicine Unit, Universidad Politécnica de Madrid, Madrid, Spain

Christian Hervé Laboratoire d'Éthique Médicale et Médecine Légale, Faculté de Médecine de l'Université René Descartes, Paris, France

Irene Higginson Department of Palliative Care, Policy and Rehabilitation, School of Medicine, King's College London, London, UK

Kunka D. Ignatova College of Communication and Information, University of Tennessee, Knoxville TN, US

Roberto E. Izquierdo Joslin Diabetes Center and Division of Endocrinology, Diabetes and Metabolism, SUNY Upstate Medical University, Syracuse, NY, US

J.J. Jansen Health Telematics Unit, Faculty of Medicine, University of Calgary, Alberta, Canada

Barbara Johnston California Telemedicine and eHealth Center, Sacramento, CA, US

David Kaufman Department of Biomedical Informatics, Columbia University, New York, NY, US

Toshio Kishimoto Welfare Systems Research Laboratory, Okayama, Japan

Rita F. Kobb Office of Care Coordination, Veterans Health Administration, Lake City, FL, US

Joseph C. Kvedar Partners Telemedicine and Department of Dermatology, Harvard Medical School, Boston, MA, US

Nancy Lugn Perceptive Informatics, Boston, MA, US

Philip C. Morin Joslin Diabetes Center and Division of Endocrinology, Diabetes and Metabolism, SUNY Upstate Medical University, Syracuse, NY, US

Hiroshi Nakamoto Department of Medical Engineering and Systems Cardiology, Kawasaki Medical School, Kurashiki, Japan

Laurie Neander At Home Care Inc., Oneonta, NY, US

Michael Nebel KfH Nierenzentrum Koln-Merheim, Cologne, Germany

Shigeru Ohta Department of Health Informatics, Kawasaki University of Medical Welfare, Kurashiki, Japan

Catherine Ollivet L'association France-Alzheimer Seine-Saint-Denis, Le Raincy, France

Vedran Ostojić Department for Clinical Immunology and Pulmonology, Internal Medicine, 'Sveti Duh' General Hospital, Zagreb, Croatia

Walter Palmas Department of Biomedical Informatics, Columbia University, New York, NY, US

Herschel Peddicord III Honeywell HomMed, Milwaukee, WI, US

Luca Quareni QBGROUP spa, Padua, Italy

Vincent Rialle Laboratory TIMC-IMAG UMR CNRS 5525, Faculté de Médecine de Grenoble, Grenoble, France

Marcia Reissig Partners Home Care, Waltham, MA, US

Simon Robinson Empirica Communications and Technology Research, Bonn, Germany

Pierre Rumeau Federation of Geriatrics and Institut Européen Télémédicine, Toulouse University Hospital, Toulouse, France

Simonetta Scalvini Fondazione Salvatore Maugeri IRCCS Cardiology Division, Gussago/Lumezzane (BS), Italy

Paul A. Scuffham School of Medicine, Griffith University, Queensland, Australia

Yoshimitsu Shinagawa Department of Health Informatics and Biostatistics, Oita University of Nursing and Health Sciences, Oita, Japan

Susan G. Slater ViTel Net, McLean, VA, US

Justin Starren Department of Biomedical Informatics, Columbia University, New York, NY, US; Department of Radiology, Columbia University

Karl A. Stroetmann Empirica Communications and Technology Research, Bonn, Germany

Veli N. Stroetmann Empirica Communications and Technology Research, Bonn, Germany

Karen R. Thomas Oxford HealthCare, Springfield, MO, US

Andrea Tura ISIB-CNR, Padua, Italy

Ruth S. Weinstock Joslin Diabetes Center and Division of Endocrinology, Diabetes and Metabolism, SUNY Upstate Medical University, Syracuse, NY, US; Department of Veterans Affairs, VA Medical Center, Syracuse, NY, US

Lynn M. Whitten Regional Palliative and Hospice Care Service, Calgary Health Region, Calgary, Alberta, Canada

Pamela Whitten Department of Telecommunication, Michigan State University, East Lansing, MI, US

Christy M. Williams Partners Telemedicine and Department of Dermatology, Harvard Medical School, Boston MA, US

Richard Wootton Centre for Online Health, University of Queensland, Royal Children's Hospital, Brisbane, Queensland, Australia

Emanuela Zanelli Fondazione Salvatore Maugeri IRCCS Cardiology Division, Gussago/Lumezzane (BS), Italy

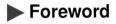

Foreword

From 1946 to 1964, the United States experienced a phenomenal growth in the number of babies born – some 77 million. These 'baby boomers' are fast approaching their sixties and, actuarially speaking, will live to the age of 85 years. This presents significant challenges for the healthcare industry. Shortages in the numbers of nurses and doctors to care for these baby boomers represent an additional cause for concern. For those of us in the homecare and hospice community, this is not surprising news, and many in the field have already embraced a 'high tech, high touch' approach to their operations.

Without losing the essential 'customer first' mindset, homecare and hospice agencies have been integrating technology into their care services, knowing that such important complementary tools help them to provide high-quality care at reasonable cost. This will be particularly important for the fast approaching surge of the aging population. New technologies are the answer to many of the vexing problems that face this industry. We view home telehealth in a positive light, as it enables caregivers, and those who employ them, to provide high-quality care to a large number of people who would not otherwise have access to it.

Technology positively affects healthcare in at least four ways. The first is at the 'point of care'. Rather than legal pads or clipboards, today's technologically aware physicians carry personal digital assistants (PDAs) or laptops. These devices enable the compilation of electronic health records (EHRs), which can be shared among multiple providers. One day, each of us may carry our own EHR as a microdot on our driver's licence or credit card, and this will give each practitioner we visit automatic access to our complete medical history. If we meet with an accident, essential personal health information will be immediately accessible to paramedics and emergency physicians, saving lives and unnecessary costs. Such tools will also allow the seamless integration of patient information among hospitals, physician specialists, and home care and hospice agencies. The importance of swift implementation of EHRs can be seen in the difficulty and frustration that healthcare providers and patients experienced in the aftermath of Hurricane Katrina, when medical records were not available.

The second way that technology affects healthcare is through telehealth. Telehealth, telemedicine or e-medicine refers to medical care delivered by telecommunications, including the Internet. This enables doctors and nurses to see, hear and talk to patients, take their vital signs and even conduct laboratory tests – all at a distance. It also allows for greater efficiency, increasing access to care in remote regions at lower costs. Telemonitoring devices give patients, their families and their practitioners the satisfaction of knowing that high-quality healthcare is being delivered on a daily basis. It also enables transparency, so that effective monitoring of costs for specific care and services is automatically documented, minimizing fraud and abuse, as well as costly investigations into such crimes.

The third aspect is through adaptive devices that diminish disability, making it possible for elderly individuals or those with disabilities to remain at home (or to help them leave home and become more fulfilled, productive members of society). This category includes the smart house, the lounge chair that tracks vital signs and the eyeglasses that prompt the wearer when they forget someone's name. Prototypes of equipment are also in development (and some are already in use), such as robots that carry out daily tasks for elderly people, robotic arms and legs that help people with disabilities live independently and robots designed to help deliver personal care to individuals who are infirm.

The fourth way is through advanced data management hardware and software that help industry to streamline their operations and to provide more efficient and effective services. A nice illustration of this concept is the story I like to tell about Southwest Airlines – a company whose software has helped them achieve great efficiency by tracking and lowering their costs and knowing where they stand at the close of business each day. This gives them speed and a vital competitive advantage. Such capacities are now available in the healthcare arena.

This book comes at a pivotal time in history. The new technology-based paradigm for healthcare and aging in place will bring huge benefits to patients, families, medical providers, caregivers and governmental agencies, as well as third-party payers. The authors have extensive expertise on this subject in general and in specific academic areas. This book will serve to advance medical technology in all parts of the world, and I wish all concerned every success in their endeavours.

Val J. Halamandaris
President and CEO,
National Association for
Homecare and Hospice,
Washington, DC, US

Preface

This is the eighth book in the Royal Society of Medicine's series of multi-author books on telemedicine topics. It is designed to provide examples of best practice. The book's predecessors are:

- *The Legal and Ethical Aspects of Telemedicine*, BA Stanberry, 1998
- *Introduction to Telemedicine*, R Wootton and J Craig (eds), 1999
- *Teledermatology*, R Wootton and AMM Oakley (eds), 2002
- *Telepsychiatry and e-Mental Health*, R Wootton, P Yellowlees and P McLaren (eds), 2003
- *Telepediatrics: Telemedicine and Child Health*, R Wootton and J Batch (eds), 2004
- *Teleneurology*, R Wootton and V Patterson (eds), 2005
- *Introduction to Telemedicine, second edition*, R Wootton, J Craig and V Patterson (eds), 2006

The present volume describes how telemedicine can be applied to the care of patients at home. Home telehealth is being practised in many parts of the world, and the book's contributors, who come from 10 countries on four continents, reflect this. All have practical experience, many are practising clinicians and most have published in detail on their respective subjects. The book presents the experience of practitioners across a wide range of applications of telemedicine in home healthcare.

Recent years have seen a growth in home telehealth activity. Reports of the first randomized, controlled trials are beginning to appear, and it is clear that the discipline will form an important part of future home care. Therefore, the time seems to be right to try and distil the early experience of home telehealth practitioners into book form. It is a pleasure to acknowledge the contribution of Honeywell HomMed LLC, iMetrikus Inc and VitelNet, prominent American suppliers of home telehealth systems and services, towards the cost of producing the book.

The aim of the book is to show how telemedicine can be applied to home care and to challenge clinicians to consider it in their everyday working practice. Although it is most relevant to practising clinicians, many chapters will be of interest to health service managers, planners and information technology staff. We think that anyone involved in telemedicine will find the material interesting, because much of it is relevant to other fields, rather than simply to home care.

This book is divided into four sections:

- a section dealing with the basics
- a section dealing with techniques
- a section describing applications
- a section concerning the future.

The emphasis is on the utility of the discipline, rather than on the technology itself. We therefore have deliberately kept the technical information to a minimum. (Readers who are anxious for more may consult previous books in the series.) We hope that in the broad spectrum of ideas expressed in this book, everyone will find something of relevance to their individual practice. We hope you enjoy reading it.

Richard Wootton
Brisbane, Australia

Susan L. Dimmick
Knoxville, US

Joseph C. Kvedar
Boston, US

April 2006

▶1

Introduction

Richard Wootton, Susan L. Dimmick and Joseph C. Kvedar

Introduction

The world's population is aging. In Japan, for example, a quarter of the population will soon be older than 65 years (Fig. 1.1). As we age, the incidence and prevalence of chronic illness continue to rise. Furthermore, elderly patients typically have multiple chronic diseases (Fig. 1.2). This is one reason why expenditure on healthcare is skewed: in most healthcare delivery systems, 5% of patients are responsible for 50% of costs.[1] These patients are at the heart of the looming crisis in healthcare costs that is beginning to occupy the policy discussions of most governments in the industrialized world. The economic consequences of chronic diseases are even more serious in the developing world: 80% of deaths from chronic disease occur in low- and middle-income countries, and World Health Organization estimates suggest that losses of national income will amount to billions of dollars (Fig. 1.3).[2]

We must find a more compelling way to care for these patients – a strategy that maintains or increases quality and access, while decreasing cost. The challenge is complicated by the supply and demand curve in healthcare. The number of chronically ill people increases each year. For example, in the US, the number of Medicare

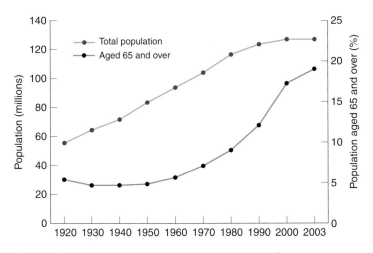

Fig. 1.1. Proportion of the Japanese population older than 65 years[10]

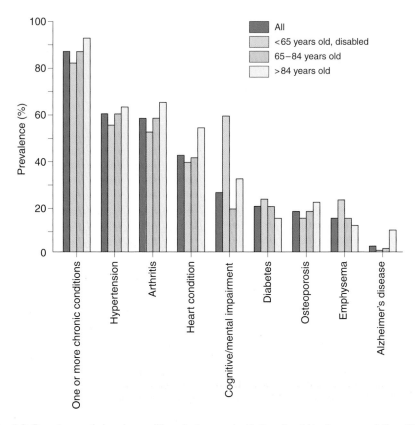

Fig. 1.2. Prevalence of chronic conditions in the non-institutionalized Medicare population, 2002. Heart condition is defined as a diagnosis of angina, hardening of arteries, myocardial infarction, congestive heart failure or problem with heart valves or heart rhythm. Cognitive/mental impairment is defined as a diagnosis of mental retardation, mental disorder or Alzheimer s disease or having memory loss that interferes with daily activity[11]

beneficiaries is steadily increasing (see Fig. 1.4) (Medicare is a social insurance programme that provides healthcare for almost 42 million elderly and disabled Americans). At the same time as demand is rising, apparently inexorably, there are global provider shortages. In the US, the mean age of nursing professionals is 42 years. There is already an acute nursing shortage, and there is no realistic prospect that this will change in the short term.[3] Documentation that relates to physician shortage is harder to find, but most medical deans, for example, believe that a physician shortage is looming.[4]

Dramatic increases in the numbers of chronically ill patients in the face of shrinking provider numbers and significant cost pressures mean that a fundamental change is required in the process of care. Several imperatives are born of this impending crisis. One is the need to provide patients with feedback systems that will allow them to self-manage more effectively. A second is to create models in which population-based care

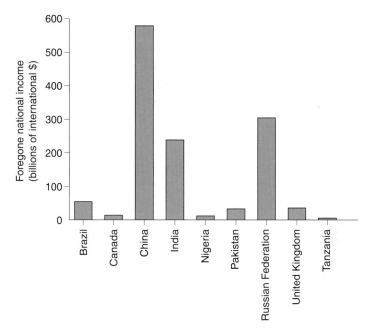

Fig. 1.3. World Health Organization's estimates of foregone national income due to heart disease, stroke and diabetes in selected countries, 2005–15 (billions of constant 1998 international dollars).[2] An international dollar is a hypothetical currency that is used as a means of translating and comparing costs from one country to another, using a common reference point (the US dollar). An international dollar has the same purchasing power as the US dollar has in the United States

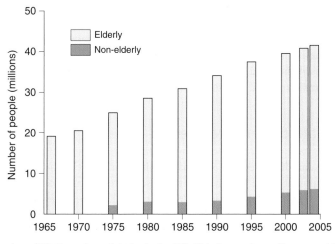

Fig. 1.4. Number of Medicare beneficiaries in the US. Elderly people are those aged 65 years and over. Non-elderly disabled people include those with end-stage renal disease[11]

is practised and rewarded financially. The one-to-one model of care, especially the transaction-based care model currently employed in the US, is outmoded. A third imperative is to move care out of institution-owned physical spaces. Today's healthcare leaders are gravely concerned that they will not be able to continue to service demand by constructing more buildings.

All the above factors combine to create a serious situation for healthcare planners around the world. They also, however, create the opportunity for innovation in the process of care.

Home telehealth

Home telehealth has no generally accepted definition. Clearly the term is intended to indicate the use of telemedicine techniques in a non-institutional setting – that is, at home or in an assisted-living facility. Such telemedicine techniques are normally divided into those that involve videoconferencing and those in which patients are monitored in some way. Overlap exists between the categories.

Home telehealth systems combine a number of interesting attributes. Physiological monitoring leads to richer data and therefore to improved decision making. Giving patients access to their own physiological data leads to improved self-care. In some cases, patients are so enthusiastic that they purchase the equipment with their own money. It is also worth noting that technologies are available to support home telehealth:

- cheap, accessible computing
- always-connected consumers (mobile phones and the Internet)
- wireless sensors that can be worn and require low power.

The use of home telehealth thus allows patients to be monitored at home, nurses to visit in person less often and better management of chronic disease. This brings cost savings if unnecessary visits can be avoided – either by the provider to the home, or by the patient to a physician's office or a hospital emergency room. There may be subsidiary benefits in the form of earlier detection of problems – and thus earlier initiation of treatment – and improved patient education. The latter may produce better medication compliance and lead to improved lifestyle choices.

Present state of home telehealth

The last few years have seen an increase in the number of manufacturers of home telehealth equipment in the US (mainly) and elsewhere. An increase has also occurred in the number of home telehealth episodes. During 2001–03, the number of Medicare home health users increased to 2.6 million and the number of episodes rose to 36 million. At the same time, the average number of visits per episode fell slightly to 17.3 (Chetney R, personal communication, 2005). Thus there are signs that interest in home telehealth is awakening. Recent data show that 20% of American-based home health agencies employ some kind of telehealth in their day-to-day operations and another 20% plan to offer telehealth services in the next 12 months (Flynn J, personal communication, 2005). As healthcare costs continue to rise steeply, payers (that is, governmental payers and large employers) have begun to look at creative solutions. A recent White House conference on aging concluded that technology could be used to improve the aging experience in America. It also called for the removal of barriers to and creation of incentives for the deployment of existing and future telehealth technologies.[5]

Patients are eager to embrace technology as part of their care. No evidence shows that elderly people, for example, are technophobic. In a recent poll for Harris Interactive/*Wall Street Journal*, 87% of chronically ill patients who were online had looked for healthcare information on the Internet.[6] A study of elderly patients in rural eastern Tennessee noted that patients and caregivers found substantial benefit in using two-way videoconferencing and remote monitoring. The key was to keep the telehealth technology as similar as possible to the domestic technologies with which the patients were familiar – the telephone and the television.[7]

Providers are cautiously adopting home telehealth. The nursing profession was the first group to embrace home telehealth, and primary care providers are now beginning to dip a toe into the water. Specialists and hospitals will no doubt follow in due course. Some preliminary evidence shows that home telehealth can reduce healthcare utilization, and hence costs, although definitive studies are awaited.[8]

The field is blossoming, but decision-makers continue to seek definitive data on outcomes and cost-effectiveness before making large investments. Important principles in the introduction of any new technique in medicine are that the outcomes should be the same or better than conventional practice and that the costs should be the same or preferably lower. As this book shows, evidence on these points is beginning to emerge in various areas of home telehealth.

Why a book on home telehealth?

Home telehealth depends on technology, although it is very important to recognize that the technology is only one component of a successful home telehealth programme. This book therefore mentions the technology but does not dwell on it. As in much other telemedicine work, the human and organizational factors will ultimately determine success or failure.[9] The experience reported in this book shows clearly that the success of home telehealth rests as much on the behaviour of the providers and patients as it does on the underlying technology. The American Telemedicine Association has drawn up guidelines for home telehealth (Box 1.1), and, properly, the criteria that relate to technology are but one aspect of the whole.

The history of telemedicine has been bedevilled by loose terminology that, some observers feel, has not helped its cause. What began originally as 'telemedicine' successively has become 'telehealth', 'online health', 'e-health' and so on. In this book, different contributors use slightly different terms to describe their home telehealth experience, depending on their local environment. Although the editors

---

Box 1.1. Excerpts from the American Telemedicine Association's home telehealth clinical guidelines[12]

Patients
- Informed written consent must be obtained before starting home telehealth
- An assessment should be conducted to determine access to utilities and safety concerns appropriate for the installation of the equipment
- Patients (or their designated caregiver) must demonstrate their ability to use and maintain the equipment according to the agency's policy
- The first and last home visit to the patient's home must be in person and not through a video visit

Providers
- A physician order to integrate home telehealth into the plan of care must be obtained
- The agency personnel who provide home telehealth must document each video visit in the patient's chart
- Changes in the frequency of video visits are to be treated like changes in other parts of the plan of treatment and should be approved by the physician
- Patients must be given clear written instructions as to whom to call in case problems arise

Technology
- The technology used should be based on the patient's clinical and functional needs
- Home telehealth equipment should be checked for accuracy against standard devices on installation
- Safety instructions should be given to patients and reviewed on installation and at future times as necessary
- Instructions on whom to call for patient questions and concerns regarding equipment must be provided to patients and agency staff

---

have tried to reduce the number of terms used, we deliberately have not enforced a uniform terminology throughout, in recognition of these local differences.

It is the editors' intention that this book should serve two purposes. It is a state-of-the-art review of home telehealth in the early twenty-first century. It also should provide a reference and a high-level operations manual. Readers should feel more comfortable about implementation of home telehealth applications after reviewing chapters of specific interest to them.

The first two sections of the book describe the nuts and bolts of successful planning for the implementation of telehealth – business models, evaluation strategies and an up-to-date literature review all are included here. In addition, a wide variety of home telehealth techniques are described, including wound management, smart homes and the role of telehealth in quarantine. The third section is application oriented. This section uses a disease-state-oriented approach to illustrate the application of home telehealth technologies in practice. The book concludes with a glimpse of what the future may hold.

We hope you enjoy reading the work reported in this book and benefiting from the experience of others.

References

1   Berk ML, Monheit AC. The concentration of health care expenditures, revisited. *Health Aff (Millwood)* 2001;**20**:9–18.
2   World Health Organization. *Preventing chronic diseases: a vital investment.* Geneva: World Health Organization, 2005. Available at: www.who.int/chp/chronic_disease_report/contents/en/index.html (last accessed 8 January 2006).
3   Buerhaus PI, Staiger DO, Auerbach DI. Implications of an aging registered nurse workforce. *JAMA* 2000;**283**:2948–54.
4   Cooper RA, Stoflet SJ, Wartman SA. Perceptions of medical school deans and state medical society executives about physician supply. *JAMA* 2003;**290**:2992–5.
5   Center for Aging Services Technologies (CAST). *Statement from Eric Dishman, Chair, Center for Aging Services Technologies, about the outcomes of the White House Conference on Aging.* Washington, DC: CAST, 2005. Available at: www.agingtech.org/documents/whcoa_statement.doc (last accessed 8 January 2006).
6   Harris Interactive. *Harris Interactive conducts first major online study of the chronically ill.* Rochester, NY: Harris Interactive. Available at: www.harrisinteractive.com/news/allnewsbydate.asp?NewsID=20 (last accessed 12 January 2006).
7   Dimmick SL, Mustaleski C, Burgiss SG, Welsh T. A case study of benefits & potential savings in rural home telemedicine. *Home Healthc Nurse* 2000;**18**:124–35.
8   Galbreath AD, Krasuski RA, Smith B, *et al.* Long-term healthcare and cost outcomes of disease management in a large, randomized, community-based population with heart failure. *Circulation* 2004;**110**:3518–26.
9   Wootton R, Craig J, Patterson V. *Introduction to telemedicine.* London: Royal Society of Medicine Press, 2006.
10 Japan Aging Research Centre. *Aging in Japan.* Tokyo: Japan Aging Research Centre, 2003. Available at: www.jarc.net/aging/03oct/index.shtml (last accessed 8 January 2006).
11 Cubanski J, Voris M, Kitchman M, *et al. Medicare chartbook.* Washington, DC: Henry J. Kaiser Family Foundation, 2005. Available at: www.nahc.org/MedicareChartbook05.pdf (last accessed 14 January 2006).
12 American Telemedicine Association. *Home telehealth clinical guidelines.* Washington, DC: American Telemedicine Association, 2002. Available at: www.atmeda.org/ICOT/hometelehealthguidelines.htm (last accessed 8 January 2006).

Section 1: Basics

►2

Outcomes

Susan G. Slater, Laurie Neander and Dottie Fazenbaker

Introduction

Home telehealth has been claimed to provide the same or better clinical results than conventional care, improved access, increased cost-effectiveness and better patient self-management. How do we know whether these claims are true? The answer lies in comparing the outcomes of care delivered by home telehealth with those when healthcare is delivered by conventional methods. In healthcare, outcomes are those results that occur after an intervention is made. The intervention can be formal, as in a controlled study, or informal, as in the customary delivery of care in a real-world setting. Outcomes research 'evaluates the impact of healthcare (including discrete interventions such as particular drugs, medical devices, and procedures as well as broader programmatic or system interventions) on the health outcomes of patients and populations. It may include evaluation of economic impacts linked to health outcomes, such as cost-effectiveness and cost utility.'[1]

Outcome indicators

In home telehealth, a range of outcome indicators may be used (Box 2.1). A well-accepted outcome is based on an accumulation of evidence. Evidence is established by choosing outcome indicators that are valid and reliable. Validity means that the indicator measures what it is intended to measure. Reliability means that the indicator produces the same results repeatedly under similar circumstances.

The Canadian telehealth outcomes indicators project was initiated to overcome a major barrier to the broad adoption of telehealth in Canada. The barrier was the lack of standardized and measurable outcome indicators to demonstrate the value of telehealth applications. The project goal was to use a national consensus-building process to develop outcome measures in four areas of telehealth evaluation: quality, cost, access and acceptability. These themes were first identified in an Institute of Medicine report about factors relevant to the evaluation of telemedicine programmes.[3]

In the Canadian project, there was general agreement that a telehealth outcomes development (TOD) model would assist in the evaluation of a diverse group of telehealth projects. The model includes, among other things, indicators, measures and tools (Table 2.1). These can be used to evaluate the four areas of quality, cost, access and acceptability (Tables 2.2–2.5, respectively).

Box 2.1. Case study – Dorothy

Dorothy spent her 81st year averaging one hospitalization per month for complications related to congestive heart failure. But she spent her 82nd year at home, using telehealth equipment that kept her connected to her healthcare team (Fig. 2.1). While in her home, Dorothy could interact with clinicians in much the same way as if she was in a clinic or emergency room. This made it possible to detect any change in her condition quickly.[2] Nearly three years later, Dorothy had had no hospitalizations related to congestive heart failure.

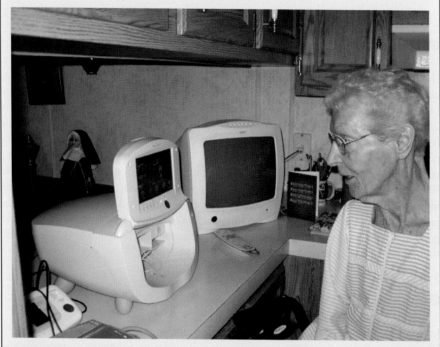

Fig. 2.1. Patient using telehealth equipment (Turtle 600 and ViTel Net) at Home Care, Oneonta, NY, US

Comment

Several outcomes were evident for Dorothy. The clinical outcome was reduced hospitalizations. The quality-of-life outcome was being able to remain in her home as well as participating in her own care. The quality-of-care outcome was more rapid access to her clinicians.

Table 2.1. Indicators, measures and tools from the Canadian Telehealth Outcomes Development model

Indicators	Measures	Tools
Quality of life	Morbidity	Minnesota Living with Heart Failure Questionnaire
Quality of care	Number of hospitalizations	Caregiver Burden Inventory
Timeliness	Length of stay	Short-Form McGill Pain Questionnaire
Availability	Distance to nearest facility	

Table 2.2. Potential outcome indicators and measures for the area of quality from the Canadian Telehealth Outcomes Development model

Outcome indicator	Outcome measure
Quality of life	• Limitations in physical activities because of health problems
	• Limitations in usual role activities because of physical health problems
	• Bodily pain
	• General health perceptions
	• Vitality (energy and fatigue)
	• Limitations in social activities because of emotional problems
	• Limitations in usual role activities because of emotional problems
	• Mental health (psychological distress and well-being)
Health status	• Changes in morbidity
	• Population perspective on changes to health status – that is, client assessment

Table 2.3. Potential outcome indicators and measures for the area of cost from the Canadian Telehealth Outcomes Development model

Outcome indicator	Outcome measure
Equipment	• Installation
	• Equipment and depreciation costs
	• Software
	• Service charge
	• Maintenance costs
Patient/itinerant clinician travel	• Average cost per trip to healthcare centre
Communication	• Line fees
	• Installation of integrated services digital network (ISDN) line
	• Long-distance connection
	• Data transmission costs
	• Mobile phone usage
	• Modem costs
Administrative	• Administrative expenses
	• Supplies
Staffing	• Salaries and wages
	• Fees for service
	• Hospital personnel costs

Table 2.4. Potential outcome indicators and measures for the area of access from the Canadian Telehealth Outcomes Development model

Outcome indicator	Outcome measure
Utilization of healthcare services	• Length of hospital stay
	• Number of emergency visits
	• Number of hospitalizations
	• Number of physician visits
Timeliness of care	• Length of wait to see a healthcare worker
(this is most easily identified as	• Length of wait for specialist care, such as magnetic resonance
relevant to the clinical setting)	imaging
Availability	• Distance to the nearest healthcare facility
	• Rural versus urban, and distance to nearest healthcare facility in each setting
	• Category of nearest facility – hospital or clinic; primary, secondary or tertiary care

Table 2.5. Potential outcome indicators and measures for the area of acceptability (satisfaction) from the Canadian Telehealth Outcomes Development model

Outcome indicator	Outcome measure
Rate of use	• Clinical – number of consultations per month
	• Research –number of meetings per month
	• Education – number of sessions per month
	• Administrative – number of meetings per month
	• Mixed – total number of events per month
Convenience	• Number of trips avoided
Client satisfaction	• Global impressions of telehealth
	• Technological performance
	• Exchange of knowledge
	• Physical presence
	• Confidentiality

Quality of life

The indicators, measures and tools described above can be used to demonstrate the value of home telehealth programmes. Evidence showing that this method of delivering healthcare is the same as or better than current methods is essential if the technique is to be adopted more widely.

A primary target audience for home telehealth is the chronically ill. Bayliss *et al* noted that 'the goal of caring for persons with chronic medical conditions is frequently to maximize quality of life, rather than to cure illness.'[4] One of the most frequently cited benefits of home telehealth is that individuals who want to stay at home can do so longer by using remote monitoring, for example. Using the guidelines discussed in the Canadian model, an acceptable indicator would be quality-of-life (QoL) benchmarks before and after remote monitoring is begun. A suitable measure of QoL would be the number of days an individual was able to cook a meal. An appropriate QoL tool would be the international Activities of Daily Living (ADL) scale.

QoL is the ability of individuals to enjoy their lives in a fulfilling manner. For some people, this could be retaining physical functionality, experiencing physical and emotional enjoyment, or continuing to live at home. Healthcare workers are often called on to evaluate a person's QoL, and these evaluations contribute to the execution of their plan of care. A standard QoL measure evaluates a patient's ability to perform activities of daily living, such as:

• the ability to take a shower or bathe without significant symptoms of heart failure (for example, shortness of breath)
• the ability to make a meal
• the ability to eat a meal
• the ability to dress
• the ability to walk to and use the toilet.

Another outcome tool, the International Classification of Functioning, Disability and Health, is becoming accepted as a standard for measurement of functional status – ranging from no impairment in functional status or activities of daily living to complete impairment or dependency for activities of daily living. Porell and Miltiades showed an association between the degree of functional decline and limited access to healthcare services among elderly patients with one or more chronic healthcare conditions.[5] On the basis of this association, it might be concluded that the use of telehealth would create better access and perhaps lead to the kind of professional and social support that would help patients to bolster their functionality and consequently their ADL scores.

In addition to physical functioning, outcomes measured in QoL surveys also include health status, depression and self-care. Several QoL outcome tools have been developed and tested for validity. One tool that is commonly used for assessment is the Short Form 36 (SF-36) questionnaire.[6] This has 36 questions and is a generic measurement that does not target any specific age group, disease group or treatment group. The SF-36 is useful for comparisons in groups of patients with specific diseases and problems, such as cardiovascular disease, chronic obstructive pulmonary disease, depression and transplantation.

A shorter version of the tool, the Short Form 12 (SF-12), comprises 12 questions from the SF-36 tool. Both versions have been found to be very helpful in surveys of general and specific populations and have been documented in nearly 4000 publications. More information pertaining to these forms, such as validity and reliability, can be found on the SF-36 website.[6]

Patients with chronic medical conditions commonly have additional comorbid conditions that can affect their QoL (Box 2.2). It is important to evaluate QoL with comorbidity, because the subjective assessments of QoL correlate with mortality, job loss and many other measurable outcomes. Many factors contribute to patients' perception of their overall QoL. One factor is the social support received. Several caregivers may be involved in delivering care, such as a spouse, or another relative or significant other.[7] Support is important: many patients with complex chronic diseases have depression and have a need to feel supported.

One of the primary goals of home telehealth is to identify early exacerbations of patient conditions, especially for patients with chronic conditions, such as heart failure, diabetes and depression. Using telehealth, subtle changes in a patient's condition that indicate deterioration of health status may be identified. Home telehealth monitoring therefore is integral to an early and effective response to the decline of those with chronic healthcare conditions.

A 24-month longitudinal study of the effect of telehealth for individuals with heart failure demonstrated significantly reduced hospital admissions (63% decline) and readmission rates (75% decline).[8] In addition, when hospitalization was required, the average length of stay was significantly shorter for those served by home telehealth.[9] A six-month study of home telehealth for 15 patients with heart failure in Colorado showed a 90% reduction in hospital admissions, a 100% reduction in emergency hospital visits and a 50% reduction in the agency's staffing costs because of a decrease in the number of home visits.[10]

The US Department of Veterans Affairs was an early adopter of home telehealth in an effort to reduce emergency care and rehospitalizations. In total, 92 patients with a new or unstable diagnosis of heart failure were studied. Marked reductions in blood pressure, body weight and shortness of breath ratings were seen for those monitored daily by telehealth. In addition, in comparison with the previous year, the total inpatient hospital days were reduced by 80%, and only 31% of those hospitalizations were directly attributable to heart failure.[11]

Unlike traditional home healthcare, home telehealth monitoring increases the number and frequency of patient assessment days. Routine monitoring of real-time patient physiological information enables home visiting that is based on clinical need, early identification of deteriorating clinical values, enhanced clinical decision-making and avoidance of the progression of illness.

Box 2.2. Case study – Andy

Andy was a 93-year-old gentleman who suffered from a multitude of health problems: heart failure, chronic obstructive pulmonary disease, history of myocardial infarction, renal failure, colon cancer with metastasis to the bone, neurogenic bladder, anaemia and hypertension. With acute exacerbations of heart failure, Andy was hospitalized for two lengthy periods during the six months before home telehealth was initiated. After admission to telehealth in 2003, Andy required only two hospitalizations for the period June 2004–April 2005. The first admission was unrelated to his cardiac condition, being the result of a need to surgically repair a strangulated bowel secondary to metastatic disease. The second admission was for acute exacerbation of heart failure because of a failure to respond to treatment with diuretics at home.

After Andy's final discharge from hospital, the home telehealth nurse noted significant instability in his condition through daily telehealth monitoring. Data changes were communicated promptly to his physician, and frequent adjustments of his medication became necessary. On the basis of the trends in his telehealth data, standing orders for medication adjustments were implemented.

Despite Andy's advanced age and deteriorating condition, only one unscheduled home nursing visit was required while he was on telehealth, and he required only one rehospitalization for treatment of his cardiac disease. Without telehealth, the physician, nurse and patient agreed that the subtle changes in Andy's condition would not have been identified early enough to adjust the treatment plan and avoid recurrent hospitalizations.

Comment
The patient and caregivers were pleased with telehealth monitoring as it 'alleviated many worries'. On many occasions, Andy had been known to contact the telehealth nurse after working hours to report a perceived decline in his respiratory status. By remote monitoring, the nurse was able to verify that Andy's blood oxygen concentration was in acceptable limits and alleviate his concerns (Fig. 2.2). This contributed to enhanced self-management of Andy's chronic disease. The physician also noted a marked decrease in the number of 'panic calls' and firmly believed that the remote monitoring had not only decreased cost to the healthcare delivery system but, perhaps more importantly, had also improved Andy's quality of life by enabling him to remain in his preferred setting – at home.

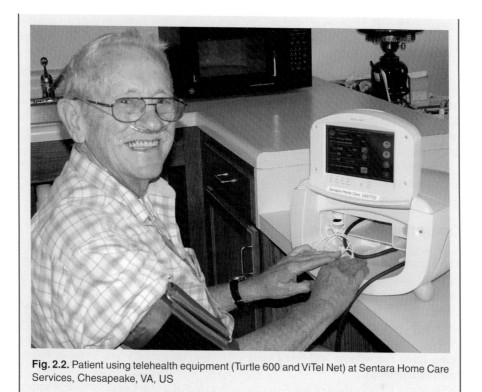

Fig. 2.2. Patient using telehealth equipment (Turtle 600 and ViTel Net) at Sentara Home Care Services, Chesapeake, VA, US

Risk adjustment

In the US, government regulations require Medicare-certified home healthcare agencies to collect data on all patients enrolled in public payer programmes. This information is reported to the Centers for Medicare and Medicaid Services (CMS). The instrument/data collection tool used to collect and report performance data is the Outcome and Assessment Information Set (OASIS).

The data collected are used for risk adjustment, benchmarking and consumer reporting. As healthcare shifts to a payment-for-performance model based on outcome measures, it is becoming clear that variations among patient characteristics, organizational practice patterns and provider behaviours contribute to variations in the results reported. Recognizing the importance of adjusting for these variations, the health data analysis company Strategic Health Programs (SHP) collected and analysed OASIS data from homecare agencies for a 27-month period ending in March 2004. The company compared 14 488 patients who had been remote monitored at home with 235 994 patients who had received usual care. The patients had at least one of the following diagnoses: congestive heart failure, coronary artery disease, diabetes, chronic obstructive pulmonary disease or asthma. There were significant comorbidities. The pattern of comorbidity was not the same between the two groups, however, necessitating a risk adjustment (by severity stratification) to compare patients with similar diagnostic profiles.

The analysis showed a smaller number of acute care rehospitalizations among telemonitored patient groups than those not monitored.[12] In patients with congestive heart failure, hospitalizations were seen in 10.1% of non-monitored patients and in 6.2% of monitored patients; emergency care visits were seen in 8.8% and 4.5%, respectively. Similar reductions were observed in patients with diabetes, coronary artery disease and chronic obstructive pulmonary disease.

The SHP risk-adjusted outcomes study clearly shows that diabetes and heart failure are chronic diseases that can be managed successfully by home telehealth.

Operating outcomes

The Kaiser Permanente telehealth project showed a 33–50% decrease in cost of care delivery and increased patient satisfaction.[13] Part of the cost savings were due to a significant decrease in the nursing time required: an average of 15–20 minutes for a telehealth visit and 45 minutes plus travel time and mileage to conduct a direct in-home visit. Net savings of $70–80 per visit have been shown elsewhere.[14] The capacity to visit more patients without additional nurses – or to increase the number of patients being cared for without additional staff – is likely to be very important in future healthcare delivery.

The Pennsylvania Home Care Association conducted a study to determine whether a link exists between the use of telehealth and home-care nurse satisfaction, staff retention and improved productivity.[15] Early data showed improvements in all three domains in agencies that had adopted home telehealth. For example, the 23 agencies that used telehealth had 15 patients per registered nurse, whereas the 11 agencies that did not use telehealth had 11 patients per nurse.

The traditional model of home healthcare service delivery, in which clinicians have to drive substantial distances to isolated rural homes to provide healthcare services, is expensive, inefficient and unsustainable. Results show that telehealth enables a home healthcare agency to increase its census without additional nursing staff – enhancing its capacity to do more with less. Clinically indicated direct home visits effectively supplement telehealth visits, thereby reducing cost, improving the productivity of nurses and increasing the availability of nurses for patients with complex acute care needs who require the provision of direct in-home services.

Potential variability in outcomes reporting

A number of variables in operating environments have the potential to affect telehealth outcomes. To reduce differences between providers and decrease variability in outcomes reporting, organizations that use telehealth equipment should consider standardizing their approach. Factors for consideration include:

- Effective use of telehealth equipment: Acute exacerbation of disease is not something that occurs only during the working week. To demonstrate the value of telehealth, access to remote monitoring must occur on a routine and daily basis. This will allow the detection of subtle changes in patients' conditions and early intervention, with the potential to avoid hospitalization. Web-based applications facilitate remote or off-site clinician monitoring and improved access to patient data.
- System interoperability: Integration of telehealth applications and electronic patient records is essential to achieve improved operating efficiencies, shared decision-making between providers, improved patient–provider communications, secure messaging between care providers and system-generated reports based on standardized methodologies to determine outcome.
- Timely placement of monitors: Early identification of patients suitable for telehealth monitoring is required. Once identified, there must be timely installation of the necessary equipment in the patient's home.
- Technology flexibility: A combination of video and non-video monitors must be available to suit specific groups on the basis of diagnostics, age, dependency, functional ability and illness.
- Clinical continuity: Continuity is required to:
  - maintain consistency in methods of patient education
  - maintain consistency of data flow or communications between the patient and providers
  - facilitate rapport with a predominantly elderly population that is participating in a 'technology-based environment'
  - maintain consistency of record-keeping and outcome reporting.
- Patient education: Standardized education is important to ensure appropriate use of the monitoring equipment and to optimize patient knowledge about effective disease-management and hospital-avoidance strategies. Daily telemonitoring should be a component of the patient's morning routine.

Conclusion

The importance of demonstrating outcomes for telehealth interventions cannot be overstated. It is also essential to have appropriate tools to measure them. For example, timeliness of care (that is, length of time before a healthcare provider can be seen) may be used as an indicator of access to healthcare. Indicators and measures already in use are the preferred way to develop standard evaluation tools for telehealth. This is not to say that innovation in telehealth evaluation should be discouraged, but it is time to move from the 'starting from scratch' approach of studying telehealth to building on the work of others.

The key to the acceptance of telehealth as standard practice lies in peer-reviewed publications that provide proof that home telehealth is the same as or better than traditional home health practices. A body of evidence is certainly developing, but better controlled studies will be required to fully understand telehealth's effectiveness in creating better quality of life/care, access and acceptability at the same or lower cost. Studies must use common definitions, indicators, measures and tools before conclusions can be reached about telehealth outcomes.

Further information

Centers for Medicare and Medicaid Services. *Home health quality initiatives: overview.* Baltimore, MD: Centers For Medicare and Medicaid Services, 2005. Available at: www.cms.hhs.gov/HomeHealthQualityInits/ (last accessed 20 December 2005).

Ministry of Health and Long-Term Care. *Health outcomes for better information and care.* Toronto: Ministry of Health and Long-Term Care, 2002. Available at: www.health.gov.on.ca/english/providers/project/nursing/overview/overview.html (last accessed 20 December 2005).

Slater SG. What does it take to implement a telemedicine program in your home care agency? *Home Health Care Manage Pract* 2001;**13**:322–5.

References

1 Scott RE, McCarthy GF, Jennett PA, *et al. National Telehealth Outcome Indicators Project [NTOIP] – Project information document and a synthesis of telehealth outcomes literature.* Calgary: Health Telematics Unit, University of Calgary, 2003. Available at: www.md.ucalgary.ca/Medicine/Centres/TeleHealth/NTOIP/_resources/InformationDocument.pdf (last accessed 20 December 2005).

2 Moore RS. *Telehealth programs: introducing the basics.* Marietta, GA: Patient Safety and Quality Healthcare, 2005. Available at: www.psqh.com/janfeb05/viewpoint.html (last accessed 20 December 2005).

3 Field MJ, ed. *Telemedicine: a guide to assessing telecommunications for healthcare.* Washington, DC: National Academy Press, 1996.

4 Bayliss EA, Ellis JL, Steiner JF. Subjective assessments of comorbidity correlate with quality of life health outcomes: initial validation of a comorbidity assessment instrument. *Health Qual Life Outcomes* 2005;**3**:51.

5 Porell FW, Miltiades HB. Access to care and functional status change among aged Medicare beneficiaries. *J Gerontol B Psychol Sci Soc Sci* 2001;**56**:S69–83.

6 Ware JE. *SF-36® health survey update.* Lincoln, RI: QualityMetric, 2002. Available at: www.sf-36.org/tools/sf36.shtml (last accessed 20 December 2005).

7 Strickland OL, Dilorio C. *Measurements of nursing outcomes, volume 3: self-care and coping.* New York: Springer Publishing Company, 2003.

8 Lehmann C, Giacini JM. Telehealth and disease management: 2004. *Remington Rep* 2004;**12**:14–18.

9 Roglieri JL, Futterman R, McDonough KL, *et al.* Disease management interventions to improve outcomes in congestive heart failure. *Am J Manag Care* 1997;**3**:1831–9.

10 American Association for Homecare. *Telehealth success stories.* Alexandria, VA: American Association for Homecare, 2005. Available at: www.aahomecare.org/associations/3208/files/TELEHEALTH%20STUDIES%20MAY%2013%20REVISION.pdf (last accessed 27 December 2005).

11 Schofield RS, Kline SE, Schmalfuss CM, *et al.* Early outcomes of a care coordination-enhanced telehome care program for elderly veterans with chronic heart failure. *Telemed J E Health* 2005;**11**:20–7.

12 Rosenblum B, Schabert V, Davis N. *Independent analysis of monitored/non-monitored patients.* Santa Barbara, CA: Strategic Healthcare Programs, 2004. Available at: www.hommed.com/data/_pdfs/shp_2004_07_01.pdf (last accessed 27 December 2005).

13 Johnston B, Wheeler L, Deuser J. Kaiser Permanente Medical Center's pilot Tele-Home Health Project. *Telemed Today* 1997;**5**:16–17,19.

14 Kinsella A. Telehealth opportunities for home care patients. *Home Healthc Nurse* 2003;**21**:661–5.

15 Pennsylvania Home Care Association, Pennsylvania State University. *2003–2004 telehealth project evaluation year two: the impact of telehealth on nursing workload and retention.* Lemoyne, PA: Pennsylvania Home Care Association, Pennsylvania State University, 2004. Available at: www.pahomecareresource.org/documents/evaluation2.pdf (last accessed 20 December 2005).

▶ 3

Economic evaluation

Paul A. Scuffham

Introduction

Economics is the study of people with choice. When there is choice, decisions must – and will – be made. Policy decisions on whether to provide healthcare services are influenced by a number of questions, such as: 'Is it feasible to provide the service?', 'Is providing a service by telemedicine acceptable to the public?', 'What are the alternatives?', 'How does the service under consideration compare with the alternatives?' and 'What are the costs and expected health benefits of the service being considered and the alternatives?' Decision rules are necessary for a transparent and consistent approach to making public policy. Resources – such as people, time, facilities, equipment and knowledge – are scarce. Inevitably, demand for goods outstrips resources available to produce goods and services at any point in time. That is, society's ability to supply goods and services is finite, and, thus, healthcare has to compete for public funds with other services such as education and justice.

Health economics is about applying economic theory to problems in healthcare. In the spectrum of health economics, economic evaluation is the branch used to facilitate decisions on how to allocate scarce resources efficiently between different, competing, interventions. Economic evaluation is concerned with systematically assessing the costs and benefits of the intervention being considered and comparing these with the costs and benefits of the alternative interventions. Typically, proposed new healthcare interventions compete for funding with other existing healthcare interventions. The purpose of undertaking an economic evaluation is thus to determine whether the new intervention represents good value for money.[1] Because of the accelerating introduction of new medical technologies, healthcare policy makers require evidence about the expected benefits from healthcare spending and whether the benefits justify the costs. The approach to undertaking an economic evaluation is the same whether it is applied to the medical devices in a clinical trial, a community nursing intervention or home telemedicine. Several well-known guidelines and checklists for economic evaluation specify the approach and key factors that should be addressed.[2,3] This chapter presents the main features of economic evaluation applied to telemedicine, drawing on examples from a study of teledentistry[4] and other analyses.

Economic evaluation methods

The aim of economic evaluation is to determine the most efficient intervention of those being compared. The most efficient intervention is the one with which the greatest output can be obtained for the least input. In other words, the intervention that produces the greatest health benefit for the lowest cost is the most efficient. To make meaningful comparisons, we must focus on efficiency at the margin rather than the average – that is, what are the additional costs for an additional unit of health benefit (i.e. effect)? This is known as incremental analysis and is reported as the incremental cost-effectiveness ratio (ICER). The ICER is calculated as:

$$ICER = \frac{Costs_{new} - Costs_{comparator}}{Effects_{new} - Effects_{comparator}}$$

Four main forms of economic evaluation exist: cost-minimization, cost-effectiveness, cost-utility and cost-benefit analysis. Each deals with costs in the same manner, but they differ on how health benefits are measured (Boxes 3.1 and 3.2).

Selecting the main comparator

In undertaking an economic evaluation, the first step is to formulate a well-defined question that can be answered. Then, the next step is to select the most appropriate comparator from a list of alternatives. In a clinical trial, the most appropriate comparator may be a placebo control group; in the delivery of healthcare services, the

---

Box 3.1. Types of economic evaluation

Cost-minimization analysis (CMA) is the process of identifying and measuring costs for a specific intervention or service and the alternatives. The benefits expected from the intervention and the alternatives must be assessed and deemed as identical. For example, the efficacy of two pharmaceuticals may be shown to be equivalent in a head-to-head clinical trial. In this case, the pharmaceutical with the lowest cost will be the most efficient. In telemedicine, the investigator often assumes equivalence between health outcomes from telemedicine and the comparator without undertaking a head-to-head or controlled trial. Because of the assumed equivalent outcomes, cost-minimization analysis is often used (see Box 3.2).

Cost-effectiveness analysis (CEA) is similar to CMA, but differences in health benefits are measured. Health benefits may be measured in natural units (such as deaths, hospitalizations or clinical events), a composite of these natural units or a score on a disease-specific or general health status instrument.

Cost-utility analysis (CUA) is similar to CEA; however, health benefits are measured on a preference-based scale. Preference-based scales value the trade-offs people are prepared to make to avoid or change health states. These trade-offs may be elicited through economic experiments with hypothetical scenarios, using techniques such as the time trade-off or standard gamble. However, several instruments have been developed using these techniques, which allow measurement of health state that is then transformed to a utility score. The most widely used is the EQ-5D,[5] which measures 243 health states.[6]

Cost-benefit analysis (CBA) is similar to CEA and CUA, but health benefits are measured in monetary values. Measurement of health outcomes in monetary terms is difficult, however, so this approach is used rarely.

Box 3.2. Example of cost-minimization analysis

In a study of teledentistry in Scotland,[4] two scenarios were compared:
- a scenario in which a specialist visits remote areas periodically
- a scenario in which patients attend the hospital as needed.

Teledentistry consultations were established with a specialist restorative dentist in a base hospital in Aberdeen and two satellite general dental practices (one in the Orkney Islands and the other in the central highlands of Scotland).

The clinical outcomes for three scenarios were assessed during this trial and deemed as equivalent; health outcomes were assumed to be equal on the basis of this finding. (There may be some differences in health outcomes; for example, in current practice, patients were required to travel three hours by road from the central highlands and substantially longer from the Orkneys, and travel has risks of injury and death.)

When outcomes are identical, the incremental cost-effectiveness ratio (ICER) reduces to incremental costs (IC = $costs_{new}$ − $costs_{comparator}$), and a cost-minimization analysis (CMA) is conducted.

The costs per patient for that study are shown in Table 3.1.

Table 3.1. Costs per patient in a study of teledentistry in Scotland

Type of care	Total costs per patient (£)	Incremental cost (£)
Teledentistry	430.94*	
Outreach visits	281.30†	149.64**
Hospital visits	442.60‡	−11.66††

* a.
† b.
‡ c.
** (a − b).
†† (a − c).

Thus, the incremental cost of teledentistry was £149.64 compared with outreach visits and saved costs compared with hospital visits.

---

most appropriate comparator may be current practice (that is, the proportionate mix of practices currently in use), the practice that is most likely to be replaced from the new intervention or the practice that is most widely used. Different countries have different requirements. For example, the National Institute for Clinical Excellence (NICE) in England and Wales requires 'best alternative practice',[7] whereas the Pharmaceutical Benefits Advisory Committee (PBAC) in Australia requires 'the practice that is used by the largest number of patients' as the main comparator.[8] The main comparator should therefore be selected with the target audience in mind.

Measuring resources and costs

An essential component of an economic evaluation is the estimation of costs. The key issues of costing are determining what costs should be included in the evaluation and how costs should be collected and measured. Determining the range of costs to include – and how these should be measured – depends on the perspective chosen for the study.

Perspective

A number of different perspectives may be used for an evaluation. The broadest is that of society as a whole. This perspective should reflect the true opportunity costs to society, including production losses, value of leisure time lost and the value of life lost. The methods for valuing production, leisure and life are controversial, however, and this perspective therefore is not used frequently. Other perspectives include the public sector (that is, costs to government), the healthcare system, a specified institution (for example, a hospital or insurer) and the patient. The perspective chosen should reflect that of the budget holder – that is, the perspective of the decision-maker who will fund the intervention. In practice, a decision on the costs to include in an analysis is constrained heavily by the availability of data.

Direct costs

Direct costs are those that are monetized: that is, costs where a transaction occurs. Direct healthcare costs typically include the cost of hospitalization, pharmaceuticals, dressings, equipment and facilities. Direct non-health costs that are associated with healthcare but not necessarily incurred by the healthcare provider include patient travel costs (this often is a key factor in the cost-effectiveness of telemedicine). These costs have two primary components – the quantities of resources used and the monetary value of the resources. The quantities of resources can be counted for the intervention and the main comparator: for example, the number of visits to a general practitioner (GP). These resources consumed can then be valued at their unit costs. Estimating and presenting resources and costs separately is advantageous in the sense that the applicability of resource use and costs can be assessed for different settings. For example, the frequency of visits to GPs varies greatly between urban and rural areas.

One costing issue in the evaluation of healthcare programmes is how to deal with the initial set-up costs required, which in some cases may be substantial. A distinction must be made between initial costs and operating costs. Operating costs are largely variable costs; they vary with throughput, such as the number of patients. Each unit of throughput may incur a given cost (Box 3.3). These costs may be averaged over all patients; however, throughput capacity, and consequently costs, are generally 'lumpy': that is, there is a maximum limit before more resources are required, such as employing another staff member, purchasing an additional scanner or, in the case of telemedicine, purchasing another network connection.

Initial set-up costs

Telemedicine programmes often require a relatively large initial expenditure for video equipment and telecommunications to establish a service. These are usually an important feature in evaluating telemedicine services. Initial costs are normally categorized into capital items (that is, assets) and non-capital items (for example, staff time for training). These costs may be classed as sunk costs and, if so, they will be one-off costs that can be omitted from the analysis of an existing service. If a decision is to be made about establishing a new service, however, these costs should be included.

Box 3.3. Calculating direct costs

The perspective used in the teledentistry study described in Box 3.2 was that of costs to society. The study therefore included costs to the National Health Service (NHS), out-of-pocket costs to the patient and costs to the dentist not reimbursed from other sources. The costs below are summarized from detailed information about travel distance for the patient, the dentist's time and NHS procedure costs. (Note: These direct costs are the variable costs and exclude the *pro rata* costs for capital items (see Box 3.5).)

Table 3.2. Direct costs in a study of teledentistry in Scotland

Type of direct cost	Cost (£)		
	Teledentistry	Outreach visits	Hospital visits
Patient			
Diagnosis and treatment plan	29.50	–	–
Travel costs	4.39	8.24	–
Dental practitioner costs			
Pre-consultation	38.35	9.17	9.17
Consultation	38.74	–	–
Post-consultation	4.32	–	–
NHS costs			
Pre-consultation costs	8.07	–	–
Consultation costs	73.98	54.50	54.50
Post-consultation costs	25.74	18.17	18.17
Nurse and administration costs	0.20	3.69	3.69
Diagnostic images	7.38	0.88	0.88
Patient travel and accommodation	–	–	250.64
Total	230.69	94.64	337.04

– No costs.

Box 3.4. Annuitizing capital costs

Annuitization is the process of converting an initial capital outlay into an annual equivalent cost for the useful life of the asset. The process requires the mathematical formula below, in which E = annual equivalent cost, K = initial capital outlay, S = salvage value at the end of the period, t = period of time, r = discount rate and A = annuity factor.

$$E = \left(K - \frac{S}{(1 + r)^t} \right) * \frac{1}{A}$$

The discount rate indicates how costs (and benefits) occurring at different times are evaluated (see Box 3.8). For capital items, the discount rate is the rate at which the value of property is reduced. The governments of some countries have set discount rates for the evaluation of public investment projects; the rate often follows the long-term interest rate for government bond issues. The annuity factor for use in the above formula, is in turn given by:

$$A = \frac{1}{r} * \left(1 - \left[\frac{1}{(1 + r)^t} \right] \right)$$

The annual equivalent cost (E) can be multiplied by the years of interest, such as the years of follow-up in a study. For example, a piece of equipment with an initial cost (K) of $50 000 has a life (t) of 10 years, depreciates (r) at 10% annually (the discount rate) and has zero salvage value at the end of 10 years. The annuity factor is 6.14 and the annual equivalent cost is $8137. If this equipment was used for three years in a study, the total equivalent cost is $24 412.

Box 3.5. Total fixed costs in connecting two satellite units to a base hospital for teledentistry

The fixed costs for the teledentistry project included the purchase of several capital items (Table 3.3). These items all had a life of four years before replacement would be needed (or substantially improved technologies are available), and the salvage value at the end of that period would be 10% of the initial value (except for the ISDN connection, which has a zero value). The depreciation rate used was 6%.

In addition, line rental is an annual cost rather than a capital item (i.e. it is not an asset). This cost is independent of patient throughput and therefore is included as a fixed cost.

Table 3.3. Fixed costs in a study of teledentistry in Scotland

Item	Cost by location (£)			
	Satellite 1	Satellite 2	Base hospital	All
Videoconferencing unit	860	860	1660	3380
Camera and software	1396	1396	1396	4188
Imaging equipment	1176	1176	–	2352
ISDN connection	199	199	199	597
Total capital costs	3631	3631	3255	10517
Annual equivalent cost of total capital costs	969	969	870	2808
Line rental	552	552	552	1656
Total annual equivalent fixed costs	1521	1521	1422	4464

Capital items have a value over a predetermined period – their 'lifetime'. These items might be sold at a future date or scrapped at the end of their life. Non-capital costs are incurred at the outset and should be included in the financial year in which the costs were incurred. The costs of capital items should be spread over the life of the item through a process known as annuitizing (Boxes 3.4 and 3.5).[9]

Indirect costs

Indirect costs are those that are not directly monetized: that is, there is no transaction. Examples of these costs include reduced efficiency when at work (decreased productivity), absenteeism due to illness, lost production from premature death, voluntary work, unpaid care (for example, by family members) and lost leisure time. There are three approaches to valuing these indirect costs: human capital, friction cost and willingness-to-pay (WTP).[9–11]

The human capital approach values people according to what they can produce for the economy. The present value of future earnings is calculated from market wages (and discounted) to express lost production (and other non-paid output) in monetary terms (Box 3.6). For example, if an office worker who earns $40 000 annually ($200 per day) is off work for 10 days with influenza, the value of lost production is calculated as $200 × 10 = $2000.

The friction cost approach is a modification of the human capital approach. Where the human capital approach uses the full period of illness or death until the end of the

---

Box 3.6. Calculating indirect costs in teledentistry

Indirect costs for the teledentistry project were calculated, using the human capital approach, as the total time away from work for a dental consultation. Table 3.4 shows the values when a mean wage of £10.27 per hour was used.

Table 3.4. Value of work lost in a study of teledentistry in Scotland

Care approach	Mean work lost (hours)	Value of lost production (£)
Teledentistry	2.1	21.68
Outreach visits	1.7	17.40
Hospital visits	10.3	105.56

---

age of gainful employment (or contribution to the economy), the friction cost approach shortens this period until the position in question is filled. This approach takes the narrowest view by valuing lost production as the losses between the start of the illness or death up to when a replacement is found and employed. This period can be very short for a workforce that requires unskilled labour – especially when there is an excess supply of labour (that is, unemployment exists). For example, if the office worker in the above example is part of a large pool of office workers, they may be replaced in the first hour when they do not show up for work. The associated friction cost would be a maximum of $200/8 hours = $25. This approach gives the lowest value to indirect costs. When highly skilled labour must be replaced, however, the period to finding a replacement and training that person could be longer than the period of illness. For example, if the office worker who has influenza for 10 days is a company director who earns $400 000 annually ($2000/day), the time to find and recruit a replacement is likely to be longer than 10 days, by which time the executive with influenza will have recovered and returned to work. As such, the friction cost will be $2000 × 10 days = $20 000. In these cases, the friction cost and human capital approaches have the same values.

The WTP approach is used to determine the maximum amount of money an individual (or society) is willing to pay to gain a particular benefit, such as to avoid or reduce the risk of death and/or illness. This is done prospectively, by using economic experiments (typically contingent valuation) with trained interviewers to elicit preferences and values, or retrospectively, when values are deduced by drawing conclusions about behaviour (this is known as revealed preference). For example, if a government decided to spend $200 million to prevent influenza and the programme is expected to avert a total of two million cases of influenza, the WTP value to government of averting a case of influenza is $100 ($200 million/two million cases). Individuals may have different values if asked prospectively. For example, an individual may be willing to spend $75 to reduce their risk of contracting influenza from one in 10 to one in 15; the individual's WTP value to avoid influenza is $375 ($75 divided by 1/5). The WTP approach needs to be explicit about what is being measured and what is not. Although WTP values implicitly include values around losses of future income, they may include many other attributes related to the individual's perceptions of risks and values that are not measured explicitly. Caution must therefore be exercised when this approach is used.

Measuring outcomes for economic evaluation

Health outcomes are generally measured in clinical trials, observational studies, cohort studies, before and after studies, and so forth. Depending on the design of the economic evaluation and the audience, some outcome measures may need to be transformed into a single index measure, such as a quality-of-life index.

Direct outcomes

Health effects may be measured in natural units (such as deaths, hospitalizations or clinical events), a composite of these natural units or a score on disease-specific or general health status instruments such as the Short Form 36 (SF-36). Other outcome measures commonly used include life-years and dichotomous outcomes such as non-responder/responder, successfully treated, disease-free survivors or satisfied with service. These measures can then be used in a cost-effectiveness analysis (CEA).

Composite outcome measures

The range of composite outcomes reported in the literature is vast. Most are disease specific and based on validated disease-specific instruments (for example, the Psoriasis Area Severity Index, which combines affected skin surface with intensity of disease). Others combine a range of disease-specific events that the investigator decides upon (for example, major adverse cardiac events may include death from any cause, cardiac death, acute myocardial infarction, revascularization procedures, angina, symptomatic stenosis and subclinical stenosis). Comparison of one outcome measure with another thus requires consistent definitions of the outcome used.

Other outcomes include disability-adjusted life-years (DALYs), in which weights, obtained from two panels of 17 clinicians (in total) in the Netherlands, are placed on various health states to provide an index of disability. Quality-adjusted life-years (QALYs) use a similar approach to DALYs but are superior, as the weights used for QALY calculations are based on preferences of the public to calculate years of healthy life. Instruments with preference weights for calculating overall utility scores measure health states. These instruments are easy to use and most require only a few minutes to complete. The most widely used is the EuroQoL-5D (EQ-5D); other instruments include the Assessment of Quality of Life (AQoL), Health Utilities Index Mark 3 (HUI3) and 15-dimension Health State Descriptive System (15D). The Short Form 6D (SF-6D) is a recent addition to the list of instruments and is a preference-based algorithm developed to convert scores from the SF-36 and SF-12 into utility scores, thus allowing QALYs to be calculated.

Utility scores are on a cardinal scale (full health = 1.0 and dead = 0.0; Box 3.7. (Note that there can be health states worse than dead, such as permanent vegetative states or being confined to bed with extreme pain or discomfort plus extreme anxiety). These scales enable direct and indirect comparisons across all healthcare

---

Box 3.7. Some utility weights obtained from administering the EQ-5D to cardiac patients[12]

Health-related quality of life was not measured in the teledentistry project. Table 3.5 shows health-related quality of life scores for cardiac patients with ischaemic heart disease – one group underwent percutaneous coronary intervention (PCI) and had a stent implanted, and the other group underwent coronary artery bypass surgery.[12] The quality of life was measured on a cardinal scale (0 = dead; 1.0 = best imaginable health state). These scores are sometimes referred to as utility weights or tariffs. In this example, the EQ-5D QoL questionnaire was used and scored according to the weights derived from time trade-off experiments in the British population.

Table 3.5. Health-related quality of life scores for cardiac patients with ischaemic heart disease

Time point	Percutaneous coronary intervention (stent)	Surgery
Baseline (pre-intervention)	0.69	0.68
One month after intervention	0.84	0.78
Six months after intervention	0.86	0.86

To calculate quality-adjusted life years (QALYs), these weights need to be multiplied by the length of time in each health state. The weight for six months after intervention could be multiplied by the remaining life expectancy. For example, assuming patients who survive surgery live for five years, surgery patients accrue one month at 0.68, five months at 0.78 and four years and six months at 0.86 = $(1 \times 0.68) + (5 \times 0.78) + (54 \times 0.86) = 51.02$ quality-adjusted life months = 4.25 QALYs (undiscounted).

---

interventions. From April 2004, NICE required all appraisals of health technologies to report an economic evaluation using QALYs.[7] Preference weights are obtained in economic experiments using preference elicitation methods – typically these are the time trade-off, standard gamble or discrete-choice experiments, but sometimes a visual analogue scale is used. (Note that NICE requires utility to be elicited using a time trade-off, standard gamble or discrete-choice experiment; a visual analogue scale is not acceptable.[7])

Other factors

Clinical trials, including trials of telemedicine, tend to be conducted for relatively short periods. They often end before all beneficial and detrimental effects and costs have been incurred. A full economic evaluation should estimate the costs and effects for the intervention and its main comparator for the expected duration that effects and costs might be incurred. This usually requires some extrapolation and modelling to project future costs and effects – unless all costs and effects are observed during the trial. A common approach to modelling in economic evaluations is the use of Markov-chain models.[13] These are used to model the time in various health states, with transitions from one health state to another on the basis of a set of probabilities.

Costs and utility weights can be assigned to each health state, and Monte Carlo simulations can be conducted relatively easily in some of the specialist software packages available (for example, TreeAge Pro, see www.treeage.com).

Discounting

The timing of costs incurred and benefits received is a matter of importance. That is, we generally prefer to receive benefits earlier and incur costs later. For example, we prefer to receive goods now and pay for them at some stage in the future, such as by using a credit card. Similarly, we prefer to obtain beneficial health effects now (such as from a curative intervention) and pay for them in the future rather than paying for a preventive programme from which the benefits are not obtained until some later time. Economists call this preference for receiving benefits now rather than in the future a positive rate of time preference. In order to reflect our positive rate of time preference, costs and effects are converted from expected future values into present values through a process of discounting (Box 3.8).[14] Discount rates for use in economic evaluation are usually set by health technology assessment agencies. The UK rate is 3.5% for both costs and effects; in the US, Australia and most of Europe, the rate is 5%. Higher discount rates give lower weights to costs and effects occurring in the future. The literature on whether the discount rate should be the same for both costs and effects is large.[13] It is often useful to present effects and costs undiscounted, as well as discounted, so that policy-makers can see the absolute costs and effects irrespective of when these occur.

Box 3.8. Discounting

If the capital equipment in the teledentistry project is to be replaced four years after purchase, we might expect the cost to be close to the current purchase price of the equipment – that is £3361 at each satellite. If we expect to incur this cost again in four years' time, using a 5% annual discount rate, the present value (PV) is given by:

$$PV = \frac{FV}{(1 + r)^t} = \frac{3361}{(1 + 0.05)^4} = 2987$$

If the discount rate is increased to 10%, the PV = £2480, or if the time we expect to incur that cost is increased to 10 years, the PV = £2229.

The same discounting process is used for health outcomes that occur in the future.

Allowing for uncertainty

All costs and effects are subject to some uncertainty because of a whole variety of factors (for example, some estimates may be imprecise). The most common approach for addressing uncertainty is to conduct a sensitivity analysis. Perhaps the most useful is a one-way sensitivity analysis, in which one parameter at a time is varied over a range of values to assess the effect on the results from changes in that parameter. All key parameters may be varied over the expected feasible range (for example, the lower and upper confidence limits) or by a given percentage (for example, ±30%). The latter approach is useful for identifying the factors that have the greatest effect on the results.

The former approach, however, is useful for estimating the likely range in which the true ICER lies.

Other approaches include multi-way sensitivity analysis (in which two or more parameters are varied together) and probabilistic sensitivity analysis (in which values are drawn randomly in a series of simulations from distributions assigned to each parameter).[13] The NICE now requires probabilistic sensitivity analysis to be undertaken in all appraisals,[7] so the use of this approach is growing considerably.

Scenario analysis is related to sensitivity analysis. Scenarios can be developed by changing several parameters to represent a particular population subgroup, indication for treatment or restriction on access. For example, the effects of restricting the use of a high-cost drug to a subgroup of patients who might benefit the most can be estimated.

Presenting results

Results should report the costs and health effects for the intervention and the comparator, incremental cost, incremental effects and ICER in a table. In addition, the numbers of events for both intervention and comparator groups should be presented.

Visually, results should be presented in a cost-effectiveness plane (Fig. 3.1), which is a graph of the incremental effects (horizontal axis) and incremental cost (vertical axis). For points that fall in the lower right (southeast) quadrant, the new intervention has more health effects and at lower cost than the comparator; such interventions will

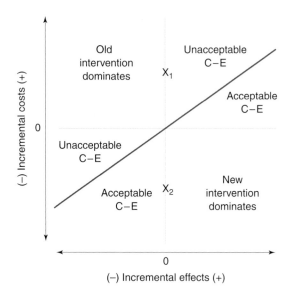

Fig. 3.1. The cost-effectiveness plane: X_1 and X_2 show the incremental costs of teledentistry compared with specialist outreach visits and patient hospital visits respectively. The diagonal line indicates an implicit cost-effectiveness acceptability threshold.

always be preferred over the comparator and are said to dominate. Points in the opposite quadrant (northwest) are said to be dominated by the comparator, as the new intervention has inferior health effects and higher cost. The comparator will always be preferred in this quadrant. The remaining quadrants are where decisions about value for money occur. In the northeast quadrant, the new intervention has better health effects but at a higher cost than the comparator, whereas the opposite occurs in the southwest quadrant (it is relatively rare for new interventions to fall in this category).

Presenting sensitivity analysis results

A simple way of displaying the results from a one-way sensitivity analysis is to use a 'tornado' diagram (Fig. 3.2). This is a visually convenient approach to ranking the factors that have the greatest to smallest effect on the ICER results.

More complex analyses require correspondingly more complex methods of presentation. Probabilistic scenario analysis is already required by NICE (and sooner or later, it is likely that all economic evaluations will need something similar to quantify uncertainty). Scenario analyses can be tabulated in the same format as the main results. If probabilistic sensitivity analysis is undertaken, the simulation results should be used to construct 95% confidence intervals for the incremental costs and incremental effects, and the 95% confidence ellipse should be included in the cost-effectiveness plane. Because the ICER is a ratio, it has a non-normal distribution with discontinuities at the boundaries (that is, where incremental costs or effects equal zero). The usual approach to estimating a confidence interval for the mean, therefore, is to use the BCa bootstrapping method.[15] In addition, cost-effectiveness acceptability

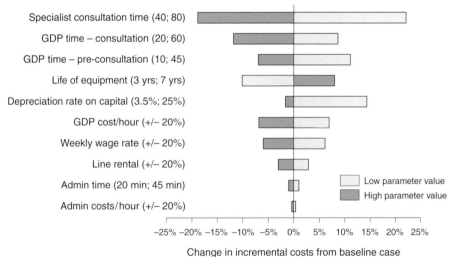

Fig. 3.2. Example of a tornado diagram – incremental costs of teledentistry versus outreach visits

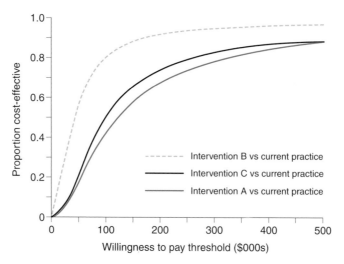

Fig. 3.3. Cost-effectiveness acceptability curves

curves (CEAC) should be presented. In these graphs of the ICERs constructed from the simulations, ICERs are ranked and are presented with the ICER on the horizontal axis and the percentage on the vertical axis.[13] These graphs depict the joint distribution of the uncertainty in the ICER, which means that policy-makers can assess visually the probability (proportion of simulations) that the ICER is below the threshold of what they are willing to pay for a one-unit gain in health benefit (Fig. 3.3). For example, the implicit thresholds of acceptability are about £30 000 per QALY gained in the UK and around $70 000 per life-year gained in Australia.[16]

Budget impact

Results should also be scaled up from a trial to address the question of 'What if the telemedicine intervention was generalized to a larger population?' That is, during a telemedicine trial, the service may be offered to selected patients and/or in selected locations. If the criteria for accessing telemedicine were relaxed, or if the service was extended to other locations, an estimate of the expected costs (and effects) is needed. If the service is extended to a wider group of patients in the same location, the cost will be only marginal (that is, the costs of extra patients), as additional investments in capital will be small or non-existent. If the service is to be extended to other locations, however, additional costs might include additional satellite systems without needing to expand the base system. In both cases, the average cost will be lower than those from a trial.

Scaling up of costs should include estimates of the uptake of the new technology and the reduction in existing practice over the forthcoming years. A suggested rule of thumb is to use a time horizon of five years for the budget impact assessment.

Conclusion

A principal aim of telemedicine in the home (or elsewhere) is to improve access to healthcare services. In the process, telemedicine should produce savings in time and travel costs. However, whether these savings are greater than the set-up and operating costs of a service and whether the health outcomes obtained from telemedicine are better than, equal to or inferior to conventional healthcare services must be taken into account. The demands for high-quality and scientifically sound approaches to economic evaluation have increased substantially over recent years. This demand for higher quality has been fuelled by improvements in technology (such as increased computer processing capacity for simulations), substantial advances in the methods of economic evaluation and the requirements of health technology appraisal agencies for explicit quantification of uncertainties in the costs and effects of an intervention, as well as estimates of the effect that this uncertainty may have on their decision-making.

Very few rigorous economic evaluations of telemedicine interventions have been undertaken (see Aoki *et al*[17] for a good example). Most have used a cost-minimization approach, with assumptions that health outcomes are identical for the intervention and control groups. Often the perspective of costs is narrow or poorly defined. Thus, costs and potential cost-savings may be underestimated. When an economic evaluation is undertaken, it is important to include measures of patient outcomes such as health-related QoL. Health-related QoL can be captured during a trial using instruments such as the EQ-5D, which take less than one minute to complete. Therefore, health-related quality of life outcome measures should be included wherever possible. In addition, patient/consumer satisfaction/convenience may be highly important; the value of this may be elicited using a willingness-to-pay/contingent valuation study.

Healthcare policy-makers at the national and local levels need sound information on the costs and benefits before they can make decisions about whether to assist or fully fund a telemedicine service. In addition, policy-makers need to make decisions on whether a given sum invested in telemedicine is likely to produce greater benefits than an investment of the same value in another (competing) service or intervention. These decisions on the best value for health expenditure can be made only with adequate and robust information from a full economic evaluation.

Further information

Drummond M, McGuire A, eds. *Economic evaluation in health care*. Oxford: Oxford University Press, 2001.

Drummond MF, Sculpher MJ, O'Brien BJ, *et al. Methods for the economic evaluation of health care programmes*. Oxford: Oxford University Press, 2005.

Gold MR, Siegel JE, Russell LB, Weinstein MC, eds. *Cost-effectiveness in health and medicine*. New York: Oxford University Press, 1996.

Kernick D, ed. *Getting health economics into practice*. Oxford: Radcliffe Medical Press, 2002.

References

1 Kernick D. An introduction to health economics. In: Kernick D, ed. *Getting health economics into practice.* Oxford: Radcliffe Medical Press, 2002.
2 Siegel JE, Weinstein MC, Torrance GW. Reporting cost-effectiveness studies and results. In: Gold MR, Siegel JE, Russell LB, Weinstein MC, eds. *Cost-effectiveness in health and medicine.* New York: Oxford University Press, 1996.
3 Drummond MF, Jefferson TO. Guidelines for authors and peer reviewers of economic submissions to the BMJ. *BMJ* 1996;**313**:275–83.
4 Scuffham PA, Steed M. An economic evaluation of the Highlands and Islands teledentistry project. *J Telemed Telecare* 2002;**8**:165–77.
5 Greiner W, Weijnen T, Nieuwenhuizen M, *et al.* A single European currency for EQ-5D health states. Results from a six-country study. *Eur J Health Econ* 2003;**4**:222–31.
6 EuroQol Group. EuroQol – a new facility for the measurement of health-related quality of life. *Health Policy* 1990;**16**:199–208.
7 National Institute for Clinical Excellence. *Guide to the methods of technology appraisal.* London: National Institute for Clinical Excellence, 2004. Available at: www.nice.org.uk/page.aspx?o=201974 (last accessed 9 November 2005).
8 Commonwealth Department of Health and Ageing. *2002 Guidelines for the pharmaceutical industry on preparation of submissions to the Pharmaceutical Benefits Advisory Committee.* Canberra: Commonwealth Department of Health and Ageing, 2002. Available at: www.health.gov.au/internet/wcms/publishing.nsf/Content/health-pbs-general-pubs-guidelines-content.htm-copy2 (last accessed 4 January 2006).
9 Drummond MF, O'Brien B, Stoddart GL, Torrance GW. *Methods for the economic evaluation of health care programmes.* Oxford: Oxford University Press, 1997.
10 Koopmanschap MA, Rutten FF, Van Ineveld BM, van Roijen L. The friction cost method for measuring indirect costs of disease. *J Health Econ* 1995;**14**:171–89.
11 Jones-Lee MW. Paternalistic altruism and the value of statistical life. *Econ J* 1992;**102**:80–90.
12 Serruys PW, Unger F, Sousa JE, *et al.* Comparison of coronary-artery bypass surgery and stenting for the treatment of multivessel disease. *N Engl J Med* 2001;**344**:1117–24.
13 Briggs A. Handling uncertainty in economic evaluation and presenting the results. In: Drummond M, McGuire A, eds. *Economic evaluation in health care.* Oxford: Oxford University Press, 2001:172–214.
14 Lipscomb J, Weinstein MC, Torrance GW. Time preference. In: Gold MR, Siegel JE, Russell LB, Weinstein MC, eds. *Cost-effectiveness in health and medicine.* New York: Oxford University Press, 1996.
15 Efron B, Tibshirani RJ. *An introduction to the bootstrap.* London: Chapman and Hall, 1993.
16 National Health and Medical Research Council. *How to compare the costs and benefits: evaluation of the economic evidence.* Canberra: National Health and Medical Research Council, 2001. Available at: www.nhmrc.gov.au/publications/synopses/cp73syn.htm (last accessed 4 January 2006).
17 Aoki N, Dunn K, Fukui T, *et al.* Cost-effectiveness analysis of telemedicine to evaluate diabetic retinopathy in a prison population. *Diabetes Care* 2004;**27**:1095.

►4

Patient and provider satisfaction

Pamela Whitten and Alicia Bergman

Introduction

Home telehealth is a fast-growing segment in the field of telemedicine. Research and evaluation of telehealth services delivered to patients in their homes have mirrored the scope and types of research conducted for the field of telemedicine as a whole. In general telemedicine research, one of the most commonly studied variables is satisfaction.[1]

It is worthwhile studying how users of telemedicine feel about it for a variety of reasons, some of which are intuitive and some of which have been documented in general health research. First, there is some indication that patients who express satisfaction with aspects of their healthcare will demonstrate higher levels of compliance. This in turn produces positive health outcomes. Just as important is the growing notion that patients are partners in healthcare. As Whitten and Mair have pointed out,[1] this new mode of interaction via technology merits serious study in the realm of satisfaction to better understand how communication (and thus relationships) between providers and patients is affected. In some segments of healthcare delivery, we are also witnessing the transformation of healthcare from a sellers' market to a consumers' market. In this case, satisfaction contributes to the definition of quality and affects client retention. Finally, there is the ideological reason that, in a democratic society, patients and providers should have the right to influence decisions that affect them. A better understanding of satisfaction allows us to work towards ensuring a high quality of life – not only for the recipients of telemedicine healthcare but also for those providing it. The measurement of both patient and provider satisfaction realizes the principle of community participation in healthcare.

Patient satisfaction

Most research has found that satisfaction with home telehealth from the perspective of patients is overwhelmingly positive. This includes studies of home telehealth for elderly patients and outpatient management of those with cancer or congestive heart failure.[2,3] Patient satisfaction with home telehealth spans the different types of services offered as well as the specific diseases being treated,[4] and it echoes findings of high patient satisfaction in telemedicine in general. For example, satisfaction and even preference for paediatric home telehealth have been expressed by parents with children who have serious healthcare needs.[5]

Patients have expressed high satisfaction with regard to a number of different aspects of home telehealth. Satisfaction with the ease of use as well as the abilities of the telehealth technology has been found across various contexts.[6–8] The improved access to healthcare that telehealth facilitates has been especially popular with patients; the peace of mind that 24-hour and/or immediate access to healthcare provides pleases many patients in otherwise very stressful situations.[8] One study found that elderly patients preferred more frequent home videoconsultations and less frequent home visits by nurses.[9] Another study illustrated how telenursing patients discharged from hospitals with ostomies as a result of cancer treatment not only found the care to be more accessible and preferable to waiting for face-to-face visits, but also felt that the telenurses had more understanding of their conditions. In this particular

---

Box 4.1. Michigan Home Health Agency experience with home telehealth

Marquette Home Health, a healthcare organization in Michigan's Upper Peninsula region, uses home telehealth to deliver services (Fig. 4.1). From 2001–03, researchers from Michigan State University evaluated the home telehealth services being provided to patients with diabetes, chronic obstructive pulmonary disease, congestive heart failure and stroke.[23] Most patients found their chronic diseases easier to manage with home telehealth and 76% said they wanted to use it again in the future. Other advantages listed by patients included increased access to healthcare, convenience and savings in terms of travel and time.

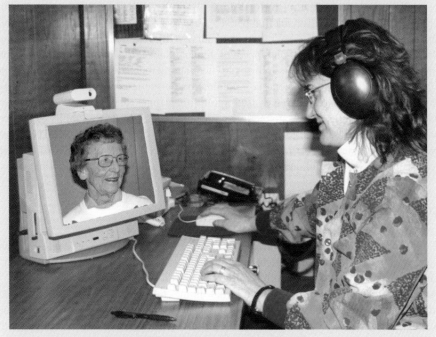

Fig. 4.1. Marquette home health nurse providing teleconsultation to a patient in rural Michigan

case, the patients were more comfortable with the information given to them about ostomies.[2] Another study showed that the more often telehealth technology was used, the more positively it was viewed by the patients.[6] Marquette Home Health is a home telehealth provider that has documented positive overall perceptions with telehealth (Box 4.1).

On the rare occasions where patient satisfaction (or aspects of satisfaction) with home telehealth has emerged as questionable, researchers have linked the satisfaction results with explanatory variables. For example, when patients who participated in a general practice out-of-hours co-operative reported dissatisfaction with their telephone consultations, it was mainly due to frustration over not knowing whether an accurate diagnosis could be made by telephone or the feeling that they were wasting the doctor's time. The researchers felt that these complaints could easily be mitigated by ensuring that patients were better informed beforehand about what services they could expect from this type of healthcare service.[10] In another study in which patient satisfaction was high, the authors concluded that patient location and their perceptions of the quality of the communication encounter were important predictors of patient satisfaction with home telehealth services.[11]

Although patient satisfaction has been reported to be high to extremely high in most home telehealth studies,[4] measures are often limited to general levels of satisfaction rather than patient satisfaction being broken down into specific ranges or categories. For instance, patient satisfaction with the technology or the overall home telemonitoring system is commonly used to elucidate satisfaction.[12] This may be because many studies aim to investigate multiple aspects of home telehealth applications and not just satisfaction per se.[13] Taking a more multi-faceted approach to the construct of satisfaction, Whitten et al surveyed home telehealth patients over a three-year period as a part of an Upper Michigan Telehealth Network initiative.[14] The measure of overall satisfaction in this study was supplemented by areas of assessment such as ease of use of equipment, communication during teleconsultation and quality of care. Other researchers have used multidimensional scales and multiple-item satisfaction measures (e.g. satisfaction with helpfulness or dependability of office staff), as well as satisfaction differences in system characteristics.[6,8,11] The most commonly used data collection strategies for studies of patient satisfaction with home telehealth are surveys and questionnaires, followed by experiments and clinical trials.

Provider satisfaction

Satisfaction on the part of providers in home telehealth is an area studied less than patient satisfaction. Moreover, data from provider satisfaction has been more varied.[4] However, there have been general findings of high levels of provider satisfaction.[7,16] Administrators and staff have found that home telehealth is cost-effective and improves patient and disease management,[3] as well as reducing hospital admissions and emergency room visits.[16] Worker satisfaction has also been shown to be high, with no significant differences found between home telenurses and nurses among the general population.[17]

In contrast, however, some studies have noted the difficulties of overcoming preconceived notions that providers have about the technology involved with home telehealth, despite already being involved in successful applications. A recent study of providers' satisfaction with the telehospice highlighted the providers' tendency to act as gatekeepers of the new technology and new ways of providing care. As gatekeepers, they often control whether a patient will even be offered telehealth. Some of the concerns included questions about worker autonomy and even mileage reimbursement.[18] Other studies have pointed out the difficulties of establishing the value of and commitment to new home telehealth technologies among providers, despite initial enthusiasm regarding their experiences. Some researchers have concluded that in order for this to change, a commitment to the use of home telehealth must come from the top of the organization.[19]

Other provider concerns with home telehealth have centred on the perceived limitations of the technology to facilitate clinical considerations. For example, the more muted enthusiasm on the part of nurses in one study was thought to be due to their perception that it is necessary to be present in person to observe the patient's surroundings, skin colour, wound healing and so on.[15] In another study, most providers (92%) thought that the televisits conducted would have been better if done in person.[20] Finally, some results on provider satisfaction have been mixed. The providers studied in one sample felt that the telehospice technology they used increased access and efficiency to care as well as reducing costs; however, perceived weaknesses concerned the difficulty of persuading patients and families to use the telehospice, having less intimacy with patients and limiting patients' stays.[21]

The data-collection strategies used for assessing provider satisfaction have mostly been interviews, surveys or questionnaires. In addition, satisfaction of providers in the home telehealth context is often only one result in studies that set out to investigate multiple things.[6,9,16] This is similar to research in patients. Finally, few studies have broken down provider satisfaction into more detailed components.[7]

Summary of satisfaction results

Evaluation activities in home health indicate that patients consistently report high levels of satisfaction with telemedicine across a range of applications – from paediatric home care to services for adults with diabetes (Table 4.1). Data indicate enhanced levels of perceived satisfaction with increased use. In addition, patients report positive perceptions in regards to ease of use and the enhanced access home telehealth offers.

Studies about health providers' satisfaction with home telehealth are less common than studies about patients' satisfaction. Many publications have reported high general levels of satisfaction (Table 4.1). A handful of studies that have delved more deeply into perceptions, however, indicate that this issue may be a little more complicated for providers because of their role as gatekeepers, general work-related expectations and scepticism about the technology and the range of appropriate applications.

Data from research studies on patients and providers provide information to inform

Table 4.1. Summary of satisfaction studies

Study	Type of condition/ consultation	Findings
Bohnenkamp et al, 2004[2]	Cancer (new ostomies)	Patients perceived telenurses as more knowledgeable and accessible; combining traditional and telehealth visits was judged the best approach
Chae et al, 2001[11]	Elderly home health services patients (various conditions)	Patient satisfaction was greater in home than nursing home applications; quality of communication was important in patient satisfaction
Dick et al, 2004[5]	Paediatric (e.g. cardiac, respiratory and otolaryngology)	Patient satisfaction the same for traditional and home telehealth; parents expressed strong preference for home telehealth
Johnston et al, 2000[8]	Heart failure, chronic obstructive pulmonary disease, diabetes, cancer and wound care	High patient satisfaction, effective quality of care and potential for cost savings
Kerner et al, 2004[15]	High-risk pregnancy	High patient satisfaction
Kobb et al, 2003[16]	High-risk/-cost Veterans (e.g. heart failure and diabetes)	High patient and provider satisfaction; improved perception of physical health
Lehmann and Giacini, 2004[3]	Congestive heart failure	Patients found care better due to monitoring of vital signs and connectivity with nurses. Administrators found lower labour costs and improved patient and disease management
Nanevicz et al, 2000[12]	Heart failure	High patient and provider satisfaction with system. Improved patient quality of life and understanding of preventive measures
Rosser et al, 2000[13]	Post-laparoscopy	High patient satisfaction. Postoperative evaluations similar to standard evaluations
Schlachta-Fairchild, 2002[17]	Telenurses	Work satisfaction the same as for traditional nurses
Wakefield et al, 2004[9]	Geriatric volunteers (≥70 years)	Patients preferred more frequent video visits to less frequent home visits. Nurses' clinical considerations made them less enthusiastic
Whitten et al, 1998[21]	Hospice	Providers noted increased access and efficiency but found difficulty persuading patients, providers and families to use telehealth
Whitten et al, 2005[18]	Hospice	Providers acted as gatekeepers. Concerns about job autonomy and mileage reimbursement

policy and business decisions regarding home telehealth. As the section below illustrates, however, flaws in the research place some limitations on the generalizability of the results.

Satisfaction studies must address relevant issues

The quest to study satisfaction in healthcare is not limited to telehealth; however, traditional healthcare studies that examine satisfaction are often riddled with problems that compromise generalizability. Telehealth satisfaction studies commonly suffer from the same difficulties. One problem with satisfaction research in general telemedicine, as well as in home telehealth, concerns shortcomings of methods. Studies demonstrate over-reliance on small convenience samples. It is not uncommon, even in peer-reviewed publications, for information about selection criteria to be absent. Data-collection instruments typically are untested for validity. Strategies for measuring satisfaction in home telehealth need to be standardized to facilitate broad conclusions about home telehealth.

Perhaps the most significant problem in satisfaction research concerns the very construct itself. The meaning of the term varies widely from individual to individual. Some researchers define satisfaction as meaning adequate care, whereas others interpret it to mean less than adequate care or care that could be done better.[22] Unfortunately, 'satisfaction' as a construct is often not defined at all or is simply employed in very different ways across studies. For example, some researchers employ the concept of satisfaction to indicate acceptance. Satisfaction for these researchers was just one aspect of an entirely different construct. This is not simply an argument about semantics. When researchers use multiple and inconsistent interpretations, interpretation of their findings becomes very difficult.

We all agree intuitively that it is worthwhile gathering data that enable us to understand how both patients and providers feel about home telehealth. It is important for descriptive purposes to help us explain how and why it is used, and it is important for enabling us to enhance and improve care delivered in this fashion. Researchers in home telehealth must recognize that the notion of satisfaction is multidimensional, is subject to contextual influences and has different meanings for different people. Broad or general research questions about satisfaction may offer only limited information to those wishing to make decisions about implementation or modification.

The most important element in achieving better understanding of patient and provider perceptions is the design of studies based on research questions or hypotheses that are pragmatic, valuable, specific and consistent with the longitudinal goals of the home telehealth programme in question. Each research project will have pertinent questions that in turn will be of interest to other projects. For example, rather than asking if a patient is satisfied with the care they received via home telehealth, researchers may delve deeper about specific aspects of that care. This means finding out if the care was delivered in a timely manner and asking about the specific content and quantity of communication interactions between the patient and provider, for example. It may also involve enquiring into specific differences in the patient's expectations, as they may be holding home telehealth to a higher (or lower) standard than conventional home care. In this way, the specific questions address actual research goals, rather than simply reflecting the general concept of satisfaction.

Conclusion

The recent growth in home telehealth activity around the world indicates that this is an area of telemedicine that meets a growing demand. Research has documented overwhelming evidence of patient satisfaction with this new way of delivering health services. Patients using the services feel safer and more secure with the increased monitoring that it facilitates, enjoy receiving more frequent (tele)visits and often feel more rapport with their nurses. Although reactions on the part of providers have been mixed, mounting evidence shows that home telehealth results in cost savings, along with improvements in patient care (for example, in efficiency, access and quality). As home telehealth becomes more widely adopted, there will probably be further improvements in provider perceptions.

Further information

Bauer JC, Ringel MA. *Telemedicine and the reinvention of healthcare: the seventh revolution in medicine*. New York: McGraw-Hill, 1999.
Whitten P, Cook D, eds. *Understanding health communication technologies*. San Francisco: Jossey-Bass, 2004.

References

1   Whitten PS, Mair F. Telemedicine and patient satisfaction: current status and future directions. *Telemed J E Health* 2000;**6**:417–23.
2   Bohnenkamp SK, McDonald P, Lopez AM, *et al.* Traditional versus telenursing outpatient management of patients with cancer with new ostomies. *Oncol Nurs Forum* 2004;**31**:1005–10.
3   Lehmann C, Giacini JM. Pilot study: The impact of technology on home bound congestive heart failure patients. *Home Health Care Technology Report* 2004;**1**:59–60.
4   Whitten P. Evidence regarding patient and provider perceptions and health indicators for telehome health. *Public Policy and Aging Report* 2004;**14**:19–21.
5   Dick PT, Bennie J, Barden W, *et al.* Preference for pediatric telehome care support following hospitalization: a report on preference and satisfaction. *Telemed J E Health* 2004;**10** (Suppl 2):45–53.
6   Finkelstein SM, Speedie SM, Potthoff S. Telehome care: healthcare for the elderly via telemedicine. *Medinfo* 2004;1592.
7   Whitten P, Collins B, Mair F. Nurse and patient reactions to a developmental home telecare system. *J Telemed Telecare* 1998;**4**:152–60.
8   Johnston B, Wheeler L, Deuser J, Sousa KH. Outcomes of the Kaiser Permanente Tele-Home Health Research Project. *Arch Fam Med* 2000;**9**:40–5.
9   Wakefield BJ, Holman JE, Ray A, *et al.* Nurse and patient preferences for telehealth home care. *Geriatric Times* 2004. Available at: www.geriatrictimes.com/g040427.html (last accessed 18 January 2005).
10 Payne F, Shipman C, Dale J. Patients' experiences of receiving telephone advice from a GP co-operative. *Fam Pract* 2001;**18**:156–60.
11 Chae YM, Heon LJ, Hee Ho S, *et al.* Patient satisfaction with telemedicine in home health services for the elderly. *Int J Med Inform* 2001;**61**:167–73.
12 Nanevicz T, Piette J, Zipkin D, *et al.* The feasibility of a telecommunications service in support of outpatient congestive heart failure care in a diverse patient population. *Congest Heart Fail* 2000;**6**:140–5.
13 Rosser JC Jr, Prosst RL, Rodas EB, *et al.* Evaluation of the effectiveness of portable low-bandwidth telemedical applications for postoperative follow-up: initial results. *J Am Coll Surg* 2000;**191**:196–203.
14 Whitten P, Eastin MS, Davis S. Telemedicine in the Michigan Upper Peninsula region: an evaluation of the first five years. *J Telemed Telecare* 2001;**7**:288–99.
15 Kerner R, Yogev Y, Belkin A, *et al.* Maternal self-administered fetal heart rate monitoring and transmission from home in high-risk pregnancies. *Int J Gynaecol Obstet* 2004;**84**:33–9.
16 Kobb R, Hoffman N, Lodge R, Kline S. Enhancing elder chronic care through technology and care coordination: report from a pilot. *Telemed J E Health* 2003;**9**:189–95.
17 Schlachta-Fairchild L. Telehealth practice in home care: synopsis of the 2000 US telenursing role study. *Caring* 2002;**21**:10–13.

18   Whitten P, Doolittle G, Mackert M. Providers' acceptance of telehospice. *J Palliat Med* 2005;**8**:730–5.

19   Hayes RP, Duffey EB, Dunbar J, *et al.* Staff perceptions of emergency and home-care telemedicine. *J Telemed Telecare* 1998;**4**:101-7.

20   Demiris G, Speedie S, Finkelstein S. A questionnaire for the assessment of patients' impressions of the risks and benefits of home telecare. *J Telemed Telecare* 2000;**6**:278–84.

21   Whitten P, Cook DJ, Doolittle G. An analysis of provider perceptions for telehospice. *Am J Hosp Palliat Care* 1998;**15**:267–74.

22   Collins K, O'Cathain A. The continuum of patient satisfaction – from satisfied to very satisfied. *Soc Sci Med* 2003;**57**:2465–70.

23   Whitten P, Davis S. Value added of telehome care for COPD and CHF patients in Michigan's Upper Peninsula. *Telemed J E Health* 2003;**9** (Suppl 1):S64–5.

▶5

Business models and return on investment

Herschel Peddicord, Karen R. Thomas and Allyson M. Beach

Introduction

Telemonitoring has been used successfully in the management of chronic diseases such as congestive heart failure, diabetes and chronic obstructive pulmonary disease. A two-year study in the US found that patients with chronic diseases who were monitored remotely used fewer high-cost resources, such as the emergency room or hospitalizations, than patients who were not monitored.[1]

Chronic diseases are generally manageable if the clinician has adequate information to make clinical interventions. Daily monitoring of heart rate, body weight, blood pressure, oxygen saturation, blood glucose and peak flow rates can provide early warning of changes in a patient's condition. For example, in a patient with congestive heart failure, responding to subtle changes early in a decompensation episode means the patient can be treated using simple drugs (such as furosemide), avoiding the need for the hospital attendance that usually follows an exacerbation of the condition. Such savings form the basis for return-on-investment calculations in the use of home telehealth and telemonitoring services.

Return on investment

'Return on investment' has no generally accepted definition. It is a slightly vague term that is taken to mean the monetary benefits derived from having spent money on developing or revising a system. That is, the return on investment is a measure of an organization's profitability: how much profit or cost saving is realized for a given use of money. This is one aspect of a formal health economics analysis – that is, it reflects the provider's viewpoint, not the patient's or society's (see Chapter 3).

In the US, both hospitals and home health agencies are reimbursed on an episodic basis for care provided. They are paid a predefined sum for an episode of care, regardless of the length of the episode or the actual cost incurred. This creates a powerful incentive for hospitals and home health agencies to increase efficiency. In contrast, physicians are reimbursed on a transactional basis, according to the volume of care provided. Their incentive is to provide more care. This unbalanced alignment of incentives is a potential deterrent to the widespread adoption of home telehealth and telemonitoring.

The return on investment for telemonitoring will be different depending on the setting in which it is used:

- hospitals
- managed care/insurance
- home health agencies.

Hospitals

Hospitals have the potential to realize a significant return on investment from home telehealth. For example, consider the cost of treating a patient with congestive heart failure (CHF). The average cost for an admission for CHF is $7200, while the average reimbursement from Medicare for that admission is $4300 (2005 Medicare fee data). Therefore, patients who frequently decompensate and require readmission cost hospitals large amounts of money – on average, hospitals lose $2900 per admission. In the US, acute heart failure is one of the most common causes of hospital admission. In 2003, there were 1.1 million admissions.[2]

This large discrepancy between the cost of providing hospital care and the governmental reimbursement for it prompts the question: Why would a hospital not invest in telemonitoring to improve outcomes and reduce costs? The answer is complex, but hospital managers have a number of issues to consider:

- Would a simple telephone call work as well and cost even less? (In fact, comparative trials of telemonitoring versus nurse telephone calls have produced equivocal results.[3])
- Will physicians accept a new care delivery strategy and use it?
- Is it better for the hospital to invest in advanced diagnostic imaging technology or a surgical suite enhancement rather than new and perhaps riskier technology such as telemonitoring?

In general, the American hospital sector still bases its investment strategy on revenue enhancement rather than efficiency gains. This behaviour is beginning to change because of the US government's experiments with reimbursement models, which involve sharing financial risk with providers. Two Medicare programmes – Medicare Health Support and Care Management for High Cost Beneficiaries – are in the early phases of implementation. Through these programmes, more than 250 000 patients will be cared for using a risk-sharing model rather than a traditional fee-for-service model. Both programmes make explicit recommendations to participating providers to use telemonitoring. Hospital managers will be watching carefully as these trials move forward.

Telemonitoring of the acutely ill, if properly implemented, could theoretically allow earlier discharge, because patients would be monitored at home. When hospitals are paid on a set fee-for-patient basis, early discharge will reduce costs and provide an opportunity for streamlined bed management. When clinically appropriate, patients can be discharged to a home health agency that can provide care and monitoring services. In practice, this coordination between home-care agencies and the acute care sector is uncommon at present.

Telemonitoring may also produce cost savings for hospitals because of the Medicare reimbursement model. After a patient has been admitted to hospital for CHF, Medicare will not reimburse for any readmission under the same diagnosis in 30 days. Therefore, it is in the interests of the hospital to ensure that the patient is cared for in an appropriate setting and that readmission is prevented. With telemonitoring, stable but high-risk patients can be released from hospital earlier and can be evaluated continuously in their home for the remainder of the 30-day period. This provides additional assurances to help prevent readmission in the 30-day time frame.

For hospitals, the factors in the return on investment include:

- telemonitoring equipment costs of $60 per month
- hospital readmission cost of potentially $7200
- savings due to earlier discharge: cost savings of $800–1000 per day (difference between the actual cost and Medicare reimbursement)
- potentially increased nurse retention as a result of reduced case loads.

Managed care/insurance

Patients in managed care and insured populations include:

- acutely ill patients who require constant surveillance and care
- sick chronically ill patients who can become ill quickly if not properly monitored
- well chronically ill patients whose disease state will decline over time to a more serious condition
- the overall well population.

Acutely ill patients represent about 1% of the managed care population but account for 28% of the total costs of healthcare.[4] Sick chronically ill patients, who are teetering on the edge of acute care, represent 15–20% of the managed care population but account for 50% of the total costs of healthcare. The remaining patients represent 80% of the population and account for 20% of the total costs of healthcare. The greatest potential for cost saving lies with the acutely ill and sick chronically ill patients, who represent 16–21% of the total population but account for nearly 80% of the total costs of healthcare.[5]

Congestive heart failure

Managed care organizations and disease management groups can provide improved care through telemonitoring, with potential cost savings, especially in the most expensive patient subgroups. For example, a case manager may observe an increase in body weight and blood pressure and a decline in oxygen saturation in a patient with congestive heart failure. The case manager could then contact a local home-care agency and request a visit to the patient's home for a physical assessment. After contacting the patient's physician, an in-home injection of furosemide could be arranged, which might avoid an expensive hospital emergency room visit and perhaps hospitalization. The factors in the return on investment include:

- $150 to administer an injection of furosemide in the home versus $1200 for a visit to the hospital emergency room for the same purpose
- telemonitoring equipment costs of $60 per month versus $4500 per day for hospitalization.

Note that despite the nursing and telemonitoring costs, organizations can still accrue significant savings.

Diabetes

Chronically ill patients are high users of emergency care, inpatient care and physician time. Telemonitoring can give an organization that manages cases a more timely way of educating patients about best practices in disease management. In traditional case management, informational brochures and pamphlets are mailed to patients regularly, perhaps every three to four weeks. With telemonitoring, education about lifestyle choices can occur more immediately and have greater chance of success (Box 5.1).

As well as more rapid intervention, telemonitoring may produce more accurate data than can be obtained by patient self-reporting. Although few patients are intentionally deceptive, there is room for incorrect information in self-reporting. In the example below (see Box 5.1), Ms Brown might not remember to include carrot cake in her daily diabetic food diary. She might have learned how to step on her scale 'just right', so that any weight she gained in the previous week does not show up. Patients generally mean well and may think they are pleasing the physician if they simply write the same blood glucose reading for three days in a row when they forget to carry out the test. Telemonitoring is the most accurate tracking method available – apart from 24-hour hands-on nursing care. More accurate records mean better and more efficient care and cost savings.

The factors in the return on investment for Ms Brown include:

- accurate reporting prevents an acute episode, potentially saving $4500 per day in hospital costs
- immediate intervention in lifestyle choice prevents costly relapses
- immediate intervention prevents a condition from requiring a physician visit, potentially saving $50 per visit
- the patient becomes more involved in their own care, motivating improvement and lowering costs for multiple acute episodes.

Obstetrics

Preventive care is an emerging component of healthcare across the globe. Providers and insurers alike are beginning to recognize that prevention is better than cure. One area in which this is obvious is prenatal care. Women with a high-risk pregnancy are more likely to deliver prematurely and have higher hospital costs. Their infants are more likely to have birth defects, low birth weight and cognitive impairment.

Box 5.1. Case study – diabetes monitoring

Ms Brown is a 34-year-old woman with diabetes. Her glucose levels have been inconsistent over a three-day period. In typical case management, there is no way of knowing that Ms Brown is having trouble managing her blood glucose unless she sees a doctor or becomes acutely unwell. By the time the episode has occurred, the cost of managing it could be substantial, and the opportunity for prevention will have passed.

If Ms Brown is recording and transmitting her glucose levels using a telemonitor (Fig. 5.1), her nurse will know that the values are out of the acceptable range and can contact her to discuss her concerns. When the nurse speaks to Ms Brown, she may learn that the patient has not been following her diet. This is the best time for intervention and behaviour modification: the readings are outside limits, the nurse finds the cause and then takes the opportunity to discuss why dietary change is important.

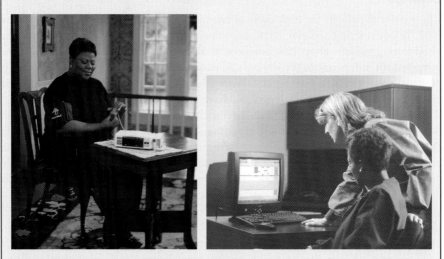

Fig. 5.1. Diabetes monitoring (Honeywell HomMed)

Comment
Telemonitoring allows more rapid intervention. Action can be more relevant when done in a timely manner. Ms Brown can better understand cause and effect, because a nurse manager has taken the time to explain, at an appropriate time, that dietary choices will affect her disease.

Depending on the time of year of birth, these infants may require palivizumab injections ($1000 each) for prevention of respiratory syncytial virus – a respiratory infection that causes colds in healthy adults and children but can be deadly for premature infants. Prevention of premature births is in the interests of the managed care or insurance organization in order to reduce future costs.

Telemonitoring can be used in patients with gestational diabetes, pre-eclampsia and other conditions that previously required long-term hospitalization. Remote monitoring allows bed rest at home rather than in a hospital ($800/day not including tests), and a change in condition can alert the doctor to any potential problems. A visit

---

Box 5.2. Case study – pre-eclampsia

Mrs Smith is 30 weeks pregnant when she develops pre-eclampsia – a disorder that can occur during pregnancy and affects both mother and unborn baby. Pre-eclampsia affects 5–8% of all pregnancies. It is a rapidly progressive condition characterized by high blood pressure, swelling and the presence of protein in the urine. Hypertensive disorders of pregnancy complicate 10% of all pregnancies in the US (360 000 women) at a cost of more than $8000 per case.[6]

The traditional course of action might call for Mrs Smith to spend the next 12 weeks in hospital on bed rest to try to ensure her baby makes it to 39–42 weeks. At $800 a day (room cost alone), the insurance or managed care organization might pay $67 000 to hospitalize Mrs Smith. Her obstetrician suggests keeping Mrs Smith in a nearby hotel (or her home, if appropriate) and using a telemonitor to evaluate her condition. At $45/day for the hotel room and $10/day all-inclusive monitoring costs, Mrs Smith's care now costs $4620 for the 12-week period. Mrs Smith's baby is more likely to go to full term than without monitoring, so the costs of palivizumab may be unnecessary, as will be the long-term costs related to premature birth.

Comment
Avoidance of the hospital costs of monitoring and conducting telemonitoring out of hospital result in savings of more than $62 000.

---

to the doctor's office may be somewhat costly, but it will be less expensive than a trip to the hospital emergency room or an extended stay in hospital. Some organizations have experimented with monitoring in a facility near the hospital (such as a Ronald McDonald House or nearby hotel), which keeps the patients close to hospital but frees up hospital beds and nurses, while lowering costs (Box 5.2).

The factors in the return on investment for Mrs Smith (see Box 5.2) include:

- $62 000 cost savings on a 12-week hospitalization
- $6000 cost savings in palivizumab injections for a premature baby
- $75 000 average cost of neonatal intensive care for a premature baby
- lifetime of health-related costs avoided because the baby went to full term or near full term
- hospital beds and nursing staff freed for acute care patients.

Summary

Telemonitoring is not appropriate for every condition and every patient, and compliance is a key factor. For patients who qualify for telemonitoring, however, the potential savings for managed care organizations are substantial.

Home health agencies

Home-care agencies may achieve efficiencies by using telemonitoring to avoid unnecessary home visits. In conventional practice, home visits are conducted according to a predetermined schedule. The use of telemonitoring allows a more efficient case management model of care. In this model, a clinician (usually a registered nurse) can review dozens of patients each day and assign the proper staff to the patients who need a visit that day. It is not unusual for one nurse to manage as many as 60 patients with the assistance of less-skilled nurses and physical therapists.[7] The registered nurse makes visits only to the most serious cases and primarily acts as a case manager – directing care where and when it is needed. The result is an overall reduction in visits by the registered nurse, which therefore reduces the cost per episode (Box 5.3).

Other evidence for efficiency gains due to home telehealth comes from a large survey in Pennsylvania. Information was collected from 33 home health agencies that had been using telehealth for periods of two years or more; about one-third of the agencies had not implemented telehealth.[8] The average number of patients per nurse was lowest in the agencies that had not used telehealth and was highest in the agencies that had used home telehealth for longest.

In the Pennsylvania survey, some home health agencies used relatively simple forms of telemonitoring, while others used interactive video. The average equipment costs were therefore quite high. It was perhaps unsurprising that the average cost per telehealth visit was $183, while the average revenue per visit was only $170. However, the analysis suggested that a reduction of 5% in actual home visits would be enough to recoup the investment in home telehealth.[9]

Acute care is more manageable when home health agencies can obtain data on vital signs at regular intervals. Many monitoring systems can be programmed to ask for readings several times a day, so that data capture can be scheduled according to the physician's orders. However, home telehealth equipment should not be viewed as a replacement for human contact and intervention. The most successful models of telemonitoring include intensive patient management and communication. An agency cannot simply place a monitor in the home and assume that the patient will improve. Interaction, instruction and cooperative care are essential components in a successful telemonitoring programme.

Compliance may also be a concern in the case of certain acutely ill patients. If such patients are unable to perform the basic skills that telemonitoring requires, or they

---

Box 5.3. Case study – home health agency

Sentara is a community, not-for-profit healthcare organization in southeast Virginia and northeast North Carolina. It operates more than 70 care-giving sites, including six acute care hospitals (with a total of >1500 beds), seven nursing centres and three assisted living centres. In 2004, Sentara conducted 1100 home telehealth visits and telemonitoring.

The company recently examined the results of its telehealth intervention for its patients with congestive heart failure. In 68 patients with heart failure older than 65 years with a New York Heart Association ranking of 3 or 4, a 72% decrease in readmissions to Sentara hospitals over a two-year period was seen (Chetney R, personal communication, 2005).

Comment
The reduction in hospital admissions resulted in large savings to the Sentara organization.

have no support system to help them, telemonitoring might be inappropriate until the patient's condition improves. It is crucial to choose patients for whom this type of care is appropriate.

The factors in the return on investment include:

- fewer nursing visits, reducing costs to the agency (for example, because fuel and vehicle costs are lower)
- the level of care is increased because more patients can receive regular care
- nurse retention is improved, along with their ability to care for more patients.

Partnerships

Home health agencies partnering with insurance and managed care companies will enjoy a greater return on investment from telemonitoring their chronically ill patients. As in the acute care model, fewer nursing visits mean direct cost savings for the agency. The benefits to both managed care organizations and home health agencies are strikingly similar in the chronic care model. Management of disease state and education about disease process are critical components of gaining control over both the illness and the costs to treat that illness. Comorbidities often come into play with the chronically ill as well. Many patients who have CHF are also diabetic, and many patients with chronic obstructive pulmonary diseases first would have been diagnosed with asthma. Educating the patient on potential disease progression is relevant to the prevention of disease progression.

An important factor in telemonitoring of chronically ill patients is knowledge of the appropriate length of time to conduct the monitoring. To achieve optimum outcomes and cost-effectiveness, most patients will not need to be monitored indefinitely. The true goal of telemonitoring is to improve health and the patient's 'ownership' of their health.

The factors in the return on investment include:

- fewer nursing visits and lower costs
- as the patient's condition improves, less care is needed; monitoring costs become negligible and patient care becomes highly profitable.

Conclusion

Telemonitoring, when used appropriately, lends itself to deployment in a number of settings. These applications generate savings by reducing healthcare utilization and preventing or delaying exacerbations of acute and chronic illnesses. The population that benefits from telemonitoring ranges from the very young to the very old and from pre-eclampsic mothers to the elderly with New York Heart Association stage 4 CHF. Although more research is needed to quantify the return on investment from telemonitoring in hospitals, managed care organizations and home health agencies, preliminary results are very encouraging. The ultimate return on investment is achieved by using telemonitoring to bring together the physician, hospital, home-care agency, managed care company and patient to provide prompt, efficient and cost-effective healthcare.

Further information

American Telemedicine Association. *Home telehealth is an effective and efficient approach to delivering home care*. Washington, DC: American Telemedicine Association, 2005. Available at: www.atmeda.org/news/mediaguide/home telehealth.htm#4 (last accessed 15 January 2006).

Honeywell HomMed website. Available at: www.hommed.com (last accessed 15 January 2006).

References

1 Rosenblum B, Schabert V, Davis N. *Independent analysis of monitored/non-monitored patients*. Santa Barbara: Strategic Healthcare Programs, 2004.
2 Agency for Healthcare Research and Quality. *Healthcare cost and utilization project (HCUP)*. Available at: hcup.ahrq.gov/HCUPnet.asp (last accessed 15 January 2006).
3 Jerant AF, Azari R, Nesbitt TS. Reducing the cost of frequent hospital admissions for congestive heart failure: a randomized trial of a home telecare intervention. *Med Care* 2001;**39**:1234–45.
4 Sipkoff M. Health plans begin to address chronic care management. *Manag Care* 2003;**12**. Available at: www.managedcaremag.com/archives/0312/0312.kaiserchronic.pdf (last accessed 15 January 2006).
5 Partnership for Solutions. *Chronic conditions: making the case for ongoing care*. Baltimore, MD: Johns Hopkins University, 2002. Available at: www.partnershipforsolutions.com/DMS/files/chronicbook2002.pdf (last accessed 15 January 2006).
6 Preeclampsia Foundation. *Statistics*. Bellevue, WA: Preeclampsia Foundation, 2005. Available at: www.preeclampsia.org/statistics.asp (last accessed 15 January 2006).
7 Brown R, Schore J, Archibald N, *et al. Coordinating care for medicare beneficiaries: early experiences of 5 demonstration programs, their patients, and providers. Appendix a.* Princeton, NJ: Mathematical Policy Research, 2004. Available at: www.mathematica-mpr.com/publications/PDFs/bestpracconga.pdf (last accessed 15 January 2006).
8 Pennsylvania Homecare Association and Pennsylvania State University. *2003–2004 telehealth project evaluation, year two: the impact of telehealth on nursing workload and retention.* Available at: www.pahomecare.org/evaluation2.pdf (last accessed 15 January 2006).
9 Pennsylvania Homecare Association and Pennsylvania State University. *The Financial Viability of Telehealth and Telehealth's Impact on Home Health Nurses: Telehealth Project Evaluation Year 3.* Available at: www.pahomecare.org/telehealth_evaluation_report_year3.pdf (last accessed 15 January 2006).

▶6

The evidence base

Mark Bensink, David Hailey and Richard Wootton

Introduction

Continued advances in science and technology, and general improvements in environmental and social conditions, have increased life expectancy around the world. As a result, a growing proportion of the world's population is elderly. Over the last 50 years, the number of people aged 60 years or over has tripled, and is expected to triple again to almost two billion by 2050.[1] Along with this increase in life expectancy has come an increase in the prevalence of chronic diseases, such as cardiovascular disease, cancer and diabetes. Chronic disease has become the major cause of death. By the end of 2005, it is estimated that 60% of all deaths will be due to chronic diseases,[2] accounting for 46% of the global burden of disease.[3]

The economic burden of chronic disease is profound. The World Health Organization has calculated the cost of deaths from heart disease, stroke and diabetes in international dollars – a hypothetical currency that facilitates comparisons between countries. The losses in national income for 2005 were estimated to be $18 billion in China, $3 billion in the Russian Federation, $1.6 billion in the UK, $1.2 billion in Pakistan and $1.2 billion in Canada.[2] The increasing burden of disease on healthcare resources, together with the demographical and epidemiological changes that are taking place, provide a powerful incentive to care for patients in their homes where possible.[4]

Provision of care directly to the home offers a number of alternatives to traditional care. It can offer a substitute for acute hospitalization, an alternative to long-term institutionalization, a complementary means of maintaining individuals in their own community[4] and an alternative to conventional hospital outpatient or physician visits. Provision of care in the home using telehealth will be important, therefore, for the future delivery of health services – if it can be considered a plausible alternative to conventional methods.

Literature review

Home telehealth is an area of increasing interest to providers and consumers alike, but what is known about it? In what areas has home telehealth been investigated? What is the evidence of benefits, costs and acceptance by users to support its implementation?

To answer these questions, we conducted a systematic review of the literature. We examined articles in which a home telehealth intervention had been compared with a non-telehealth alternative in terms of administrative changes, patient management decisions, patient outcomes, economic impact, or social impact on patients or carers, or both. The articles were drawn from a search of computerized literature databases, including Medline, CINAHL, EMBASE, PsycINFO, Allied and Complementary Medicine, and Rehabilitation and Physical Medicine. We used search terms such as telehomecare, remote consultation, home health care and home monitoring. This resulted in a large number of potential reports (over 9000). Once duplicates and articles without abstracts were removed, the abstracts of 2636 references were reviewed. From these, 103 controlled studies, which reported outcomes of home telehealth applications in a scientifically valid manner, were identified and reviewed.

Progress in home telehealth

Reports of controlled investigations into the use of telehealth in home healthcare first appeared in the literature in the early 1980s. Early studies investigated the use of the telephone for counselling hypertensive patients; for educating, counselling and monitoring patients after a heart attack; and for supporting patients after heart surgery. Since then, the number of controlled studies published has increased progressively, reflecting the increased interest in home telehealth (Fig. 6.1).

The most common areas of investigation have been the management of chronic diseases: diabetes, heart failure and other cardiac disease (including post-myocardial infarction rehabilitation, coronary artery bypass grafting and arrhythmia). The general area of mental health has also been a frequent area of investigation, with studies on home telehealth applications for more specific conditions such as depression, obsessive compulsive disorder and substance abuse. Other areas include care for the

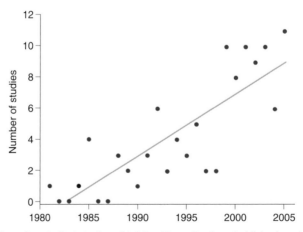

Fig. 6.1. Number of controlled studies of telehealth applications published each year from 1981 until mid-2005 (*n*=103). The line shown is a linear regression

elderly, support for caregivers of home-care patients, smoking cessation support, arthritis, hypertension, asthma and cancer (Fig. 6.2).

The studies identified were undertaken in 14 countries. Three-quarters of the studies were from the US, with Canada, the UK and Japan accounting for another 14%. Other countries included Israel, France, Germany, Argentina, Greece, China, Denmark and Japan (Fig. 6.3), with one multicentre study undertaken in the UK, Germany and Netherlands combined.[5]

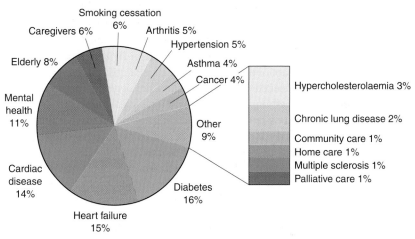

Fig. 6.2. Conditions or areas of healthcare considered in home telehealth studies (n=103)

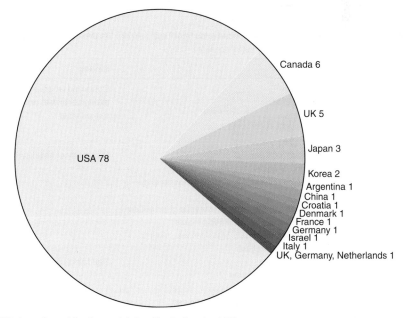

Fig. 6.3. Location of the home telehealth studies (n=103)

Characteristics of the research

Most studies (95%) reported investigations in terms of patient outcomes (evaluations pertinent to the condition being studied, such as blood pressure for hypertension or level of functioning for cardiac disease). Administrative changes were considered in two studies and social outcomes in one. A high proportion of the reports were of feasibility or short-term studies. This is to be expected in the early stages of evaluating a new telemedicine application. Table 6.1 summarizes the recommended stages in any telemedicine evaluation.

Although establishing the safety and feasibility of home telehealth is essential, what has been relatively neglected to date is economic evaluations of home telehealth applications. The literature review showed that less than 20% of papers published had incorporated any sort of economic analysis. Evidence of cost-effectiveness is perhaps the persuasive argument needed to motivate healthcare decision-makers and could be a catalyst for the widespread implementation of home telehealth.

More than 80% of studies reported the outcomes of randomized, controlled trials (RCTs) – the gold standard for medical and health research. This contrasts with the research being undertaken in other areas of telehealth, such as teleradiology and teledermatology,[7] which generally have a much lower proportion of RCTs. Non-randomized designs included non-randomized, controlled trials, cohort studies and case-control studies, which provide different (weaker) levels of evidence.[8] Only half of these trials were large trials (with more than 50 patients in each arm) which may be partly the result of difficulties in designing, running and ensuring the methodological

Table 6.1. Stages of telemedicine evaluation (adapted from Taylor, 1999[6]). An evaluation is a description or assessment to answer a question or set of questions

Questions	Components*	Setting
Is it safe?	Equipment Data transmission Data retrieval Data viewing Training requirements	Controlled laboratory-style experiments with or without real patients
Is it feasible?	Organization of service Provision of equipment where required Competent clinicians both to send and receive information Practicality of required procedures in given setting Acceptability to clinicians and patients Identification of human, organizational, legal or financial complications	Pilot study or small-scale trial
Is it effective?	Quality of care Health status of patients Economics	Randomized, controlled trial
Is it sustainable?	Monitoring the effects of long-term use	Long-term studies

* Including but not limited to listed components.

rigour of home telehealth research. These are challenges that will have to be addressed in future studies.

What sort of home telehealth is being practised?

Almost half of the home telehealth applications combined some form of patient monitoring with patient counselling – the process of listening to someone and giving them advice about their problems.[9] An example of this is the transmission of electrocardiographic data during home exercise after myocardial infarction and subsequent telephone counselling on exercise adherence.[10] Fifteen per cent of studies involved active patient monitoring without the delivery of counselling or education via the home telehealth device: for example, the transfer of blood glucose levels for physician analysis from a combined glucometer and modem device.[11] In 12 studies, videoconferencing was used as a substitute for face-to-face home visiting. Only three studies involved the use of a call centre that patients rang for advice.

More than half of the studies involved nurses providing or facilitating care with support from physicians or care teams. Physicians were providers in 13% of studies and mental health professionals in 7%. Other studies used automated systems for data collection, non-medical staff or technicians, case managers, counsellors or care teams. The professional who provided home telehealth care was unspecified in 10 studies.

What technologies are being used?

In examining the technologies being used in home telehealth, it is worth distinguishing between the physical device being used with the patient and the telecommunications medium being used for data transmission. The ordinary home telephone was the primary communications medium used in more than half of the studies (Table 6.2). The telephone was also used for audio communication and was combined with additional devices such as glucometers, sphygmomanometers, electrocardiographs

Table 6.2. Summary of technologies used in home telehealth studies

Device	Number of studies
Telephone alone	59*
Telephone combined with additional device	13
Videophone	8†
Composite device without videophone‡	12
Composite device with videophone	4
Computer	5
Mobile phone	1
Still image videophone	1

* Seven studies used the home telephone interfaced with a computer or automated system in the hospital.
† Two studies compared videophone, telephone and face-to-face intervention groups.
‡ Composite devices were those that provided a number of different functionalities, such as voice communication and measurement of blood pressure, pulse oximetry or blood glucose.

and pulse oximeters for transferring data over the ordinary home telephone line in an additional 13 studies (13%). Most home telehealth devices communicated via the ordinary telephone network (91%). The infrastructure was unspecified in six studies (6%). One study used mobile phones for data transmission. Only one paper reported using a videophone that required digital lines.

Only three of the studies used the Internet. In one study, the patient interfaced directly with the Internet; for the other two studies, information provided via telephone was automatically collated by a computer and uploaded to an Internet page for viewing by a health professional. The small number of Internet applications is the result of selecting studies that compared a home telehealth alternative to a non-telehealth alternative. Fourteen studies that used the Internet compared a home telehealth intervention with another home telehealth intervention: for example, Internet-delivered therapy versus telephone-delivered therapy. In addition, 11 studies that used the Internet compared a home telehealth intervention with a wait-list control group rather than an active non-home telehealth alternative. As the use of the Internet increases in home telehealth, it can be assumed that research into its use will move beyond feasibility testing to investigations of its place in routine care delivery.

Home telehealth – where is the evidence?

Most studies reported that the home telehealth alternative had advantages over the non-telehealth alternative studied (Table 6.3). This provides reasonable evidence for the feasibility of home telehealth as a delivery mechanism. It also provides indirect assurance about safety, although few studies carried out formal assessments of safety. Thus, the first two stages of evaluation seem to have been dealt with (see Table 6.1).

Different study designs provide different strengths of evidence. Large RCTs, such as that described in Box 6.1, are indubitably more convincing than anecdotal case reports. To take into account the strength of the evidence, a design score (Table 6.4) was assigned to each study identified in the literature review (see Hailey *et al*[7] for more information about design scoring). This allows the results from different applications of home telehealth to be compared, albeit in a rather approximate way, as no account has been taken of how the studies were performed. The design scores show that there is more evidence in support of certain conditions than others (see Fig. 6.4): stronger evidence for the value of home telehealth is available for diabetes, heart failure, cardiac disease and mental health than for the other 12 areas.

Table 6.3. Summary results of the home telehealth practice investigations

Result category	Number of studies
Home telehealth practice had advantages over alternative approach	81
Home telehealth practice had advantages over alternative approach, but there also were some disadvantages	7
Unclear whether home telehealth practice had advantages; further work probably needed	14
Alternative approach had advantages over home telehealth practice	1

Box 6.1. An example of home telehealth research, the DIAL trial was a randomized trial of telephone intervention in patients with chronic heart failure[12]

Objective To determine whether a centralized telephone intervention reduces the incidence of death or admission for worsening heart failure in outpatients with chronic heart failure.

Design Multicentre, randomized, controlled trial.

Setting 51 centres in Argentina (public and private hospitals and ambulatory settings).

Participants 1518 outpatients with stable chronic heart failure and optimal drug treatment randomized, stratified by attending cardiologist, to telephone intervention or usual care.

Intervention Education, counselling and monitoring by nurses through frequent telephone follow-up in addition to usual care, delivered from a single centre.

Main outcome measure All cause mortality or admission to hospital for worsening heart failure.

Results Complete follow-up was available in 99.5% of patients. The 758 patients in the usual care group were more likely to be admitted for worsening heart failure or to die (235 events, 31%) than the 760 patients who received the telephone intervention (200 events, 26.3%) (relative risk reduction = 20%, 95% confidence interval 3 to 34, p=0.026). This benefit was mostly due to a significant reduction in admissions for heart failure (relative risk reduction = 29%, p=0.005). Mortality was similar in both groups. At the end of the study, the intervention group had a better quality of life than the usual care group (mean total score on Minnesota Living With Heart Failure Questionnaire 31 vs 35, p=0.001).

Conclusions This simple, centralized heart failure programme was effective in reducing the primary end point through a significant reduction in admissions to hospital for heart failure.

Table 6.4. Study design scoring

Study design	Study design score
Large randomized, controlled trial (at least 50 participants in each arm)	5
Small randomized, controlled trial (less than 50 participants in each arm)	3
Non-randomized, controlled, prospective trials	2
Non-randomized, controlled, retrospective trials	1

Although patient numbers are incorporated into the study design score, the calculation of design score alone does not reveal the whole picture. The number of study participants has a large influence on the ability of any trial to reliably detect a treatment effect. The larger the number of participants, the greater the statistical power of the study.[13] Fig. 6.5 provides an additional picture of the conditions investigated, taking into account the total number of participants involved in the studies in each area. With this perspective, the application of home telehealth to smoking cessation emerges as an additional area for which evidence of clinical effectiveness exists.

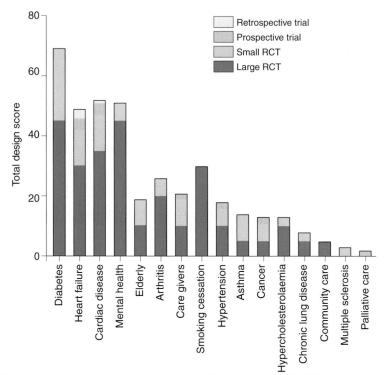

Fig. 6.4. Study design scores for areas investigated in home telehealth trials

Although only six studies in smoking cessation were identified, the large numbers of participants involved in four of these (a total of nearly 10 000 patients) gives increased confidence in the evidence of treatment effects. These trials compared self-help quit guides, standard care, and quit guides plus a number of telephone counselling sessions after quitting.[14–17]

The future

A growing body of evidence supports the application of home telehealth to different conditions. Evidence exists for the clinical effectiveness of home telehealth in smoking cessation, diabetes, cardiac disease, heart failure and mental health. Most of these applications have used the ordinary home telephone network as a simple, cheap and readily available communications infrastructure. More evidence is needed from large RCTs with appropriate rigour and quality. Economic evaluations will be essential to provide high-quality evidence of the cost-effectiveness of home telehealth before its widespread adoption.[18–23] In addition, long-term studies of applications are required to gain a better understanding of the true effectiveness of home telehealth and to demonstrate its sustainability.

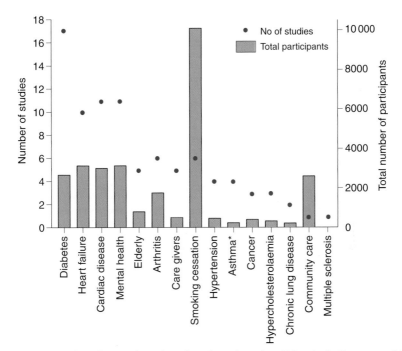

Fig. 6.5. Number of studies conducted, and total number of participants, in the areas of home telehealth identified in the literature review. Some data on numbers of participants were missing for two studies in asthma

Acknowledgement

This work was funded in part by the Australian Government Department of Veterans' Affairs.

Further information

American Telemedicine Association. *Home telehealth toolkit*. Order form available at: www.atmeda.org/news/newres.htm (last accessed 21 December 2005).

Hailey D. The need for cost-effectiveness studies in telemedicine. *J Telemed Telecare* 2005;**11**:379–83.

Kinsella A. *Home telehealthcare: process, policy and procedures*. Kensington, MD: Information for Tomorrow, 2003.

References

1   United Nations. *World population ageing: 1950–2050*. New York: United Nations, 2002.

2   World Health Organization. *Preventing chronic diseases: a vital investment.* Geneva: World Health Organization, 2005.

3   World Health Organization. *Facts related to chronic diseases.* Geneva: World Health Organization, 2005. Available at: www.who.int/dietphysicalactivity/publications/facts/chronic/en/ (last accessed 21 December 2005).

4   Havens B. *Home-based and long-term care: home care issues and evidence.* Geneva: World Health Organization, 1999.

5   Cleland JG, Louis AA, Rigby AS, *et al.* Noninvasive home telemonitoring for patients with heart failure at high risk of recurrent admission and death: the Trans-European Network-Home-Care Management System (TEN-HMS) study. *J Am Coll Cardiol* 2005;**45**:1654–64.

6   Taylor P. Evaluating telemedicine systems and services. In: Wootton R, Craig J, eds. *Introduction to telemedicine.* London: Royal Society of Medicine Press, 1999:105–20.

7   Hailey D, Roine R, Ohinmaa A. Systematic review of evidence for the benefits of telemedicine. *J Telemed Telecare* 2002;**8** (Suppl 1):1–30.

8   Jovell A, Navarro-Rubio M. [Evaluation of scientific evidence]. *Med Clin (Barc)* 1995;**105**:740–3 (in Spanish).

9   Cambridge University Press. *Cambridge dictionaries online.* Cambridge: Cambridge University Press, 2005. Available at: dictionary.cambridge.org/ (last accessed 21 December 2005).

10 DeBusk R, Haskell W, Miller N, *et al.* Medically directed at home rehabilitation soon after clinically uncomplicated acute myocardial infarction: a new model for patient care. *Am J Cardiol* 1985;**55**:251–7.

11 Billiard A, Rohmer V, Roques M, *et al.* Telematic transmission of computerized blood glucose profiles for IDDM patients. *Diabetes Care* 1991;**14**:130–4.

12 Grancelli H, Varini S, Ferrante D, *et al.* Randomized trial of telephone intervention in chronic heart failure: DIAL trial. *BMJ* 2005;**331**:425.

13 Wikipedia contributors. *Clinical trial.* Wikipedia, The Free Encyclopedia, 2006. See en.wikipedia.org/w/index.php?title=Clinical_trial&oldid=35552655 (last accessed 19 January 2006).

14 Orleans C, Schoenbach V, Wagner E, *et al.* Self-help quit smoking interventions: effects of self-help materials, social support instructions, and telephone counseling. *J Consult Clin Psychol* 1991;**59**:439–48.

15 Zhu S, Stretch V, Balabanis M, *et al.* Telephone counseling for smoking cessation: effects of single-session and multiple-session interventions. *J Consult Clin Psychol* 1996;**64**:202–11.

16 Rabius V, McAlister AL, Geiger A, *et al.* Telephone counseling increases cessation rates among young adult smokers. *Health Psychol* 2004;**23**:539–41.

17 Curry SJ, McBride C, Grothaus LC, *et al.* A randomized trial of self-help materials, personalized feedback, and telephone counseling with nonvolunteer smokers. *J Consult Clin Psychol* 1995;**63**:1005–14.

18 Wainwright C, Wootton R. A review of telemedicine and asthma. *Dis Manag Health Outcomes* 2003;**11**:557–63.

19 Louis AA, Turner T, Gretton M, *et al.* A systematic review of telemonitoring for the management of heart failure. *Eur J Heart Fail* 2003;**5**:583–90.

20 Hill A, Theodoros D. Research into telehealth applications in speech-language pathology. *J Telemed Telecare* 2002;**8**:187–96.

21 Hailey D, Ohinmaa A, Roine R. Published evidence on the success of telecardiology: a mixed record. *J Telemed Telecare* 2004;**10** (Suppl 1):36–8.

22 Currell R, Urquhart C, Wainwright P, Lewis R. Telemedicine versus face to face patient care: effects on professional practice and health care outcomes. *Cochrane Database Syst Rev* 2000;(2):CD002098.

23 Hailey D, Ohinmaa A, Roine R. Study quality and evidence of benefit in recent assessments of telemedicine. *J Telemed Telecare* 2004;**10**:318–24.

Section 2: Techniques

▶7

Smart homes

Vincent Rialle, Pierre Rumeau, Catherine Ollivet and Christian Hervé

Introduction

The technologies that are making the concept of 'aging in place' possible have arrived at a time when there are more and more elderly people, health expenditure is increasing and there is a growing scarcity of healthcare providers, particularly nurses. For these reasons, and because many people prefer to age in place at home, the 'health smart home' – or smart home for short – represents a potentially important development.

Smart homes (or smart houses) may be seen as environments designed for patients, but they can also be designed for people of all ages and with all kinds of special needs. There is abundant scientific literature about their potential for favouring independent living in secure conditions for frail people living alone or in institutions, and for alleviating the burden of caregivers and family members of people with cognitive impairment.[1-7]

The cost-effectiveness of the smart home has also been studied in many countries and care settings. Despite scientific publicity and commercial availability, however, smart home technologies are not often used in home care,[8] and diffusion of the concept of smart homes remains slow. The rapid evolution of the technologies that underlie the smart home has outpaced any debate about their use and possible problems about privacy, intrusiveness and control.[9] Various questions therefore arise:

- What are the capabilities of smart home technologies for those in private or sheltered housing?
- Will these capabilities be suitable for people with impaired intellectual abilities or those with other cognitive impairments?
- What ethical considerations should drive these new practices in coping with an aging population?
- Will their use cause new types of relationships to emerge among patients, physicians, caregivers and extended family members?

Growing needs

The age group of people over 80 years is the fastest growing segment of the older population.[10] In industrialized countries, 28% of the population will be over 60 years by 2025. The 'parent support ratio' (the number of oldest-old per 100 people aged

50–64 years) in industrialized countries was 10–25 in 1998; by 2025 it will be 25 in the US, 31 in France, 35 in Sweden and 42 in Japan. By 2015, there will be more people older than 80 years in developing countries than in industrialized countries.

Although cardiovascular disease remains the primary cause of death, dementia and hip fracture are the two most worrisome public health issues in the elderly population in terms of causing handicap and institutionalization. These two major age-related disorders are likely to become the main target of smart home services.

Cognitive impairment, because of Alzheimer's disease or related disorders, is a growing concern. The dementia stage of cognitive impairment causes disorders such as being lost in time and space, having difficulties with language (aphasia), having difficulties finding the right movements for an action (apraxia), being unaware of one's condition and environment (agnosia) and often serious problem-solving difficulties. Worldwide, studies show that many inhabitants of nursing and retirement homes have some kind of cognitive impairment. People with dementia need assistance at each and every moment of the day and night. Their caregivers can be so burdened by the need for around-the-clock assistance and surveillance (to prevent accidents, wandering or running away) that they can become overwhelmed by their responsibilities.

When an elderly person falls, common sense demands that things should be organized so that someone close by is alerted quickly. Unfortunately, this is not the case for many people who live alone. A fall without rescue remains a major problem for the elderly and is associated with consequences such as psychological stroke, reduced functioning, premature admission to a nursing home and drastically reduced longevity.

What is a smart home?

The 'smart' home is a term that refers to a home capable of providing intelligent interaction with the occupants by means of special electronic devices. Rapid developments in technology have allowed demonstration smart homes for healthcare to be constructed.[3,6,11] Applications have been examined in areas such as the functional health status of the elderly at home, fall detection, rehabilitation, asthma, hypertension and cardiac disease.

Smart homes for healthcare are intended to give frail elderly people (and their caregivers) security, safety and a better quality of life, while improving access to medical care without hospitalization. They are designed to help maintain the person's autonomy and independence, enhance inclusion in society[12] and avoid, reduce or postpone institutionalization. Broadly speaking, a smart home includes:

- equipment in the person's home (Fig. 7.1), such as:
  - an array of sensors (usually wirelessly) connected to a local computer to monitor, for example, activities of daily living, falls or environmental conditions
  - actuators such as motorized blinds, curtain and window openers, and electric door locks

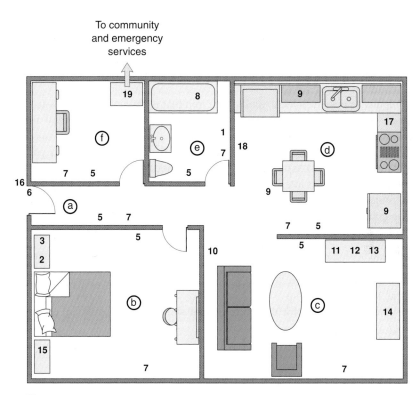

To community
and emergency
services

Biosensors

1 Bathroom scales

2 Blood pressure

3 Oximeter

Other sensors

4 Fall sensor (worn)

5 IR movement detector

6 Door contact

7 Microphones

8 Bathwater monitor

9 RFID tag for activity analysis

10 Ambient temperature

11 Programmable telephone
   with large buttons

12 Medicine reminder

13 Automatic calendar
   showing day and night

14 TV set usable for videoconferencing and telecare

15 Automatic bedroom light

16 Automatic door lock

17 Stove and oven control

18 Cooking/daily agenda display

19 Local intelligence unit

a. Entrance
b. Bedroom
c. Living room
d. Kitchen
e. Bathroom
f. Laundry

Fig. 7.1. An example of a smart home, showing an illustrative collection of sensors and devices. The local intelligence unit is responsible for handling raw sensor data, controlling devices, operating the inference engine to raise an alarm, monitoring health status, and connecting to the remote server when necessary

- perhaps robotic assistants for walking, lifting loads or cooking
- a secure Internet connection to allow the home user access to a range of information and consultation services
- an easy-to-use videoconferencing device to facilitate person-to-person communication

- a computer to provide a local intelligence unit that is connected to a remote server with a secure Internet connection; some sensors and actuators may include sophisticated communication software
- mobile, easy-to-use personal wireless terminals for caregivers, such as personal digital assistants (PDAs), smart phones and mobile computers; these devices include graphical user interfaces that allow various functions, such as access to an electronic patient record, real-time remote monitoring of sensor data, remote home context awareness, remote operation of robots and videoconferencing for person-to-person or person-to-group communication (Fig. 7.2).

Medically and socially, the smart home allows a wide range of possibilities, such as:

- injury prevention
- remote medical follow-up
- real-time data analysis for detecting critical situations or significant changes in habit

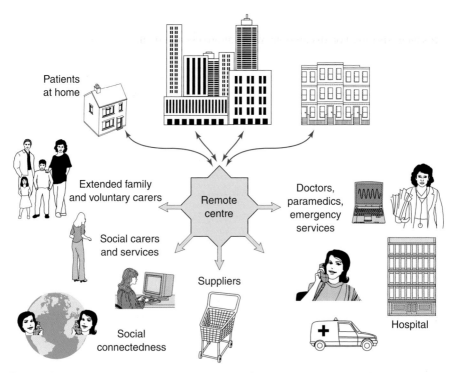

Fig. 7.2. Connection to medical, social and extended family resources and services

- help with various household tasks (such as cooking or dressing)
- sophisticated 'context awareness' of caregivers and relatives, statistical figures, social connectedness and intergenerational communication facilities
- epidemiological research on aging or handicap.

The software tools can be designed for various types of caregivers, including nurses, social workers, doctors and extended family members.

Smart home projects

Most current smart homes are demonstration flats for research and development purposes. However, the positive reports of experience attest that the technology is more than simply a theoretical concept. Smart home projects include:[13-16]

- BESTA project, Norway
- Seven Oaks project, Londonderry, Northern Ireland
- Safe-at-Home project, Northampton, UK
- Elite Care Oatfield Estates, Oregon, US.

BESTA

In the mid-1990s, eight small flats were equipped in a group-living arrangement for people with early dementia in Tonsberg, Norway[13]. The project started with a user-needs analysis based on discussions with caregivers and planners of the services in the flats. Each flat was equipped with devices such as:

- lights that automatically turned on when the resident got up at night
- alerts for staff if the resident was out of bed for more than 30 minutes at night
- heat detectors that automatically turned off cookers if they overheated or were left on because of forgetfulness
- smoke detectors to alert staff, turn on lights and unlock doors
- magnetic detectors on exit doors to alert staff (for residents at risk of wandering, especially at night).

The reported benefits were significant. For instance, the cost of the alarm installation for one person was saved in one year.

Seven Oaks project

The Seven Oaks project was a dementia-specific facility, in which innovative architecture was combined with smart home technology.[14] The facility comprised 30 single flats with integral communal facilities; 14 of the flats were equipped with various sensors that were used mostly at night to alert staff about risky situations. The sensors enabled the monitoring of room temperature, lighting, continence and falls. A local intelligence unit identified whether people were out of bed for long periods or whether they were wandering, smoking in bed or leaving water taps running. A monitoring system was capable of detecting changes in a resident's customary night-time pattern of behaviour. Ethical issues were addressed specifically, allowing the system to serve the values of dementia service and to facilitate, not substitute for, caring relationships.

Safe-at-Home project

In Northampton, the homes of 12 impaired people were equipped with automatic shut-off devices for cookers, alarms for remote care facilities and time-orientation devices. A demonstration smart house was constructed to show potential users how the technology would work in their own home.[15]

Elite Care Oatfield Estates

Elite Care Oatfield Estates is a residential care facility in Oregon, US.[1] Most of the classic smart home capabilities were implemented in a system called Creating Autonomy-Risk Equilibrium (CARE). An array of sensors showed when a resident with a risk of falls sat up during the night. In this case, the system sent an email message that lit up the call light of the nurse on duty and illuminated the suite. Both residents and staff wore credit card-sized infrared tags, which were coded to differentiate each individual in the residence and enable a computer to detect when a resident left the building (to cope with patients who wandered or ran away). The system also detected changes in behaviour patterns, regulated ambient conditions in each resident's environment and transmitted pertinent health information to predetermined recipients, such as nurses and doctors.

Other projects

Elite Care and the University of Washington also began to develop an artificial caretaker, which was based on an activity 'compass' (including a PDA, global positioning system (GPS) receiver and wireless modem) to help guide impaired people through daily routines, such as a trip to the market or a walk to the public garden. Another project dealt with an adaptive prompter that helped people with dementia focus on a task at hand and prompted them to move to the next task. For instance, it would help residents avoid the hazards of a hot stove or remind them to wear their coat when going out in the garden.

Other smart home demonstrations

Growing interest in the potential of technology for helping elderly people with disabilities – especially those with cognitive impairment and their caregivers – started in the middle of the 1990s, with several large-scale research and development projects (Table 7.1). Most of them used a collaborative analysis and design method based on strong user involvement. Other projects are listed in Table 7.2.

Finally, the Everyday Technologies for Alzheimer Care (ETAC) project, led by the American Alzheimer's Association, is worth mentioning. This consortium is developing new technologies to compensate for functional impairments, enhance care

Table 7.1. Large-scale research and development projects

Project	Country	Description
TED, 1996–9[16]	Germany, Norway, Italy, Finland, UK, Netherlands	Technology, Ethics and Dementia (TED) was a European Community-funded project aimed at providing practitioners in dementia care with guidelines on how to apply technology for people with dementia and how to make ethical decisions about their use
ASTRID, 1999–2000[17]	UK, Norway, Ireland	A Social and Technological Response to meeting the needs of Individuals with Dementia and their carers (ASTRID) was a European Community-funded project that has resulted in a detailed guide to using technology in dementia care
ACTION, 1997–2000[18]	Sweden, England, Northern Ireland, Republic of Ireland, Portugal	Assisting Carers using Telematics Interventions to meet Older persons' Needs (ACTION) is a user-focused European Union project designed to improve the quality of life and social inclusion of elderly and disabled people, and family carers of every condition by the use of information and communication technology
ENABLE, 2000–04[19]	Norway, Ireland, Finland, Lithuania, UK	The potential for home technologies to help people with cognitive impairment has been extensively investigated in this project, which aimed at 'marrying the new with the familiar'
REACH , 1995–present date[20]	US	Resources for Enhancing Alzheimer's Caregiver Health (REACH) is a National Institute of Health initiative that aims to test the effectiveness of various behavioural, environmental, social and technological interventions for improving family members' abilities to care for people with Alzheimer's disease or related disorders (www.edc.gsph.pitt.edu/REACH/)

Table 7.2. Other projects: most use similar technology (for example, passive infrared detectors) to monitor clients, such as those with dementia or Alzheimer's disease

Country	Project*
UK	Europe AID house
	Gloucester Smart House
	Dementia Friendly House
Netherlands	Smart Model House
Sweden	comHOME
France	Gardien
	Grenoble's Health Smart Home
	Smardep
	Prosafe
US	University of Rochester's Smart Medical Home
	Georgia Tech's Aware Home
	Massachusetts Institute of Technology's House of the Future
	University of Virginia's Smart Home
	Gator Tech Smart House
Canada	University of Sherbrooke's Smart Home
Japan	Smart House in Tokushima
Australia	University of New South Wales home monitoring

*Due to space constraints, the bibliographical references of the above list have been omitted, but they are available at www-sante.ujf-grenoble.fr/imtc/HSH/ (last accessed 19 January 2006).

and treatment strategies, foster independence and improve the quality of life for people with dementia and their caregivers. Somewhat similarly, the Center for Aging Services Technologies is also concerned with developing and deploying emerging technologies with a view to improving the aging experience in America.

Privacy considerations

The ease with which smart homes allow everyone and everything in a home to be observed remotely conjures up images of 'Big Brother' (as in Orwell's novel *1984*). Automatic tracking systems, motion and fall detectors, cameras and intelligent monitoring raise obvious concerns about privacy.[9,21–23] Technological innovators thus must keep a close watch on harmful or malevolent usage that might develop insidiously and jeopardize the concept of smart homes. It follows that technological innovation for home care must be rigorously framed within ethical procedures that are now well defined; for example, see Powers.[24] For instance, the agreement of the client (or the caregiver of cognitively impaired patients) is mandatory, and the cost of 24-hour technical support must be defined in the contract. Only clearly beneficial tools for the patient and immediate caregivers should be encouraged. Technology 'addiction' – or the tendency to employ technology for its own sake – must be prevented. All these considerations are closely related to the legal and ethical aspects of telemedicine.

Smart homes have to cope with the same confidentiality standards imposed on conventional medical practice. The practitioner must not betray what was disclosed to him or her as part of the medical care provided to the patient. This corresponds with the physical presence of the practitioner with the patient during the care relationship. The transmission of data from sensors in the home to a remote centre challenges this paradigm. Thus, encryption of any personal data for protection is essential, as is making sure that the data are sent with the knowledge and agreement of the patient.

Ethics

An economic model capable of achieving efficient e-health for vulnerable people depends on an 'ethical aim' capable of overcoming poverty among most elderly and handicapped people in the world. Such an aim should promote the best use of technology in the building of a society based on healthcare quality, human relationships and solidarity. A number of actions have promoted this ethical posture as part of their approach. For instance, Bjorneby and van Berlo,[21] followed by others,[7,17,25] fostered a reflection on the ethical issues raised by the use of technology with cognitively impaired people. However, for various reasons – including the lack of a clear vision of the possibilities along with economic and organizational problems – efficient devices and teleservices are used infrequently at present and are far from being widely available.

Empowerment

Smart home technologies give elderly people more responsibility for their own care, and elderly and handicapped people may become less objects of care than subjects of their gradual change of health. Popularization of smart home projects should include schemes to urge patients and caregivers to take control of the technology. Provision of user and stakeholder training is essential. Empowerment of patients and frail people at home has been achieved in a few projects. For example, for a telecare programme that was mainly based on person-to-person videotelephony, the ACTION project (see Table 7.1) resulted in a call centre that promoted the family caregivers as the experts.

Bringing generations together

People of different generations may become closer through the use of advanced information and communication technologies. For example, the 'digital family portrait' provides qualitative visualizations of a family member's daily life through a frame with iconic images that summarize 28 days of activity and various information from sensors in the home.[26] The Inter-generational Virtual Village – a largescale Canadian cross-generation videoconferencing project carried out by the Programs for Autonomy and Communication for the Elderly (PACE) 2000 Foundation – is a convincing e-inclusion and telegerontology experiment.[27] In this project, videotelephony provides people who have lost their sense of autonomy with a means of playing a valuable role in society. For example, their role might be to listen and provide advice to recent immigrants to Canada or support students in a French immersion sociology class. Another example of the use of technology to overcome frailty and isolation is the use of a communication technology provided by the Ecovip system – an ubiquitous computing approach of videotelephony for social connectedness.[28]

Conclusion

The smart home is a far-reaching concept that encompasses two distinct, although tightly bound dimensions: person-centredness for individual and familial convenience and medicosocial-centredness for social and public health policy purposes. The use of smart home technologies makes it possible to bring about a synergy in at least three kinds of intelligence:

- social services' intelligence, on which is based assistance with daily living
- family doctor's intelligence, on which is based the proximity of medical care
- hospital intelligence, on which is based acute medical care.

This promotes independent living, improves the quality of life at home, facilitates home care, tightens up human links and enhances social connectedness. Smart home technologies are invaluable tools for alleviating the care burden that rapidly develops as a result of an aging population. Because technology in itself is ethically neutral, however, it depends on technological innovators, stakeholders and users to consider unethical uses and develop a sense of responsibility. There should be a commitment to search for best practices to guide the design, evaluation and dissemination of such technology. Much remains to be done to allow smart homes to become actual and reliable supports to a healthier and happier life in a society for all.

Further information

American Alzheimer's Association website. Available at: www.alz.org/research/care/ overview.asp (last accessed 19 January 2006).

ASTRID website. Available at: www.astridguide.org (last accessed 19 January 2006).

Center for Aging Services Technologies website. Available at: www.agingtech.org (last accessed 19 January 2006).

ENABLE website. Available at: www.enableproject.org (last accessed 19 January 2006).

Gerontechnology: *Journal of the International Gerontechnology Association* website. Available at: www.gerontechnology.info/Journal/ (last accessed 19 January 2006).

Marshall M. *Dementia and technology*. London: Counsel and Care, 1997.

Programs for Autonomy and Communication for the Elderly (PACE) 2000 Foundation website. Available at: www.pace2000.org (last accessed 19 January 2006).

REACH website. Available at: www.edc.gsph.pitt.edu/REACH/ (last accessed 19 January 2006).

Weiser M. The computer of the 21st century. *Sci Am* 1991;**265**:66–75.

References

1   Gelhaus L. High-tech homes mean a brighter future for seniors. *Provider* 2002;**28**:40–2.
2   Tang P, Venables T. 'Smart' homes and telecare for independent living. *J Telemed Telecare* 2000;**6**:8–14.
3   Rialle V, Duchene F, Noury N, *et al*. Health 'smart' home: information technology for patients at home. *Telemed J E Health* 2002;**8**:395–409.
4   Stefanov DH, Bien Z, Bang WC. The smart house for older persons and persons with physical disabilities: structure, technology arrangements, and perspectives. *IEEE Trans Neural Syst Rehabil Eng* 2004;**12**:228–50.
5   Eriksson H, Timpka T. The potential of smart homes for injury prevention among the elderly. *Inj Control Saf Promot* 2002;**9**:127–31.
6   Morris M, Lundell K, Dishman E, Needham B. New perspectives on ubiquitous computing from ethnographic study of elders with cognitive decline. In: Dey AK, Schmidt A, McCarthy JF, eds. *UbiComp 2003: Ubiquitous computing: 5th International Conference, Seattle, WA, US, October 12–15, 2003, Proceedings*. Berlin, Heidelberg: Springer-Verlag, 2003:227–42.
7   Stip E, Rialle V. Environmental cognitive remediation in schizophrenia: ethical implications of 'Smart Home' technology. *Can J Psychiatry* 2005;**50**:281–91.
8   Marshall M. Technology and technophobia. *J Dementia Care* 2002;**10**:14–5.
9   Fisk MJ. Telecare equipment in the home. Issues of intrusiveness and control. *J Telemed Telecare* 1997;**3** (Suppl 1):30–2.

10   Velkoff VA, Lawson VA. *Gender and aging: caregiving.* Washington, DC: US Department of Commerce, 1998. Available at: www.census.gov/ipc/prod/ib-9803.pdf (last accessed 14 December 2005).

11   Magnusson L, Hanson E, Borg M. A literature review study of information and communication technology as a support of frail older people living at home and their family carers. *Technol Disabil* 2004;**16**:223–35.

12   Ramos LR, Xavier AK, Sigulem D. Computation and networking – compunetics – promoting digital inclusion of elderly, cognitively impaired, and Alzheimer's patients. *Gerontechnology* 2005;**3**:123–5.

13   Bjorneby S. Smart houses: can they really benefit older people? *Signpost* 2000;**5**:36–8.

14   Gibson F. Seven Oaks: friendly design and sensitive technology. *J Dementia Care* 2003;**11**:27–30.

15   Chapman A, Orpwood R. There's no place like a smart home. *J Dementia Care* 2001;**9**:28–31.

16   Bjorneby S, Topo P, Holthe T. *Technology, ethics and dementia: a guidebook on how to apply technology in dementia care.* Norway: Norwegian Centre for Dementia Research, 1999.

17   Marshall M, ed. *ASTRID: a social and technological response to meeting the needs of individuals with dementia and their carers.* London: Hawker Publications, 2000.

18   Magnusson L, Berthold H, Brito L, *et al.* ACTION, assisting carers using telematics interventions to meet older persons' needs. In: Porrero IP, Ballabio E, eds. *Improving the quality of life for the European citizen.* Ohmsha: IOS Press, 1998.

19   ENABLE Consortium. Enabling technologies for people with dementia. In: *HOPE Newsletter (Housing for Older People in Europe) November 2001.* ENABLE Consortium, 2001:16-17.

20   Eisdorfer C, Czaja SJ, Loewenstein DA, *et al.* The effect of a family therapy and technology-based intervention on caregiver depression. *Gerontologist* 2003;**43**:521–31.

21   Bjorneby S, van Berlo A, eds. Ethical issues in use of technology for dementia care. Knegsel: Akontes Publishing, 1997.

22   McShane R, Hope T, Wilkinson J. Tracking patients who wander: ethics and technology. *Lancet* 1994;**343**:1274.

23   Joy B. Why the future doesn't need us: our most powerful 21st-century technologies – robotics, genetic engineering, and nanotech – are threatening to make the humans an endangered species. *Wired Magazine* 2000;**8**:236–62. Available at: wired.com/wired/archive/8.04/joy_pr.html (last accessed 14 December 2005).

24   Powers B. Everyday ethics in assisted living facilities: a framework for assessing resident-focused issues. *J Gerontol Nurs* 2005;**31**:31–7.

25   Magnusson L, Hanson E. Ethical issues arising from a research, technology and development project to support frail and older people and their family carers at home. *Health Soc Care Community* 2003;**11**:431–9.

26   Mynatt ED, Rogers WA. Developing technology to support the functional independence of older adults. *Ageing Int* 2002;**27**:24–41.

27   Charlebois R, Côté N, O'Rourke M, *et al.* Intra- and interrater reliability of the video conference-based goniometer for active knee flexion and extension in healthy subjects. *J Rehabil Outcomes Meas* 2000;**4**:23–33.

28   Ghorayeb A, Rialle V, Coutaz J, Noury N. Breaking through the walls of loneliness and isolation by means of videophony: an ubicomp orientation and a design process based on active participation of elderly people. In: *Proceedings of the Second International Conference on Aging, Disability and Independence, St Petersburg, FL, US,* 1–4 February 2006.

►8

Wound management

Christy M. Williams, Kathy Duckett and Joseph C. Kvedar

Introduction

Wounds represent a major problem in home healthcare in the US, imposing huge economic and workforce burdens. As many as 25% of home-care referrals involve wound management. Costs of chronic wound treatment are estimated to range from $8000 to $30 000 per wound, although the payment system reimburses only about $2500 for a pressure ulcer.

About six million patients in the US have chronic wounds,[1] and many such patients are treated at home. Patients admitted to home care often suffer from problems such as dementia or immobility and, therefore, are more susceptible to developing non-healing wounds of all types, including arterial, venous and neuropathic wounds. For example, the prevalence of pressure ulcers has been reported as 17%.[2] In most cases, these patients also have multiple comorbidities, which makes the wounds much more difficult to heal once developed. This poses a burden for patients, providers and funding agencies alike. Furthermore, the population older than 65 years is projected to increase by 56% between the years 2001 and 2020.[3] An increasing number of chronic wounds are being treated in the home,[4] resulting in a substantial economic burden for the home health industry.

Specialist wound care nurses provide high-quality care and optimize the use of resources, thereby reducing healthcare costs.[5] Studies have shown that the successful healing of chronic wounds depends on consistent, skilled and community-based specialty care[6,7] and that many types of wounds heal more rapidly in home-care settings when specially trained nurses provide consultations.[8] However, only 4300 registered nurses (RNs) are certified in wound care in the US – less than 0.2% of the RNs in the country. This leaves many patients who would benefit from this expertise without access to it.

Telehealth for wound care

Telehealth has the potential to bring wound care to patients who would not otherwise have access to it and to improve their quality of care. It may also provide cost-effective solutions to home health agencies. Both store-and-forward and real-time telemedicine have been used to provide wound consultations and have been shown to be successful in pilot studies.[9,10] However, relatively few home health agencies seem to be using telehealth for wound management, or, if they are, they have not published their experiences.

Telemedicine is an alternative means of delivering the knowledge and expertise of a wound care nurse or specialist to underserved patients. As interest in telemedicine rises, increasing emphasis is placed on research validating its feasibility, quality and cost-effectiveness. The first steps have been to validate remote diagnosis and management of wounds.[11,12] For example, Wirthlin et al have shown diagnostic accuracy using a digital camera with a resolution of 756 × 504 pixels.[12] Many studies have shown proof of concept but have not evolved into sustainable services.

Mobile phone applications

Telemedicine applications require some means of data transfer. In the case of wound care, a range of telecommunications media have been employed, including high-speed digital lines,[13] the Internet (email)[14] and mobile phones.

At least three studies have shown the efficiency of image transfer through a mobile phone.[15-17] The equipment was found to be easily operated and portable, and the mean time for image upload was less than five minutes. Braun et al showed the feasibility of using the digital camera built into a mobile phone (Nokia 7650) to manage patients with lower extremity ulcers. Images of size 640 × 480 pixels were transmitted via e-mail to a wound expert. Real-time consultations were then provided by telephone. They provided data on 61 leg ulcers evaluated by three physicians. Agreement between off-site and on-site evaluation was 75%.[16] Tsai et al, evaluating 82 extremity wounds using a mobile camera phone (Panasonic GD88), found agreement ranging from 66% to 80% among surgeons.[17] Hsieh et al investigated the triaging of soft-tissue injuries with a 110 000-pixel mobile phone camera. They found that the technique was feasible but noted significant differences in treatment recommendations in 25% of the 81 digital injuries (45 patients).[18]

Home telehealth consultation system

Partners Telemedicine and Partners Home Care are organizations that provide home telehealth services in the greater Boston area. However, Partners Home Care, which serves 140 communities in eastern Massachusetts and provides more than 600 000 home visits per year, has a supply and demand problem. It provides about 500 wound care visits per day, but the organization employs only six wound specialty nurses, who cannot see that many patients themselves. Thus, not all patients who would benefit from a wound nurse's expertise have access to it. We have therefore developed a Home Telehealth Consultations System (HTCS) – a web-based system that uses store-and-forward transmission to provide specialist wound care to home health patients. We have served 203 patients since the system was introduced in 2001.

The process of obtaining a wound care consultation using the HTCS is as follows. A home health nurse (that is, not a wound specialist) takes images of the patient's wounds in accordance with an agreed protocol.[19] The camera used for this purpose is the Nikon Coolpix 950. The images are stored in a memory card, which the nurse carries from the patient's home to the home-care office. A telehealth coordinator then stores the patient information from the nurses' notes on the HTCS server and adds the images. It should be noted that this process does not use email. Data are transmitted to a secure web server using encryption (with a secure socket layer (SSL) Internet connection). Information security is necessary in most telemedicine applications, and security with email typically is not adequate.

If any problem is noted with the images, the nurse must return to the home to rephotograph the wounds or wait until the next scheduled nursing visit – either of which delays the consultation. Once all the information has been stored in the HTCS, a specialist wound care nurse evaluates the data, and enters his or her assessment and treatment recommendations. The recommendations are then implemented at the next visit to the patient's home by the home health nurse. Fig. 8.1 shows a screenshot of the user interface to the HTCS, and Fig. 8.2 is an example of a picture taken with a digital camera.

In a pilot study of the HTCS, we found good agreement between face-to-face wound assessment and telemedicine assessment, as well as a large variation in treatment plans between the registered nurse at the point of care and a remotely located wound care nurse. The results suggested that wound care specialists could improve the clinical outcomes of wounds in home health patients.[8]

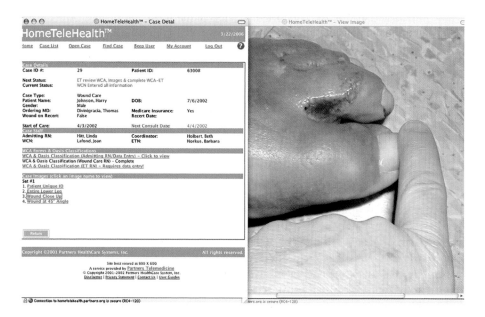

Fig. 8.1. The Home Telehealth Consultation System is a secure website that houses patient information, including wound images. Wound care nurses are able to log in to the site, review cases and images, and provide assessment and treatment recommendations that are implemented at the next patient visit by the home health nurse

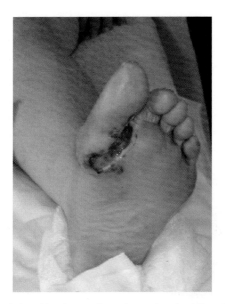

Fig. 8.2. Example of a relationship picture of an ulcer using the Nikon Coolpix 950 – the digital camera used by Partners Home Care for wound consultations

The HTCS can also be used to provide information to the patient's primary care physician or obtain consultations from wound care physicians.

New developments

In practice, there have been two main problems with the HTCS. The first involves the capture of the digital camera images: as the images and data are uploaded to the web server from an office separate from the point of care, there is a delay. This can amount to as much as five days, which increases the turnaround time of the consultations, as well as adding additional travel time for the nurses. This slows the overall process of care, thus potentially reducing patient safety.

The second problem is that the wound-imaging process typically requires two nurses in the home. This is because positioning the wound to be imaged and holding the camera is awkward for a single nurse. The need for two home nurses represents a significant barrier to the widespread adoption of the technique.

To circumvent these problems, we have developed software to capture images via a digital camera in a mobile phone (Motorola MPX220), which can also be used to send the images to the HTCS server. The entire image capture and transmission operation can thus be completed at the point of care. The smaller size and weight of the mobile phone compared with those of a digital camera enable a single nurse to hold the wound and image it without assistance. We are currently exploring the feasibility, diagnostic accuracy, participant satisfaction and efficiency (turnaround time) of the camera-phone technique. We expect this simplification of the workflow to allow the nurses to see more patients, which will improve efficiency, and enable patients to receive more rapid care. This in turn may reduce wound complications. Fig. 8.3 shows the mobile phone that we are piloting, and Fig. 8.4 shows screen shots of the image transfer application.

Our aim is a point-of-care consultation, in which the specialist can talk to the nurse while she or he is still in the patient's home and the recommendations can be implemented immediately. We anticipate that the improved efficiency will allow us to handle increased caseloads.

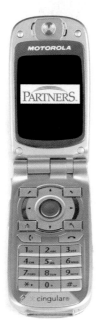

Fig. 8.3. Motorola MPX220. This device has a resolution of 1.2 megapixels and an operating system that allows for transaction control, encryption of transfer and autonomous actions

Adoption

Integrating telemedicine into home healthcare can be challenging. One reason is that home care is productivity driven, as evident by its reimbursement system. In 2000, a prospective payment system was implemented in home health in the US; this replaced the traditional retrospective cost-based payment system. In Boston, there has been only slow adoption of our telehealth wound care system. As mentioned above, the consultation process can be time-consuming, increasing the nurses' workload and interfering with their daily routines. Another reason is inherent in the type of work. The nursing profession is centred on a hands-on approach and thus information and communication technologies can be off-putting. Our eventual goal is to achieve a point-of-care wound consultation.

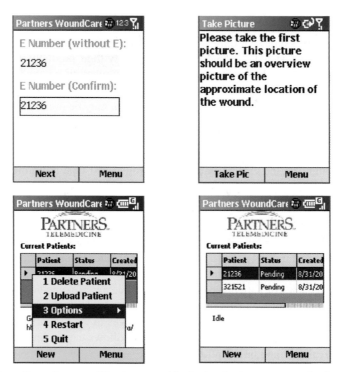

Fig. 8.4. The software in our mobile phone provides instruction to nurses on what images to take of the patient's wound, automatically repeats failed attempts to upload to the telehealth website and provides confirmation when the case has been uploaded successfully

Development of a successful programme

Implementing a successful wound care programme requires attention to four areas: the patient, the home health provider, the wound care consultant and the technology.

Patients

With respect to patients, items that must be considered include the consent process, patient confidentiality and appropriate referral to a wound care consultant. At Partners Home Care, we explain the consultation process to the patient and document their consent. We ensure patient confidentiality by observing both standard home-care practices for paper-based information and data encryption for electronic information, as described above. Additional steps are also taken to protect patient information, such as avoiding potential identifiers in the wound images. A home health agency must assess their financial and manpower resources to decide which patients will receive a consultation. At Partners Home Care, we originally sought wound care consultations for patients with complicated wounds and/or wounds refractory to standard care; currently, we are working towards obtaining consultations for all patients with wounds.

Home health providers

Home health nurses require training in the use of new technology. During the training session, the nurses are not seeing patients, so initially their productivity is reduced; however, the initial investment in training increases productivity in the long run.

Infection control is also important. A system has to be established to reduce exposure of the camera and its case to bacteria, which may be present on the wound, the wound care products and other objects in contact with the patient. We instruct the nurses only to place the camera back in its case after use. Keeping the camera clean requires setting up the wound for imaging, washing hands and changing gloves to manipulate the camera, imaging the wound and then returning the camera to its case.

Wound care consultant

Many home health agencies do not have wound care nurses on staff. A benefit of telemedicine is that it allows the remote provision of care. Home health agencies can consider collaborating with private practitioners who specialize in wound care, other home health agencies or patients' primary care physicians. Telemedicine wound care programmes offer improved communication between the home health nurse and the patients' primary care physicians. Transmitting images to the primary care physician between scheduled visits, or when problems arise, allows earlier implementation of appropriate treatment and interventions.

Technology

As technology improves, equipment has become more affordable. An image resolution as low as 756×504 pixels is sufficient for wound management.[8] Cameras with this or higher resolution are available for less than $200 (for example, the Canon SD200 PowerShot Digital Elph, which has a resolution of 3.2 megapixels). Any computer housing or transmitting electronic patient data should be secure, as previously discussed. When considering what technology to choose, we have found that ease of use is an important factor. Our current wound consultation process involves a digital camera that can be cumbersome for the nurses and sometimes involves extra steps that require additional visits to the home health office.

The future for home telehealth wound care

Technology is improving: images are getting sharper, data transmission is getting faster and costs are decreasing. We anticipate continued improvement in patient and provider confidence, more proof of positive clinical outcomes and the emergence of more positive cost-benefit analyses. The immediate future for telehealth lies in streamlining current concepts and systems. Once telehealth has been integrated successfully into the standard of care for home health agencies, we can then begin to think more broadly.

As new home health care tools become available, their effectiveness will need to be studied. For example, imagine a microscope that allows the wireless transmission of *in vivo* pathology to a remotely located dermatopathologist. The pathology report could then be given back to the healthcare provider – either via real-time or store-and-forward transmission. An important implication is the detection of non-melanoma skin cancers that mimic a chronic lower extremity wound. The current process involves a biopsy being taken and sent to a dermatopathologist for analysis; approximately one week is needed before a diagnosis is confirmed. The microscope device described above would allow visualization of pathology without the biopsy and the long wait, allowing earlier diagnosis and treatment, and reducing patient anxiety.

Certain wound characteristics, such as colour and topography, are important for accurate assessment but are difficult to capture adequately with digital imaging. Other wound characteristics, such as odour, cannot be transmitted at all using current telemedicine methods. However, odour detection and differentiation is possible using an electronic device called an electronic nose or 'e-nose'.[20,21] The e-nose has been shown to be feasible for identifying bacteria in urine.[22] The Cyranose 320 e-nose is the equipment most easily extensible to wound care. Using this, it was possible to predict six classes of bacteria with up to 98% accuracy by using a combination of three nonlinear methods of classification.[23] This may be useful in patients with *Pseudomonas* and other infections.

Other future possibilities include infrared devices to map the wound structure and biosensors to detect temperature changes (useful in cellulitis – a common complication in wounds). In a study by Braun *et al*, the lowest level of agreement was for detection of granulation tissue and necrosis.[16] Perhaps tools will be developed that can be placed over the wound and can wirelessly transmit variables such as temperature, area, percentage necrotic tissue, percentage granulation tissue and odour to a provider. Perhaps a disposable device could be embedded in the wound dressing itself. A step further might be a system in which any changes that suggest wound deterioration or lack of healing would alert the provider automatically.

Conclusion

Telemedicine for wound care is being actively investigated in home health agencies. There are still problems to be solved regarding telemedicine in wound care, but its potential is tremendous. More research in areas of clinical outcomes and cost-effectiveness is required.[24] As technology improves and becomes more user friendly, telemedicine will be more widely implemented, ultimately becoming a standard technique for delivering care. Even current technology can greatly benefit home health wound care. We have found that it is important to customize any programme to fit the needs of an individual home health agency. We believe that the technology will continue to improve to more accurately portray the clinical situation, increasing the utility of telemedicine in remote wound management and thus improving patient care.

Further information

American Telemedicine Association. *ATA special interest groups (SIGs)*. Washington, DC: American Telemedicine Association, 2005. Available at: www.atmeda.org/ICOT/icot.htm (last accessed 8 December 2005).

Milne CT, Corbett LQ, Dubuc DL, eds. *Wound, ostomy, and continence nursing secrets*. Philadelphia, PA: Hanley and Belfus, 2003.

Sauer GC, Hall JC. *Manual of skin diseases*. Philadelphia, PA: Lippincott Raven, 1996.

Wound, Ostomy and Continence Nurses Society website. Available at: www.wocn.org (last accessed 8 December 2005).

References

1   Curative Health Services Frequently Asked Questions. www2.curative.com (last accessed 8 December 2005).

2   Pressure ulcers in America: prevalence, incidence, and implications for the future. An executive summary of the National Pressure Ulcer Advisory Panel monograph. *Adv Skin Wound Care* 2001;**14**:208–15.

3   National Projections Program: Population Division. *Table 2a. Projected Population of the United States, by Age and Sex: 2000 to 2050*. Washington, DC: US Census Bureau, 2000. Available at: www.census.gov/ipc/www/usinterimproj/natprojtab02a.pdf (last accessed 8 December 2005).

4   Pieper B, Templin TN, Dobal M, Jacox A. Wound prevalence, types, and treatments in home care. *Adv Wound Care* 1999;**12**:117–26.

5   Kaufman MW. The WOC nurse: economic, quality of life, and legal benefits. *Dermatol Nurs* 2001;**13**:215–9,222.

6   Bourne V. Community nurses' views of leg ulcer treatment. *Prof Nurse* 1999;**15**:21–4.

7   Flanagan M, Rotchell L, Fletcher J, Schofield J. Community nurses', home carers' and patients' perceptions of factors affecting venous leg ulcer recurrence and management of services. *J Nurs Manag* 2001;**9**:153–9.

8   Arnold N, Weir D. Retrospective analysis of healing in wounds cared for by ET nurses versus staff nurses in a home setting. *J Wound Ostomy Continence Nurs* 1994;**21**:156–60.

9   Moore RS, Britton B, Chetney R. Wound care using interactive telehealth. *Home Health Care Manage Pract* 2005;**17**:203–12.

10 Wilbright WA, Birke JA, Patout CA, *et al.* The use of telemedicine in the management of diabetes-related foot ulceration: a pilot study. *Adv Skin Wound Care* 2004;**17**:232–8.

11 Baer CA, Williams CM, Vickers L, Kvedar JC. A pilot study of specialized nursing care for home health patients. *J Telemed Telecare* 2004;**10**:342–5.

12 Wirthlin DJ, Buradagunta S, Edwards RA, *et al.* Telemedicine in vascular surgery: feasibility of digital imaging for the remote management of wounds. *J Vasc Surg* 1998;**27**:1089–99.

13 Wilbright WA, Birke JA, Patout CA, *et al.* The use of telemedicine in the management of diabetes-related foot ulceration: a pilot study. *Adv Skin Wound Care* 2004;**17**:232–8.

14 Bangs I, Clarke M, Hands L, *et al.* An integrated nursing and telemedicine approach to vascular care. *J Telemed Telecare* 2002;**8** (Suppl 2):110–12.

15 Yamada M, Watarai H, Andou T, Sakai N. Emergency image transfer system through a mobile telephone in Japan: technical note. *Neurosurgery* 2003;**52**:986–90.

16 Braun RP, Vecchietti JL, Thomas L, *et al.* Telemedical wound care using a new generation of mobile telephones: a feasibility study. *Arch Dermatol* 2005;**141**:254–8.

17 Tsai HH, Pong YP, Liang CC, *et al.* Teleconsultation by using the mobile camera phone for remote management of the extremity wound: a pilot study. *Ann Plast Surg* 2004;**53**:584–7.

18 Hsieh CH, Tsai HH, Yin JW, *et al.* Teleconsultation with the mobile camera-phone in digital soft-tissue injury: a feasibility study. *Plast Reconstr Surg* 2004;**114**:1776–82.

19 Partners Telemedicine. *Taking clinical skin images with the Nikon Coolpix 950*. Charlestown, MA: Partners Telemedicine. Available at: www.netmedicine.org/WCPP/coolpixguide.htm (last accessed 8 December 2005).

20   Persaud KC. Medical applications of odor-sensing devices. *Int J Low Extrem Wounds* 2005;**4**:50–6.
21   Alkasab TK, Bozza TC, Cleland TA, *et al*. Characterizing complex chemosensors: information-theoretic analysis of olfactory systems. *Trends Neurosci* 1999;**22**:102–8.
22   Guernion N, Ratcliffe NM, Spencer-Phillips PT, Howe RA. Identifying bacteria in human urine: current practice and the potential for rapid, near-patient diagnosis by sensing volatile organic compounds. *Clin Chem Lab Med* 2001;**39**:893–906.
23   Dutta R, Hines EL, Gardner JW, Boilot P. Bacteria classification using Cyranose 320 electronic nose. *Biomed Eng Online* 2002;**1**:4.
24   Heinzelmann P, Williams CM, Lugn N, Kvedar JC. Clinical outcomes associated with telemedicine/telehealth. *Telemed J E Health* 2005;**11**:329–47.

▶9

Home telehealth for Veterans

Rita F. Kobb and Neale R. Chumbler

Introduction

The Veterans Health Administration (VHA) in the US Department of Veterans Affairs operates an integrated healthcare system. The changing healthcare needs of the older veteran population are representative of the healthcare requirements of the older American population in general. The VHA has experienced major organizational changes during the past decade in response to the aging of the veteran population (many of whom have disabling chronic diseases) and changes in the healthcare workforce. This has resulted in reallocation of care from inpatient settings to ambulatory care facilities and homes.[1]

Clinical interventions for chronic diseases may include a variety of strategies to help overcome related disability. Many patients do not receive appropriate interventions, which is partly the result of the inability of a poorly organized American healthcare system to meet the multifaceted demands of chronic conditions.[2] A recent Institute of Medicine report called for comprehensive system changes to provide better care and quality improvement for a twenty-first-century healthcare system. The Institute of Medicine identified care coordination as one of its 22 priority areas for national action.[3] Other priorities included strategic use of information and communication technologies and delivery of patient-centred care. To that end, the VHA launched a national initiative called care coordination, with particular emphasis on patient-centred care and the use of home telehealth to support the self-care needs of older veterans with chronic diseases.[1]

Care coordination

Care coordination can be defined as a wider application of care and case management principles to the delivery of health services using health informatics, disease management and telehealth technologies to facilitate access to care and improve the health of designated individuals and populations by providing the right care in the right place at the right time.[4] The VHA's model is referred to as Care Coordination/Home Telehealth (CCHT). The care coordination model focuses on several concepts, including:[5]

- targeting patient populations with chronic diseases (for example, heart failure,

diabetes, depression, post-traumatic stress, high blood pressure and respiratory disease)
- making the patient's home the preferred site of care whenever appropriate
- focusing on the 2% of patients who consume 20–30% of the healthcare resources
- helping veteran patients stay as independent as possible for as long as possible to avoid institutional care
- teaching veteran patients to self-manage their chronic conditions whenever possible.

Traditionally, primary care and specialist providers see veteran patients with multiple and complex health problems, who are often assigned simultaneously to several case managers. Although communication exists between departments, it can become fragmented when patients require a broad range of services. The role of care coordinator was created to manage this complex care. Care coordinators are licensed professionals with appropriate clinical, communication and critical thinking skills. The VHA's care coordinators are nurse practitioners, registered nurses, social workers, dieticians, pharmacists or rehabilitation specialists.[6] These disciplines have functioned very effectively, by collaborating with healthcare team members to improve service access and disease management, and to promote self-management and shared decision-making (Fig. 9.1).[7]

Care coordinators have created several tools to help them meet the demands of their role. For example, the patient classification system was developed to help categorize patients on the basis of complexity of care and assist with appropriate resource allocation. The tool known as ACCTS (Assessing Care Coordination and Telehealth Services) is a classification system for home telehealth, in which patients are assigned to one of five levels, depending on the complexity and types of interventions required to manage their healthcare problems (Table 9.1). Since its implementation, the tool has been used to classify thousands of patients.[8]

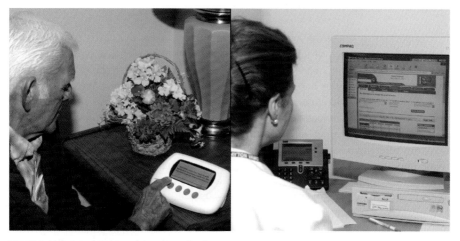

Fig. 9.1. Veteran patient and care coordinator

Table 9.1. Assessing Care Coordination and Telehealth Services (ACCTS) classification system

Level	Assessment factors	Stability of medical, cognitive, functional and social factors
1*	No encounters of any kind including telephone calls, office or home visits Monitoring information is stable with no need for intervention	Stable
2	1–2 encounters, depending on telehealth technology 1 office visit No home visits or ward visits	Require some intervention
3	3–4 encounters, depending on telehealth technology 2 office visits 1–2 ward visits No home visits	Borderline unstable
4	5–6 encounters, depending on telehealth technology 3 office visits 3–4 ward visits 1 home visit	Unstable
5†	≥7 encounters, depending on telehealth technology ≥4 office/ward visits ≥2 home visits	Significantly unstable

* Lowest complexity of care.
† Highest complexity of care.

Care coordinators have used this tool to classify specific populations, such as patients with acute heart failure and cancer patients actively undergoing chemotherapy, to differentiate the intense care needs of these groups from more chronically stable populations. In addition, the tool has helped to decide the numbers of patients per care coordinator.[9]

Role of home telehealth

It is important to select the appropriate equipment to meet the needs of the veteran population. Acceptance of technology has been viewed as a critical issue, especially among elderly people, who previously may not have been exposed to personal computers.[10–12] The VHA has experienced high satisfaction with its home telehealth devices, from both patients and providers. This includes 88–95% satisfaction for veterans using the devices, understanding how to use them and feeling that the equipment improves their healthcare. About 95% of providers have responded in favour of referring veterans to the home telehealth programme.[13,14] The VHA has also found good-to-excellent compliance rates with home telehealth devices. Compliance rates for the in-home messaging device, which was employed for veterans with diabetes, hypertension and heart failure, were 92%.[15,16]

Care coordinators believe that these satisfaction and compliance rates are so high because of the algorithm they developed to assign technology to patients (Fig. 9.2). The algorithm depends on indicators including physical and cognitive abilities such as

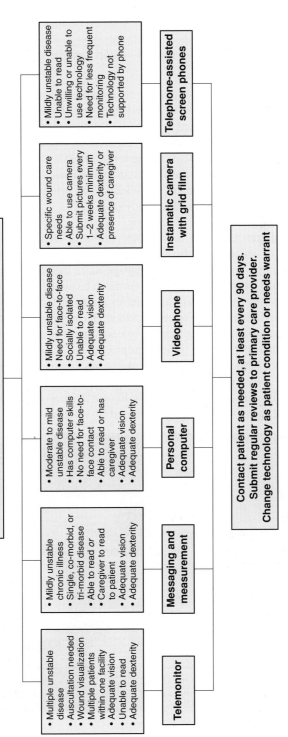

Fig. 9.2. Care Coordination Technology Assignment algorithm

manual dexterity and literacy level. Care coordinators reassess their patients quarterly.[13]

The home telehealth devices used to support care coordination can be divided into three categories:[13,14]

- **Messaging devices**: Messaging involves questions and answers that are sent daily to patients who respond to knowledge, behaviour and symptom areas. The questions are risk stratified to help triage potential problems. Messaging devices may or may not have peripheral measurement devices for vital signs, and they operate with the ordinary telephone service (public switched telephone network, PSTN). These devices are used most often for disease management and education to enhance self-management behaviours. The primary messaging device being used by veterans is the Health Buddy (Fig. 9.3).

- **Monitoring devices**: Monitoring in the VHA encompasses real-time videoconferencing, with or without peripheral measurement devices for vital signs. The monitoring devices operate via the ordinary telephone network. Monitoring is normally used to manage more medically complex patients than those managed with messaging; it may also be used for follow-up of wound care. Monitors have transducers attached to them, including a blood pressure cuff, body-weight scale, pulse oximeter, blood glucose monitor and stethoscope. Some of the monitoring devices used by veterans are shown in Fig. 9.4 and Fig. 9.5.

- **Videophones**: Like the other equipment, the videophone uses the ordinary telephone network. In contrast to the messaging and monitoring devices, however, most videophones are used for treatment and counselling of mental health disorders and do not usually have transducers attached to them. Fig. 9.6 shows an example of a videophone used by veterans.

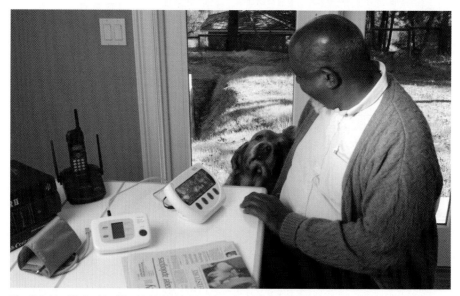

Fig. 9.3. Health Buddy (Health Hero Network)

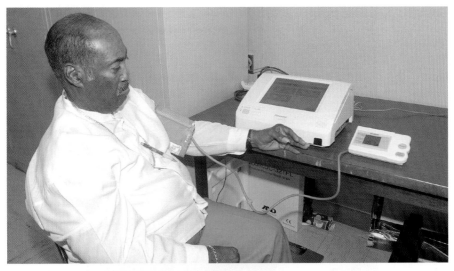

Fig. 9.4. Telemonitor (Viterion Healthcare 500)

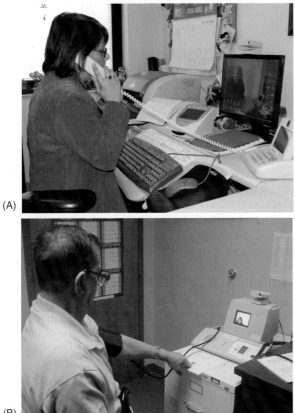

(A)

(B)

Fig. 9.5. Monitoring devices: clinician's station (American Telecare) (A) and patient's unit (Aviva 1010 SL) (B)

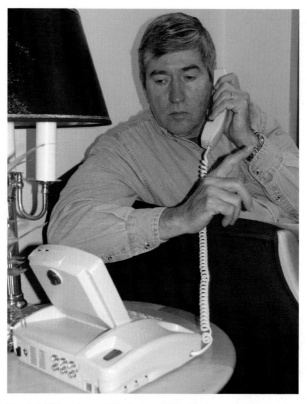

Fig. 9.6. Videophone (Windcurrent TelevYou)

Care coordinators have successfully managed their patient populations using these home telehealth devices. The case studies in Boxes 9.1 and 9.2 describe the use of a messaging device and monitor, respectively. These case studies are typical of larger groups of veterans who have experienced home telehealth in the VHA.[17]

Community care coordination service

The VHA has 21 veterans' integrated service networks (VISNs) that provide care to veterans in the US. Some are expanding rapidly: the Florida-Puerto Rico Network had a 25% increase in numbers of enrolees over two years. To meet the growing demand, a shift from institutional care to care in the community was envisaged. New healthcare models and strategies were investigated for the proposed Community Care Coordination Service (CCCS).[18]

Eight 2-year pilot projects began in 2000. The pilot projects targeted patients who were at high risk (multiple chronic diseases), had high use (two or more hospital admissions, two or more emergency room visits and 10 or more unscheduled clinic

---

Box 9.1. Case study – cancer care

Mr Nixon is a 58-year-old Vietnam veteran who was diagnosed with lung cancer. He was actively undergoing chemotherapy every three weeks and lived with his mother, who served as his informal caregiver. During the year before his enrolment in the care coordination/home telehealth cancer programme, he had 22 clinic visits and two hospital admissions. He was enrolled in the programme with the Health Buddy messaging device, which asked him about symptoms and educated him about his cancer and related issues. Five months after his enrolment in the programme, he had had no hospital admissions, three clinic visits and one emergency room visit. He had 16 telephone contacts with his care coordinator – mostly to manage his pain. Mr Nixon reported an improved relationship with his healthcare provider, who he felt was now available to answer his questions.

Comment
The role of the care coordinator was extremely important in managing the patient's pain effectively. Because of the increased communication between the care coordinator and the healthcare provider, the patient had greater confidence in the healthcare system.

Box 9.2. Case study – heart failure

Mr Patterson is a 74-year-old Korean War veteran who was diagnosed with New York Heart Association Class 4 heart failure. He also had coronary artery disease and emphysema, and lived at home alone. He was receiving continuous oxygen because of severe shortness of breath. In the 18 months before his enrolment into the CCHT programme, he had nine hospital admissions, with four of these requiring intensive care stays. He was in the emergency room at least once a month and made frequent unscheduled clinic visits in between his routine care. He was given an AVIVA 1010SL telemonitor, so the care coordinator could listen to his heart and lung sounds regularly. He had subtle symptoms that escalated quickly to become healthcare crises. Because the telemonitor gave him access to his care coordinator from home, his exacerbations were reduced significantly. In the 18 months after enrolment, Mr Patterson had two hospital admissions, no intensive care days, two emergency room visits and no unscheduled clinic visits.

Comment
Heart failure is one of the five most common diagnoses in the veteran population. It is a costly and debilitating chronic condition. Heart failure often creates significant anxiety, limited physical functioning and diminished quality of life. The CCHT programme helped patients feel in control of their health and their lives. Patients reported 92% satisfaction and indicated they felt more secure because of the care coordinator.

---

visits) and incurred high costs (greater than $25 000 in the year before enrolment). These populations would be the most likely to benefit from the intervention of care coordination and home telehealth.[18]

Initial funding of $5 million was provided for these pilot projects to prove the effectiveness of the model in improving quality of life and reducing unnecessary healthcare expenditure. The results showed that the CCCS model did benefit many patients who were frail, elderly and had complex medical situations, and encouraged independence and self-management. The care coordinator role was pivotal in organizing everything for the best possible outcome. The pilot study had a quasi-experimental design that compared the patients before and after enrolment and also included a comparison group of usual care patients. The preliminary findings showed changes in service use – for example, fewer hospital visits – from year 1 to year 2.[6]

Research on older veterans with diabetes has shown that care coordination and telehealth improved access to appropriate and timely care. Differences in the use of healthcare services, such as hospitalizations and emergency department visits, were measured in a group of 400 veterans with diabetes enrolled in CCHT and a matched comparison group of veterans who received no intervention. Twelve months after enrolment, the CCHT patients had a greater likelihood of newly scheduled primary care and special needs visits than patients in the comparison group. These newly scheduled visits enabled veterans to be treated 'just in time', with the health status monitored before health deteriorated. For example, diabetic patients in the CCHT group had significantly fewer hospitalizations than diabetic patients in the comparison group.[19]

An important benchmark of success in a healthcare system is improved quality of healthcare. The VHA performance standards include:

- 78% of patients to have current influenza and pneumonia immunizations
- 78% of patients in compliance with antihypertensive medication
- appropriate and timely communication between the patients' primary care provider and their care coordinator.

Immunization in the CCCS programme was consistent with or exceeded the VHA targets. For instance, 83% of the veterans had been immunized against influenza and 90% against pneumonia. We also found that 93% of the veterans were compliant with taking their medications. A total of 85% of primary care providers indicated that they received timely and proper communication from the care coordinators.[6]

The success of the CCCS pilot led to an expansion to new populations in the Florida-Puerto Rico Network. Since its inception, the programme has served more than 5000 veteran patients with a variety of chronic and acute care problems. The services of CCCS have been provided to chronically ill patients with hypertension, diabetes, heart failure and emphysema. Services have also been provided to populations with specialist care needs, such as those with spinal cord injury, dementia, hepatitis C, HIV, myocardial infarction, pre-diabetes, depression, schizophrenia, post-traumatic stress, stroke and amputation, and those who need palliative and cancer care.

National implementation

After the successful pilot programme in Florida-Puerto Rico, the VHA began to deploy the model nationally. A community care coordination team developed a national strategic plan with short-, medium- and long-term goals.[5] Phase 1 began in 2002, with the identification of four additional networks that replicated the model developed in Florida. These four networks received $1 million each to purchase equipment and build the necessary service infrastructure. In 2003, the next six networks also received $1 million each to initiate their care coordination and home telehealth programmes. Finally, the Office of Care Coordination funded the remaining 10 networks for implementation in 2004. As of 2005, all 21 networks in VHA have veteran patients participating in the programme.[20]

To facilitate implementation, the Office of Care Coordination tried to standardize administrative, clinical, financial and regulatory processes where possible. National codes for workload data capture were established. A national equipment contract was used to lower equipment costs (Box 9.3). This contract also laid the foundation for data integration between the home telehealth devices and the VHA's computerized patient record system. The Office of Care Coordination funded a national training centre for care coordination and home telehealth to standardize education and maintain competency for staff. This training centre's main purposes were to implement a web-based curriculum and support field staff with the implementation through distance-learning techniques. Every network in the country now uses home telehealth successfully.

The Office of Care Coordination has met its short-term census goals, having served more than 8000 patients to date. They are working on having these types of services recognized by the VHA's national reimbursement system. Populations with chronic medical disease originally targeted by earlier implementation phases have now expanded to include specialty care such as the management of pain, cancer and multiple sclerosis. A greater emphasis is also placed on the role of the caregiver and the provision of support to this individual (or individuals) in the process. The Office of

---

Box 9.3. National equipment contract

In 2003, the Office of Care Coordination began an equipment evaluation process, with a view to establishing a national equipment contract. Vendors came to the National Acquisition Center in Hines, Illinois, to compete for the business. Before the contract, the VHA regions were using various vendors to deliver home telehealth services. Once the contract was decided, only those listed in the contract were approved vendors.

The national contract has four vendors for messaging: American Telecare, Health Hero Network, Viterion Healthcare and VitelNet. It also has four vendors for telemonitoring: AMD Telemedicine, Carematix, Viterion Healthcare and VitelNet. The contract has one videophone vendor: KMEA. Before the contract, several videophones were being used, the most common being Windcurrent's TelevYou model.

Each vendor has a secure server, and all patient information is stored on that server to comply with privacy requirements. Each VHA network chose their patient populations by reviewing their usage and cost data. Many of them selected populations of patients with chronic diseases such as diabetes, heart disease and hypertension. Others focused on specialty needs such as patients in hospices and those who required palliative care. Each network is tracking outcome data on its patient population and regularly reporting this information to the Office of Care Coordination. There is a national outcome measure for average daily census, as well as a total patient census for each network. Many support mechanisms to help implementation are in place through the Office of Care Coordination, including a training centre, a help desk and annual conferences for sharing information.

Care Coordination's long-term goal is to incorporate care coordination and home telehealth into every aspect of routine patient care throughout its 21-network system. Currently, the VHA is expanding its evidence-based approach to include a greater exploration of the benefits and limitations of home telehealth.

The future

By 2010, the veteran population aged over 75 years will increase from 6.25 million to 7 million (12%). The prevalence of chronic diseases and disabling conditions will also increase.[20] Disease management programmes, many of which use home telehealth, have proliferated in the US over the past few years. Initial evaluations have found impressive reductions in service use and savings in costs.[21] To continue this expansion, studies are required of the efficacy, cost-effectiveness, facilitators and barriers to care coordination and home telehealth. It would be beneficial if these studies could be designed as randomized, controlled trials, although this is not always feasible with home-telehealth applications.[19]

The reimbursement situation for home telehealth has improved in the last three years. Forthcoming legislative changes will remove most barriers for healthcare organizations and agencies who wish to provide home telehealth services. The change that is most likely to benefit home telehealth is a new financial reimbursement model. Insurance and Medicare reimbursement for services will make it much easier for businesses to implement home telehealth successfully.

Further information

Darkins A, Cary M. *Telemedicine and telehealth: principles, policies, performance, and pitfalls*. New York: Springer, 2000.
Office of Care Coordination, Department of Veterans Affairs website. Available at: www.va.gov/occ (last accessed 13 November 2005).

References

1 Perlin JB, Kolodner B, Roswell RH. The Veterans Health Administration: quality, value, accountability, and information as transforming strategies for patient centered care. *Am J Manag Care* 2004;**10**:828–36.
2 Institute of Medicine Committee on Quality of Health Care in America. *Crossing the quality chasm: a new health system for the 21st century*. Washington, DC: National Academies Press, 2001.
3 Adams K, Corrigan J, eds. *Priority areas for national action: transforming health care quality*. Washington, DC: National Academies Press, 2001.
4 Office of Care Coordination Program Philosophy. Available at: www.va.gov/occ/ccinVA.asp (last accessed 8 November 2005).
5 Office of Care Coordination. *Strategic plan fiscal year 2005–2009*. Washington DC: Veterans Health Administration, 2004. Available at: www.va.gov/pittsburgh/vaphs_strategic_plan.pdf (last accessed 5 January 2006).
6 Meyer M, Kobb R, Ryan P. Virtually healthy: chronic disease management in the home. *Dis Manag* 2002;**5**:87–94.

7   Kobb R, Hoffman N, Lodge R, Kline S. Enhancing elder chronic care through technology and coordination: report from a pilot. *Telemed J E Health* 2003;**9**:189–95.

8   Kobb R, Hoffman N, Lodge R, *et al*. A patient classification system for home telehealth. *Telehealth Practice Report* 2005;**10**(1):2.

9   Sunshine Healthcare Network. *Community Care Coordination Service best practices report*. Bay Pines FL: Veterans Health Administration, 2003.

10 Mead S, Spaulding V, Sit R, *et al*. Effects of age and training on World Wide Web navigation strategies. In: *Proceedings of the Human Factors and Ergonomics Society: 41st Annual Meeting*. Santa Monica, CA: Human Factors and Ergonomics Society, 1997:152–6.

11 Meyer B, Rogers W, Schneider-Hufschmidt G, *et al*. Making technology accessible for older users. *SIGCHI Bull* 1998;**30**:1–7.

12 Worden A, Walker N, Bharat K, Hudson S. Making computers easier for older adults to use: area cursors and sticky icons. In: *Proceedings of CHI, 1997*. Atlanta, GA: ACM Press, 1997:266–71. Available at: www.sigchi.org/chi97/proceedings/paper/nw.htm (last accessed 5 January 2006).

13 Ryan P, Kobb R, Hilsen P. Making the right connection: matching patients to technology. *Telemed J E Health* 2003;**9**:81–8.

14 Kobb R, Hilsen P, Ryan P. Assessing technology needs for the elderly: finding the perfect match for home. *Home Healthc Nurse* 2003;**1**:666–73.

15 Huddleston M, Kobb, R. Emerging technology for at-risk chronically ill veterans. *J Healthc Qual* 2004;**26**:12–15.

16 Cherry J, Dryden K, Kobb R, *et al*. Opening a window of opportunity through technology and coordination: a multisite case study. *Telemed J E Health* 2003;**9**:265–71.

17 Meyer M, Ryan P, Kobb R, Roswell RH. Using home telehealth to manage chronic disease. *Fed Pract* 2003;**20**:24,27–30,36,41. Available at: www1.va.gov/visn8/v8/clinical/cccs/articles/UsingHome Telehealth.pdf (last accessed 5 January 2006).

18 Florida-Puerto Rico Veterans Integrated Service Network (VISN 8). *Network strategic plan*. Bay Pines, FL: Veterans Health Administration, 2001.

19 Chumbler NR, Vogel WB, Garel M, *et al*. Health services utilization of a care coordination/home-telehealth program for veterans with diabetes: a matched cohort study. *J Ambul Care Manage* 2005;**28**:230–40.

20 US Department of Veterans Affairs Strategic Plan. Available at: www.va.gov (last accessed 8 November 2005).

21 Disease Management Association of America *Disease Management Journal*. Available at: www.dmaa.org (last accessed 8 November 2005).

▶10

Home-based disease management

George Demiris

Introduction

The overall objectives of disease management are to manage chronic conditions, improve clinical outcomes and support patient–provider interactions, patient education and monitoring while allowing patients to stay at home. A disease management intervention is a 'set of coordinated healthcare interventions and communications for populations with conditions in which patient self-care efforts are significant'.[1] Disease management programmes aim to support the care plan and the provider–patient relationship by preventing deterioration and/or complications using evidence-based practice guidelines. Disease management programmes also aim to reduce the overall costs of healthcare services. Patients with chronic illnesses account for a large proportion of overall healthcare costs. An efficient disease management system should dramatically reduce medical and administrative costs.

Home care in general, and disease management programmes in particular, face several challenges, such as funding limitations, large distances that often make such care more costly for rural patients and problems with the distribution of the clinical workforce. It is a general premise that e-health applications can help solve some of these problems and enhance home-based disease management. The concept of e-health introduces new channels of communication and new kinds of transactions in healthcare. It thus alters the traditional roles of patients and providers. E-health can be defined broadly as the use of telecommunications, such as the Internet, sophisticated portable devices and new approaches to healthcare delivery and education. Thus, e-health implies a fundamental redesigning of healthcare processes based on the use of electronic communication at all levels. It potentially leads to patient empowerment.

Patient empowerment describes the transition from a passive role, where the patient is the recipient of care services, to an active role, where the patient is informed, has choices and is involved in the decision-making process. It is based on the principle that patients are entitled to access health information and determine their own choices with respect to care. Feste and Anderson have argued that the empowerment model introduces 'self-awareness, personal responsibility, informed choices and quality of life'.[2] Recent advances in telecommunication technologies have brought opportunities to enhance communication between healthcare professionals and patients. This has resulted in a shift from systems based on episodic patient encounters to systems designed to provide continuous care throughout the life of an individual. In other words, the premise of e-health is the shift from institution-centred to patient-centred information systems.

The Internet in disease management

Although information technology always seemed to be a promising tool for disease management programmes, early efforts to use it had various problems. These included attempts to integrate systems without a common protocol and developing systems with a long implementation cycle. There were also problems of higher overall costs and inconsistent performance. With the diffusion of the Internet, however, new technology that provides technically flexible applications with shorter implementation cycles is becoming available.

In the last few years, Internet technologies have been used for disease management in many clinical areas. These technologies allow patients to connect with providers, link home care with hospital and ambulatory care, facilitate transmission of monitoring data, and permit communication and collaboration between patients, caregivers, remote family members and healthcare providers. Patient education is a central component of any disease management initiative. The Internet can support patient education by providing tailored health information or automated reminders to patients and/or their caregivers. Web-based electronic health records represent a mode of enhanced communication among stakeholders that supports continuity of care. Web-based records that are accessible to patients allow them to improve self-care and disease knowledge.[3]

Virtual communities

The use of the Internet in disease management has led to the creation of so-called virtual communities. A virtual community is a social entity that involves individuals who relate to one another using telecommunication to bridge the distance between them.[4] Traditional communities are limited by factors such as their proximity, organizational structures or activities shared by the members of the community. Virtual communities enjoy interactions and exchange of information between members who may not physically meet.[4]

Virtual communities have a shared goal that provides the primary reason for being part of the community, and they engage in repeated, active participation with access to shared resources. Defined policies determine the type and frequency of access to those resources. The sustainability of the community relies on reciprocity of information, support and services among members.[5] A virtual community in healthcare is a group of people and the social structure that they collectively create based on the use of telecommunication (Fig. 10.1). The purpose of the community is education, provision of support, discussion of issues, sharing of resources, consultation with experts and sustenance of relationships beyond or without face-to-face events.[4]

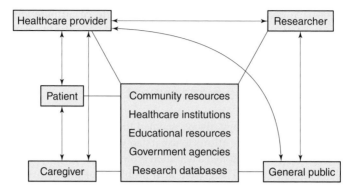

Fig. 10.1. The web and other telecommunication technologies enable numerous participants to access resources and form virtual teams and communities for the purposes of disease management interventions and research

A common reason for a virtual community is to function as a self-help group of individuals diagnosed with the same medical condition and/or undergoing similar treatment. As Finn's study showed, virtual self-help groups can provide many of the processes used in face-to-face self-help and mutual aid groups.[6] The emphasis in such virtual communities is on mutual problem-solving, sharing of information, expression of feelings, mutual support and empathy.

Technologies for virtual communities include online message boards and automatic mailing list servers for asynchronous communication and videoconferencing, and Internet relay chat, and group and private chat rooms for synchronous communication. In some cases communication is not moderated – that is, no person is responsible for reviewing and filtering messages that are inappropriate or in violation of the rules of the virtual community. In these cases, the community relies largely on the normative processes of their own internal social norms 'to define and enforce the acceptable behaviour of the community members'.[7] In other cases, a moderator will oversee the interaction between members.

In a systematic review of online healthcare communities,[8] researchers compiled and evaluated the evidence on the effects on health and social outcomes of computer-based peer-to-peer communities and electronic self-support groups. The authors concluded that there was a lack of robust evidence of consumer-led peer-to-peer communities, partly because most of these communities have been evaluated only in conjunction with more complex interventions or involvement with health professionals.[8] However, given the large number of unmoderated, web-based, peer-to-peer groups, further research is needed to assess when and how electronic support groups can be effective.[8]

Virtual communities can involve not only patients diagnosed with the same condition but also caregivers, healthcare providers and family members. The Comprehensive Health Enhancement Support System (CHESS) developed by the University of Wisconsin is a platform that provides services designed to help individuals cope with a health crisis or medical concern, but it also invites researchers to use resources and share knowledge and findings.[9] The system provides access to resources such as information, social support, and decision-making and problem-solving tools. The CHESS application and its consortia are good examples of a virtual community that serves patients' and caregivers' needs while also providing an active laboratory for research.

Advanced telecommunications enable healthcare providers to form virtual teams and interact and collaborate on cases even when separated by large distances. Many healthcare facilities lack the interdisciplinary resources required for efficient management of chronic disease. The Virtual Integrated Practice is a process that creates virtual care teams[10] to target four areas: communications, process standardization, group activities and self-management. The conditions covered by Virtual Integrated Practice are diabetes, chronic obstructive pulmonary disease and urinary incontinence. Communication among members of the virtual team is both synchronous and asynchronous. Pilot studies have demonstrated a successful integration of virtual teams into primary care practices. Virtual healthcare provider teams, in general, can ensure continuity of care, as they use a common platform for exchange of messages, opinions and resources. Such teams may be an important part of a successful disease management programme and may provide continuity of care for the patients.

Examples of e-health in disease management

Examples in which e-health has been used in disease management include:

- diabetes
- asthma
- cancer
- home monitoring.

Diabetes

Diabetes is a condition for which the Internet has the potential to support disease management. The time between sustained hyperglycaemia and observable complications can be extended, thus making a long-term programme of secondary prevention an essential part of diabetes care. McKay et al studied the development and feasibility of a website for diabetes self-management that emphasized personalized goal setting, feedback and social support, and found that patients were satisfied with the system and appreciated the social support and the availability of information.[12] The Center for Health Services Research in Detroit developed a web-based management system for diabetes care to support the routine care of patients with diabetes.[13] The system was evaluated by a non-randomized, longitudinal study. The findings suggested that web-based systems of clinical practice guidelines, patient registries and performance feedback have the potential to improve the rate of routine testing among patients with diabetes.

A European project, the Telematic Management of Insulin-Dependent Diabetes Mellitus, piloted a distributed system for the management of insulin-dependent diabetes mellitus. The aim was to use Internet technology to support healthcare providers and patients, and provide them with a set of automated services ranging from data collection and transmission to data analysis and decision support.[14] The system included a module that allowed patients to transmit data from their blood glucose monitoring device to the hospital information system. The system provided physicians with a set of tools for data visualization, data analysis and decision support, and allowed them to send messages, including therapeutic advice, to the patients.[15]

Asthma

Disease management for patients with asthma has the potential for early detection of critical situations and more rapid intervention. The Internet was employed for asthma management in the home asthma telemonitoring system,[11] which provided patients with continuous, individualized help in the daily routine of asthma self-care and coping and alerted healthcare providers if specific clinical conditions occurred.

Cancer

The National Cancer Institute Common Terminology Criteria for Adverse Events schema for seven common symptoms was adapted to a web-based patient reporting system that was accessible from computers in outpatient clinics and homes.[16] In a study by Basch et al,[16] 80 patients with gynaecological malignancies who were about to begin standard chemotherapy regimens were enrolled and encouraged to log into the system and report symptoms at each follow-up visit or, alternatively, to access the system from home. Patients were able to report symptoms experienced during chemotherapy, and their reporting often led to clinical interventions and changes in the care plan, which indicated that use of the Internet can be beneficial for the home treatment and monitoring of patients diagnosed with cancer.[16]

Home monitoring

Post-transplant care also requires monitoring of the patient's health status. Regular spirometry measurements in recipients of lung transplants are essential for early detection of acute infection and rejection of the allograft. A prospective study investigated the effects of a user-friendly, Internet-based telemonitoring system that provided direct transmission of home spirometry data to the hospital. The study showed that home monitoring of pulmonary function via the Internet in recipients of lung transplants was feasible and provided very reproducible data. However, it had 'only a mild sensitivity for the detection of acute allograft dysfunction'.[17]

The TeleHomeCare Project at the University of Minnesota included a system based on the use of low-cost, commercially available monitoring devices and an Internet application designed for patients diagnosed with congestive heart failure or chronic obstructive pulmonary disease and those who needed wound care. The system included web pages that were customized for the information needs of individual patients and included an online diary with questions to be answered each day. The latter included questions about symptoms, vital signs (such as weight, blood pressure or temperature), overall well-being and compliance with dietary guidelines. When one or more responses to these questions indicated a situation that required immediate clinical attention, alerts were triggered according to predefined rules and sent to the home-care agency staff.[18]

Ethical and technical considerations

Privacy and confidentiality

When Internet-based applications are used in healthcare, the privacy and confidentiality of individuals' health information needs to be protected. Information privacy is the patient's right to control the use and dissemination of information that relates to them, while confidentiality is a tool for protecting the patients' privacy. In the US, the Health Insurance Portability and Accountability Act (HIPAA) became law in 2000. It contains standards for the security of individuals' health information and the use of electronic signature for healthcare providers, systems and agencies. These standards refer to the security of all electronic health information and have major implications for the design and operation of applications for e-health disease management.

The use of the Internet in disease management calls for clarification of the issues of ownership of and access to monitoring data. In many web-based applications, patients record monitoring data and transmit them daily to a web server that is owned and maintained by a third party; providers are allowed to log in and access their patients' data. It is therefore necessary to control access to the data and ensure satisfactory web-based storage of the patient records.

Sociability and usability

In the context of virtual communities, the concepts of sociability and usability link knowledge about human behaviour with appropriate planning and design of online communities.[19] Specifically, sociability refers to the collective purpose of a community, the goals and roles of its members, and policies and rules defined to foster social interaction. The members' information needs can be addressed in the virtual community according to the social framework and the defined policies that govern the community. Developers and designers can influence the development trend by clearly communicating the community's purpose and policies.

Usability refers to the accessibility of the design and the specifics of an interface that lead to rapid learning, increased skill retention and minimization of error rates. The implication for virtual communities is that a usable virtual community is one in which members are able to communicate with each other, find information and navigate the community software with ease.[19]

Ensuring usability may be a problem for web-based disease management programmes. A large number of patients who require disease management are elderly, and, in some cases, they may have functional limitations. A functional limitation is a 'reduced sensory, cognitive or motor capability associated with human aging, temporary injury, or permanent disability that prevents a person from communicating, working, playing or simply functioning in an environment where other people in the population can function'.[20] Although the Internet can play a significant role in disease management, the fastest growing segment of the American population (that is, people older than 50 years) are at a disadvantage, because software and hardware designers often fail to consider them as a potential user group. Accessibility issues are important quality criteria for web-based interventions but are frequently ignored by designers and evaluators. Web-based applications that target home-care patients should aim to reach a high level of functional accessibility[21] and undergo rigorous usability tests. For that purpose, design considerations and guidelines need to be taken into account.[21]

Usability and sociability are challenges that designers of online communities have to address. These issues are not identical concepts. For example, the designers of a virtual community for patients with asthma must decide whether they should enforce a registration policy and how to define requirements for membership. These items constitute a sociability decision, as they will affect the number and type of memberships of the community and the social interactions that will occur. The design specifications for the registration procedures (for example, website layout, forms and features of functionality) are related to the software issues and constitute usability decisions. Both usability and sociability will determine to a great extent the feasibility and overall success of the virtual community.

Legal issues

The administration of virtual communities may not be straightforward, as such communities often include members from different parts of a country and in some cases even from different countries. The participation of healthcare providers may also create problems as a result of licensing issues. In the US, for example, medicine is considered to be practised at the patient's location. Thus, physicians have to be licensed to practise medicine in the state the patient is in during a teleconsultation. Another challenge is to determine the extent to which rules about the regulation of speech, which are defined by existing geographical jurisdictions, can be applied to a virtual community.

Lack of human touch

A concern with any application that involves healthcare interactions at a distance is the 'progressive dehumanization' of interpersonal relationships. Web-based disease management interventions have the potential to bridge distances and in some cases permit anonymity that may be desirable for a particular medical condition. On the other hand, such applications may lack the sense of touch and interhuman close contact that occurs in face-to-face meetings. Virtual communities represent a physically disembodied social order. Although this virtual order exists in parallel with social structures in physical space, some have argued that it will eventually compete with a structure or network of entities that occupy spatial locations.[22] In this context, the argument is that 'the fabric of human relationships and communities rests on real presences, real physical meetings and relationships'.[23] It remains to be seen whether the conventional notions of a social contract and personal rights can survive in a virtual world.

Guidelines

The concept of web-based disease management is relatively new, and no specific guidelines or regulations address some of the ethical or other considerations described earlier. The American Medical Informatics Association has provided guidelines for the electronic communication of patients with healthcare providers.[24] On the basis of these guidelines, a turnaround time for messages should be established, patients should be informed about privacy issues, and messages should be printed and included in the patients' charts. Patients must be warned not to use the online mode of interaction in an emergency and should be aware of all recipients of their messages, as well as general privacy issues.

In addition, the guidelines for the deployment of home-based telehealth applications produced by the American Telemedicine Association[25] are relevant to web-based disease management applications. The guidelines refer to technology, patients and providers. The technology criteria refer to the operation and maintenance of equipment, establishment of clear procedures, safety codes, protection of patient privacy and record security. The patient criteria involve recommendations such as the need for informed, written consent from patients, selection of patients able to handle the equipment and training. The health provider criteria refer to training issues and after-hours support. Such guidelines by professional organizations address some important concerns and provide an appropriate framework for the integration of e-health applications into the disease management process. However, many issues such as licensing, accreditation and liability have yet to be fully addressed by legislative or professional entities.

Future research and development

The field of e-health is relatively new and expanding. In order to establish evidence-based guidelines for the design and implementation of disease management applications that employ e-health, further research is required. To increase the generalizability of their findings, researchers need to document the social context and recruitment approaches in virtual communities or other web-based applications, the implied and stated rules that govern virtual communities, their rates of growth and utilization rates, the business models and the strategies that promote the applications. Cost-benefit analyses of disease management interventions will shed light on the resources required for software, hardware, training and ongoing maintenance of the applications and on their impact on clinical outcomes and utilization of health services.

The premise of e-health applications is that they lead to patient empowerment. In this context, it is important to develop assessment tools for patient empowerment. Most applications aim to empower patients; yet, measuring this effect is difficult in the absence of validated and reliable assessment tools. An assessment tool needs to be developed to cover several underlying constructs, such as disease knowledge, locus of control, trust, accessibility to services and availability of options. Such a tool used in studies after a pre–post design would show how e-health influences these underlying constructs.

Conclusion

Powerful technologies are emerging in the healthcare field. They enable people to become actively involved in disease management and prevention, and to communicate and form virtual teams and communities. This facilitates the shift from institution-centred to patient-centred or consumer-centred care. The technical, ethical and legal issues associated with web-based disease management will have to be addressed, and further research is needed to determine the effect of such applications on clinical outcomes, the overall process, and quality and access to care. As web-based applications pertaining to disease management and patient education continue to develop, all those involved – including system designers and developers, healthcare professionals, patients and patient advocacy groups – need to be prepared to take advantage of the new possibilities.

Further information

Comprehensive Health Enhancement Support System (CHESS) website. Available at: chess.chsra.wisc.edu/Chess/ (last accessed 25 November 2005).
Demiris G, ed. *E-health: current status and future trends in the EU and the US*. Amsterdam: IOS Press, 2004.
Eng TR, Gustafson DH, eds. *Wired for health and well-being: the emergence of interactive health communication*. Washington, DC: US Department of Health and Human Services, 1999.
Health e-Technologies Initiative website. Available at: www.hetinitiative.org/ (last accessed 25 November 2005).

References

1 Disease Management Association of America. *Definition of disease management*. Washington, DC: Disease Management Association of America, 2005. Available at: www.dmaa.org/definition.html (last accessed 25 November 2005).
2 Feste C, Anderson RM. Empowerment: from philosophy to practice. *Patient Educ Couns* 1995;**26**:139–44.
3 Eysenbach G. Consumer health informatics. *BMJ* 2000;**320**:1713–16.
4 Demiris G. Virtual communities in health care. In: Silverman B, Jain A, Ichalkaranje A, Jain L, eds. *Intelligent paradigms for healthcare enterprises*. Berlin: Springer, 2005:121–37.
5 Whittaker S, Issacs E, O'Day V. Widening the net: workshop report on the theory and practice of physical and network communities. *SIGCHI Bull* 1997;**29**:27–30.
6 Finn J. An exploration of helping processes in an online self-help group focusing on issues of disability. *Health Soc Work* 1999;**24**:220–31.

7   Burnett G, Besant M, Chatman EA. Small worlds: normative behavior in virtual communities and feminist bookselling. *J Am Soc Inform Sci* 2001;**52**:536–47.

8   Eysenbach G, Powell J, Englesakis M, *et al.* Health related virtual communities and electronic support groups: systematic review of the effects of online peer to peer interactions. *BMJ* 2004;**328**:1166.

9   Gustafson DH, Bosworth K, Hawkins RP, *et al.* CHESS: a computer-based system for providing information referrals, decision support and social support to people facing medical and other health-related crises. *Proc 16th Ann Symp Comput Appl Med Care* 1992;161–5.

10 Rothschild SK, Lapidos S, Minnick A, *et al.* Using virtual teams to improve the care of chronically ill patients. *J Clin Outcomes Manage* 2004;**11**:346–50.

11 Finkelstein J, O'Connor G, Friedmann RH. Development and implementation of the home asthma telemonitoring (HAT) system to facilitate asthma self-care. *Medinfo* 2001;**10**:810–14.

12 McKay HG, Feil EG, Glasgow RE, Brown JE. Feasibility and use of an Internet support service for diabetes self-management. *Diabetes Educ* 1998;**24**:174–9.

13 Baker AM, Lafata JE, Ward RE, *et al.* A web-based diabetes care management support system. *Jt Comm J Qual Improv* 2001;**27**:179–90.

14 Riva A, Bellazzi R, Stefanelli M. A web-based system for the intelligent management of diabetic patients. *MD Comput* 1997;**14**:360–4.

15 Bellazzi R, Larizza C, Montani S, *et al.* A telemedicine support for diabetes management: the T-IDDM project. *Comput Methods Programs Biomed* 2002;**69**:147–61.

16 Basch E, Artz D, Dulko D, *et al.* Patient online self-reporting of toxicity symptoms during chemotherapy. *J Clin Oncol* 2005;**23**:3552–61.

17 Morlion B, Knoop C, Paiva M, Estenne M. Internet-based home monitoring of pulmonary function after lung transplantation. *Am J Respir Crit Care Med* 2002;**165**:694–7.

18 Demiris G, Speedie S, Finkelstein SM. The nature of communication in virtual home care visits. *Proc AMIA Symp* 2001:135-8.

19 Preece J. *Online communities: designing usability and supporting sociability.* New York, NY: John Wiley & Sons, 2000.

20 Electronic Industries Alliance, Electronic Industries Foundation. *Resource guide for accessible design of consumer electronics: linking product design to the needs of people with functional limitations.* Cary, NC: Monterey Technologies, 1996. Available at: www.tiaonline.org/access/guide.html (last accessed 25 November 2005).

21 Demiris G, Finkelstein SM, Speedie SM. Considerations for the design of a web-based clinical monitoring and educational system for elderly patients. *J Am Med Inform Assoc* 2001;**8**:468–72.

22 Winner L. Living in electronic space. In: Casey T, Embree L, eds. *Lifeworld and technology.* Washington, DC: Center for Advanced Research on Phenomenology, University Press of America, 1990: 1–14.

23 Horner DS. The moral status of virtual action. In: Bynum TW, *et al,* eds. *Proceedings of the Fifth International Conference on the Social and Ethical Impacts of Information and Communication Technologies.* Gdańsk: Wydawn. Mikom, 2001.

24 Kane B, Sands D. Guidelines for the clinical use of electronic mail with patients. *J Am Med Inform Assoc* 1998;**5**:104–11.

25 Home Telehealth Special Interest Group. *Home telehealth clinical guidelines: adopted by the ATA board of directors.* Available at: www.americantelemed.org/icot/hometelehealthguidelines.htm (last accessed 25 November 2005).

▶11

Fall monitoring

Simon Brownsell and Mark S. Hawley

Introduction

The fear of falling and the consequences of an actual fall on the health and well-being of an older person are significant. Between 30% and 50% of independently living older people are fearful of falling, and this fear can decrease their quality of life and increase the speed of decline in the ability to perform activities of daily living.[1,2] About 33% of older people fall each year,[3] and the consequences of a fall to an older person can be life changing. One study even reported that 80% of women would rather be dead than experience the loss of independence and quality of life that results from a bad hip fracture and subsequent admission to a nursing home.[4] It has been suggested that the costs associated with older people who have fallen is more than £900 million per annum in the UK.[5] Consequently, many countries have developed guidance and introduced specific schemes to combat falls.[6]

Falls represent one of the major healthcare challenges that face industrialized countries throughout the world. Intervention strategies have tended to concentrate on exercise, reduction of medications and environmental modifications. Assistive technologies – such as handrails, hip protectors, walking frames and so on – are also important, but this chapter concentrates on telecare-based solutions in three categories:

- prevention: reducing the likelihood of a fall occurring
- detection: recognizing that a fall has occurred and ensuring that timely assistance is provided
- prediction: quantifying the risk that an older person may fall and therefore targeting resources to those most in need.

Fall prevention

Although exercise regimens, improved lighting and minimization of trip hazards are well-known interventions that seek to prevent falls, telecare also has a role to play – even though practitioners seem to be less aware of its potential. For people who may be considered at high risk, or who require assistance when getting out of bed, sensors placed under the mattress have been developed to identify when the user is trying to get up and raise an immediate alarm (Fig. 11.1). At this point, assistance from a nurse

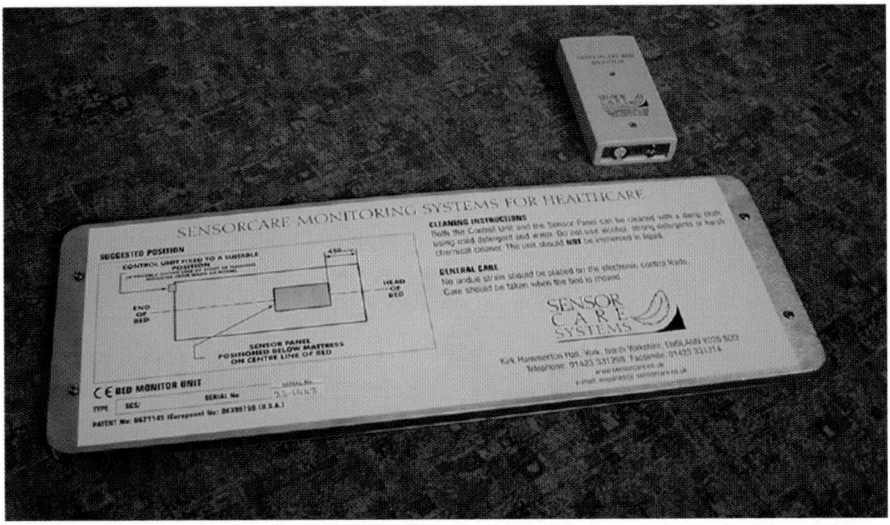

Fig. 11.1. Example of a bed sensor for the reduction of falls

or carer can be provided, which reduces the likelihood of a fall occurring. Traditionally, these devices have been used in hospital and nursing homes, from where consistently good results have been reported. A report by a commercial supplier indicated reductions of 25% in overall falls and 38% in unassisted falls (where no caregiver was present).[7] A trial at the Barnsley Hospital in the UK indicated a 28% reduction in falls and a 41% reduction of falls that resulted in injury.

Although there have been no reports of the success of using these devices in the community, scenarios for their use suggest themselves. For example, consider an older couple, where one partner is the main carer for a dependent spouse who needs help getting out of bed. Without this system, the carer would often have disturbed sleep – sleeping with 'one eye open', as it were, to provide assistance to their partner whenever it was needed. However, with the system described, the carer can sleep well, and even in a different room, knowing that as soon as their partner tries to get up, they will be woken and can provide the necessary assistance. Even in this simple scenario, there is the possibility that such a system could result in avoiding or delaying entry to institutional care.

In a variation of this technology, a timer is used; if the user does not return to bed in a set period, perhaps 10 minutes, an alert is generated. As well as being practical when a carer is in the same dwelling, such an approach also enables the system to be used by the community alarm (personal emergency response) system. However, although there are examples of its use in sheltered housing schemes and nursing homes, there seem to be few examples of it being used in the community.

Adaptations of this technology allow a lamp or the main room lights to be turned on automatically when the user gets out of bed. The rationale is that the person is more likely to fall if the room remains dark. Such an approach may be further help in the prevention of falls, but, at present, only anecdotal evidence seems to indicate this is the case. Similar functionality to the bed sensors also exists for chair occupancy.

Although not, strictly speaking, telecare, prevention strategies being developed include placing vibrating insoles in shoes. In a trial reported in the *Lancet*, it is suggested that such an approach could actually improve older people's balance and reduce the likelihood of a fall.[8] It would seem, however, that greater attention needs to be paid to verifying this strategy. A similar approach has resulted in the development of a smart ankle brace that detects an oncoming fall and triggers a vibrating sensor to help the wearer correct their movements.[9] Although developments such as these are welcome, it is likely to be some time before they are proved and in everyday use.

Fall detection

Prevention of a fall is clearly the ultimate goal, but some falls will always occur. As such, the provision of timely assistance is key, as any delay in medical treatment can lead to medical complications. This is especially true in cases when the faller is unable to get off the floor. It is thought that a prolonged lying of an hour or more occurs in about 5% of falls.[10] In such circumstances, recovery from injury may be slower than otherwise might be the case, which can compromise mobility and increase the risk of death.[11]

Anecdotal evidence also exists to show that older people with a community alarm pendant have fallen and been unable to get up, but have chosen to stay on the floor and wait for a carer to come the following morning. The reason normally given is that they did not want to be a nuisance to the control centre. One of the key benefits of telecare-based falls intervention strategies is that they can monitor for falls and almost immediately raise a call for assistance on the user's behalf. Although user choice and related ethical considerations are important, an automated approach to fall detection and early provision of assistance may have advantages in many cases.

Telecare-based fall detection systems generally fall into three main categories:

- worn devices
- lifestyle monitoring
- video analysis.

Worn devices

Automatic fall detectors have been developed by a number of companies. These devices are often worn on the waist and are about the size and weight of a pager (Fig. 11.2). When a fall is detected, a carer or the community alarm control centre can be contacted automatically, therefore removing the reliance on the user to instigate a call for assistance, which they may be unable to do. These devices commonly use a two-stage detection mechanism, with an accelerometer and tilt meter. The accelerometer is used to detect an impact greater than a given threshold, and the tilt meter determines the wearer's orientation.[12] In combination, they can reduce false alerts and maximize detection rates.

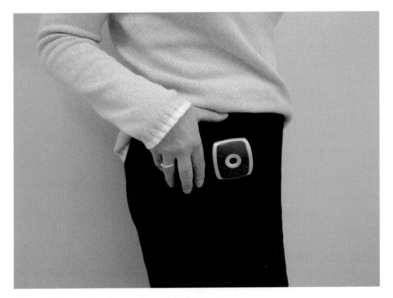

Fig. 11.2. Example of an automatic fall detector

A controlled trial in South Yorkshire, UK, investigated the effect of these detectors on fear of falling and gauged their ability to detect falls.[13] Fifty-five community alarm users, who were at high risk of falling, were recruited. The intervention group comprised 34 people who received a fall detector, and the control group comprised 21 people who did not receive a fall detector. The trial lasted for six months. No significant difference was seen between the intervention and control group (intention-to-treat analysis) on change in fear of falling assessed by the falls efficacy scale (40.3 vs 37.5; difference 2.8; 95% confidence interval –6.2 to 11.8). Differences in fear of falling between a group who wore their detector regularly (62% of the intervention group) and those who did not (38%) suggest that some people may benefit from a fall detector in terms of their fear of falling and that, conversely, others may lose confidence if provided with a fall detector. These points were supported by comments made by participants: for example, while one said, 'I would say that it's one of the best safety nets someone could have', another said, 'it made me feel vulnerable, more so than normal, because it made me more aware of the possibility that I might fall'. This has important implications if confirmed by further research, as it suggests that fall detectors should not be provided to all older people at high risk of falling but that careful assessment is crucial to determine whether provision would be beneficial.

With respect to device performance, the same study indicated that the device would mistakenly recognize a non-fall event as a fall about once per month for each user. On three occasions, falls occurred but the device failed to recognize them as falls and did not activate an alarm. On one occasion, however, a fall occurred, the detector worked appropriately and assistance was provided speedily – to the considerable relief of the user and their family. So although the evidence for a reduction in fear of falling is not, statistically, clear-cut, certain individuals can derive benefit. The user whose fall was detected commented, 'I am very pleased with it because it did what it should. It makes me feel safe.' Similar successful experiences have been reported in numerous case studies.

Despite some positive findings, certain problems remain:

- The user has to wear the device for it to be effective, which they may not want or might forget to do.
- People with physical limitations can have problems attaching or wearing the device.
- False alerts reduce confidence in the detector and can cause unease; this may result in the user declining to wear the device.
- Some falls are not detected by the device; this clearly has an impact on user safety and confidence.

An interesting development of the above approach is monitoring metabolic energy expenditure as well as falls. In a pilot study, a correlation was suggested between self-reported health status and energy expenditure. This raises the possibility that future devices may provide an independent measure of health status, as well as detecting falls, although it is acknowledged that more work is required to confirm this.[14]

The advantages and disadvantages of worn devices are summarized in Table 11.1.

Table 11.1. Worn devices are located on the body to detect a fall immediately and automatically call for assistance

Advantages	Disadvantages
Can provide immediate recognition of a fall	User must wear device for it to be effective
Small and light weight	Can be difficult to attach and wear
Relatively cheap solution	Concern over false alerts and accuracy of detection

Lifestyle monitoring

Although these systems are often called lifestyle monitoring, experience with older people suggests that such a phrase raises feelings of intrusion and that 'Big Brother' is watching me. It therefore may be more appropriate to describe these systems as 'lifestyle reassurance'. Irrespective of the name, these systems monitor the occupant's movements and look for deviations from a 'normal' pattern of behaviour, which is indicative of a potential problem. This is normally achieved by having sensors (often passive infrared (PIR) movement detectors) distributed throughout the dwelling in each room; door contacts on external doors, food cupboards and the fridge; and chair and bed occupancy sensors. Therefore, not only do these systems indirectly monitor for falls, but they also have the potential to identify a whole range of other alert conditions.

Although the worn devices described above are normally a cheap and simple option, failure to wear the device by people who are forgetful or have physical limitations makes such systems redundant. In these circumstances, it may be more appropriate to use lifestyle reassurance. It should be noted, however, that in order to reduce false alarms, lifestyle reassurance systems do not provide an immediate response when a fall occurs. Instead, they often deduce that a fall has occurred after a defined period of inactivity in a certain room. For example, a threshold may be set at one hour for the bathroom, so that an alert is generated if the user is in the bathroom for more than one hour; for the lounge, the threshold may be five hours. Consequently, if the user fell as they entered the lounge, it could be almost five hours before a call for assistance is generated. Unfortunately, no authoritative results exist about the performance of lifestyle reassurance in relation to falls, although some controlled trials are beginning to take place.[15]

Although the response from lifestyle reassurance may not be as immediate as that with worn devices, they do provide a useful safety net, and in combination with worn detectors – or the traditional community alarm pendant – could provide an effective solution. There is likely to be substantial growth and development in this area in the future, as several companies now provide, and are developing, lifestyle reassurance systems. Table 11.2 highlights some examples.

Table 11.3 summarizes the advantages and disadvantages of lifestyle monitoring.

In an attempt to derive the benefits of achieving immediate recognition of a fall without wearing a device, the Smart Inactivity Monitor using Array-Based Detectors (SINBAD) represents a hybrid of the above approaches and shows promise for the future.[16] This device uses simple infrared array technology to locate and track a

Table 11.2. Examples of companies that provide and develop lifestyle reassurance systems

Company	Website/information source
Commercially available	
ADT	www.adt.com/resi/products_services/medical_alert_systems/
Living Independently	www.quietcaresystems.com/index_fl.htm
Just Checking	www.justchecking.co.uk
Tunstall	www.tunstallgroup.com
Tynetec	www.tynetec.co.uk/assets/images/Altera_Brochure_Page_1.jpg
In development	
British Telecom	DTI. 'Nextwave Programme: A guide to NextWave Technologies and Markets.' Oct 2004:14
iControl Networks	www.icontrol.com/solutions.html
Lusora	www.lusora.com

Table 11.3. Lifestyle monitoring depends on sensors distributed around the dwelling to detect abnormal behaviour and automatically call for assistance

Advantages	Disadvantages
User does not have to wear a device or sensor	Does not provide immediate recognition of a fall
Monitors for a whole range of alert conditions	Often requires trained installers
Likely to provide a reliable safety net	Concern over false alarms and accuracy of detection

thermal target, providing information on its size, location and velocity. A two-stage process then is used to detect the fall:

- The monitor analyses target motion to detect the characteristic dynamics of any falls.
- The device monitors target inactivity and compares it with a map of acceptable periods of inactivity.

The developers suggest that the combination of fall detection and inactivity monitoring is a potentially powerful method, avoiding many false alarms by observing the activity after what looks like a fall. Trials, however, have indicated that further development is required, as only 30% of actual falls (when using actors) were detected.

Video analysis

Like lifestyle reassurance, video analysis systems seek to provide long-term analysis of behaviour changes. However, they also provide the opportunity to immediately recognize a fall.

These systems are currently at the development stage and are not yet reliable, commercially available devices. At the University of Toronto, Lee and Mihailidis have reported on a video-based system that detects 77% of actual falls and mistakenly generated false alarms on 5% of occasions.[17] However, they also reported that obstacles still needed to be overcome, such as the tracking of multiple users, falls when the user has a walking stick or Zimmer frame, and colour definition when the carpet and user's clothes are similar. Researchers at the University of Dundee and Rensselaer Polytechnic Institute are also working on such systems.[18,19] Several systems were presented at the International Expo 2005 in Japan (Fig. 11.3). Using a similar

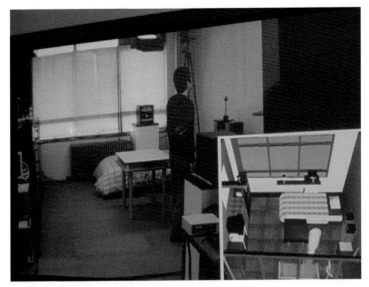

Fig. 11.3. Example of video-based tracking

Table 11.4. In video analysis, video cameras are used to track users and monitor their behaviour for immediate alert conditions and over time

Advantages	Disadvantages
User does not have to wear a device or sensor	Potential intrusion of cameras
Tracks user and provides immediate fall recognition	Need for multiple cameras to cover an entire room
Provides visual feedback to carers and assessors	Installation and need for power or data cables

approach, staff at the Carnegie Mellon University are developing a system in a nursing home environment.[20]

The advantages and disadvantages of video analysis are summarized in Table 11.4.

Fall prediction

An additional element for which telecare could be effective is in predicting falls and therefore the prioritization of resources to those most in need.

One of the key determinants of someone falling is known to be whether they have fallen in the past.[6] Telecare-based solutions can be used to gather this important information – for example, the recording of falls from the worn devices. In addition, Doughty *et al* suggested that a falls risk index could be calculated from falls history, time in bed, medication, frailty and other variables.[21] While this may be speculative at present, the use of lifestyle reassurance and video analysis does suggest that many of the indices mentioned by Doughty *et al* could be generated automatically. This represents an exciting area for development, as systems may not only respond to the occurrence of a fall but also could assist in the prioritization of falls interventions to those most at risk.

User views and telecare-based falls interventions

It has been noted that clinical observations and empirical reports point to the reluctance of many older people living in the community to adopt fall prevention behaviours. In particular, there seems to be substantial resistance to implementing recommendations about home-safety modifications and the use of assistive devices.[22] Although this may be true for assistive devices such as hip protectors – where the reluctance of users to wear such devices is well known – are these views evident for telecare?

One survey of 176 community alarm users in Birmingham, UK, indicated that 77% of users would welcome the possibility of a system that would automatically detect a fall and, if they had not regained their feet in a couple of minutes, raise an alarm. The interviews were repeated in a sheltered housing scheme in Rotherham, UK, with 27 users, where a figure of 78% was reported.[23]

An analysis with focus groups of service users ($n=34$) and providers ($n=25$) indicated a mixed response.[24] About half of the service users expressed positive views towards the detection of falls with worn fall detectors, but concerns existed about the possible accidental activation of the device and therefore 'bothering' staff who would have to respond. Service providers reported significant concerns and were generally quite negative towards the worn fall detectors. The reasons cited were the perceived difficulty in wearing the device, likely non-compliance by users and the implications to service users of false activations, which they also perceived would produce fear and anxiety in users. Providers also suggested that some users feel stigmatized by wearing a community alarm pendant and that this would increase if they had to wear the larger fall detector. However, findings from focus groups with people who subsequently do not use the technology must be treated with a level of caution. In several examples of telecare interventions in which the technology was viewed as intrusive before installation, such feelings were no longer evident at the end of the trial.

Discussion

User acceptance

At present, the understanding of the desires and wishes of users is somewhat limited. Although some attention has been given to specific telecare technologies, no attention seems to have been paid to the relative importance of telecare in overall generic falls strategies.

Each of the telecare technologies described above has different issues that need careful investigation. However, as the consequences and fear of falling for many older people are important issues, it is likely that acceptance of telecare-based falls interventions will be higher for such people. This is to be anticipated, as when the benefits (such as speed of response and security) outweigh the negative elements (such as intrusion and cost), the intervention will be accepted. However, the point at which the intervention will be viewed as beneficial is different for each user. At present, it is also unclear whether one particular type of technology is likely to be welcomed more than another. Nevertheless, a range of interventions are likely to be necessary to meet different user needs, requirements and environments.

One of the interesting conclusions from the survey of 176 users in Birmingham was that, perhaps surprisingly, nine (21%) of the interviewees who reported falling in the previous year rejected automatic fall detection. Two of the nine had fallen six times during the previous year and commented that, because they fell regularly without harming themselves, such a system would be intrusive. Some also commented that they were uncomfortable knowing that others would be informed they had fallen. This is an important consideration, as some older people worry that their carers or family members may interpret a fall as the need for entry into institutionalization. Greater understanding of the ownership and distribution of information through telecare systems needs to be explored.

Ethical issues

Many ethical issues need to be considered. Fundamentally, the user must be informed and give consent to an automatic alert being generated. Attention must also be given to the transmission of data in any such telecare system and the desire by some users for

relatives and responders not to be automatically informed if they fall. Yet, how many systems offer such an approach at the moment – even at the level of pendant activation? The use of lifestyle reassurance and especially video images brings with it additional questions, and safeguards must be put in place and agreed with users before systems become operational.

An interesting ethical dilemma concerns whether fall detection exposes the user to a new level of risk. If a user has confidence that a fall will be detected, could this result in them taking risks they previously would not have taken? For example, would a person with a detector be willing to stand on a stool and change a light bulb, thus increasing their likelihood of a serious fall? At this stage, this is simply conjecture, but such questions are important and must be studied as the field matures. Many ethical concerns can be addressed by developing detailed service plans and agreeing them with users before they receive a service.

The potential of telecare-based falls strategies

The three domains of prevention, detection and prediction are key areas that telecare could affect. As telecare-based technologies can provide effective real-time monitoring along with the gathering and manipulation of data for the benefit of their users, it is suggested that a single telecare based system could affect all three of these domains at once. Telecare therefore proposes a real tool in falls management that merits further investigation, as no other falls management strategy can cover all three domains at the same time.

Telecare technology

Much of the technology is either relatively new or in the developmental stages. As the field matures, the technology can be expected to be refined and its performance improved. There is, however, a fundamental difference between monitoring strategies, as some require the user to wear a device and others monitor the user through sensors distributed throughout the home. Both approaches have their strengths and weaknesses, as described above. What is important, however, is that service users and providers make an informed choice about the specific circumstances of the individual.

In terms of the lifestyle and video analysis systems, it would seem that video analysis functionally is the better option, because of its speed in recognizing a fall and its ability to allow carers to visually replay areas of concern. However, the acceptance, or not, of cameras in older peoples' homes is an area where greater understanding is required. Ohta *et al* suggested that cameras deprive the user of their privacy and therefore are not a desirable monitoring tool.[25] Acceptance, however, is likely to differ between older people and in different parts of the world. If older people refuse to accept cameras, or only allow them in certain rooms, the effectiveness of this approach will be heavily compromised.

Industry standards

In order to make an informed decision on which technology is suitable, performance data and evaluations are required. Even if a decision is made on the technological approach which is to be used (for example, worn detectors), a decision still has to be made about which manufacturer's equipment is most suitable. It is difficult to accurately determine an appropriate falls test structure – that is, how to quantify the variety of different ways an older person can fall and how to simulate these accurately – however, if such devices are to be adopted routinely, purchasers (and users) need an understanding of device performance. Areas of interest include the percentage of falls detected and the anticipated number of false alerts.

System level response

Telecare technologies are effective only if the system level response is appropriate, with carers and health professionals able to respond in a timely manner. Whether technology is used for prevention, detection or prediction, it must be viewed as a tool in a much larger context. The technology may indicate that someone has fallen, but the quality of the subsequent service offered by care, support and health professionals is the key to an effective system.

Limitation of the evidence

Any product or service will always have early adopters who embrace the opportunities despite a relative lack of evidence. Most people and service providers, however, require evidence of comparisons with other options before making a decision. Currently, it would seem that telecare, in the context of falls, is in the 'early adoption' stage, and the evidence is slowly growing. As the evidence grows, deployment will increase.

One of the current limitations is that few studies evaluate devices or compare different techniques. Most published studies involve only small numbers of participants or refer to technology development. Although numerous pilot studies are taking place, relatively few undergo formal evaluation or research. Where studies have reported positive results, these are often in the form of case studies, while the factors that determine a successful intervention are not reported. As mentioned earlier, in the provision of a falls-based telecare intervention, user-centred assessment may be pivotal. Analysis of the factors that result in successful and unsuccessful deployments thus would be beneficial as the evidence grows.

Conclusion

That telecare has the potential to play a significant role in strategies to manage falls is in no doubt. Telecare can be used to prevent falls and detect them when they occur and could even be used to predict people at greatest risk, thus allowing service delivery options to be prioritized. No other approach could achieve such goals with relatively cheap and simple technology. The effects that this may have on users' quality of life, security and ability to stay at home for longer could be significant, suggesting substantial benefits for users and financial savings to the health and care sector.

Nevertheless, despite these real possibilities, a note of caution must be sounded. The views of users and professionals towards a telecare-based approach need to be better understood. Much of the technology is in the developmental stage, and the technologies that are available require more formal evaluations to understand the benefits and any potential risks. However, it is evident that as the telecare field develops over the coming years, it is likely that falls are an application area in which significant progress can be made for the benefit of all.

Further information

Brownsell S, Hawley M. Automatic fall detectors and the fear of falling. *J Telemed Telecare* 2004;**10**:262–7.

Chang JT, Morton SC, Rubenstein LZ, *et al*. Interventions for the prevention of falls in older adults: systematic review and meta-analysis of randomized clinical trials. *BMJ* 2004;**328**:680.

Department of Health. *Telecare – getting started*. London: Department of Health, 2005. Available at: www.changeagentteam.org.uk/_library/docs/Housing/Telecare/Telecare_gettingstarted.pdf (last accessed 14 December 2005).

References

1   Salkeld G, Cameron ID, Cumming RG, *et al*. Quality of life related to fear of falling and hip fracture in older women: a time trade off study. *BMJ* 2000;**320**:341–6.

2   Cumming RG, Salkeld G, Thomas M, Szonyi G. Prospective study of the impact of fear of falling on activities of daily living, SF-36 scores, and nursing home admission. *J Gerontol A Biol Sci Med Sci* 2000;**55**:M299–305.

3   Department of Health. *How can we help older people not fall again? Implementing the Older People's NSF Falls Standard: support for commissioning good services*. London: Department of Health, 2003. Available at: www.dh.gov.uk (last accessed 14 December 2005).

4   Kannus P, Palvanen M, Niemi S, *et al*. Increasing number and incidence of fall-induced severe head injuries in older adults: nationwide statistics in Finland in 1970-1995 and prediction for the future. *Am J Epidemiol* 1999;**149**:143–50.

5   National Institute for Clinical Excellence. *2004/048 New guidelines for the NHS on the assessment and prevention of falls in older people*. London: National Insitute for Clinical Excellence, 2004. Available at: www.nice.org.uk/page.aspx?o=233482 (last accessed 3 October 2005).

6   American Geriatrics Society, British Geriatrics Society, American Academy of Orthopaedic Surgeons Panel on Falls Prevention. Guideline for the prevention of falls in older persons. *J Am Geriatr Soc* 2001;**49**:664–72.

7   Geffre S. *Bed alarms: investigating their impact on fall reduction and restraint use*. Tulsa, OK: Bed-Check Corporation, 2005. Available at: www.bedcheck.com/fall-prevention-study.html (last accessed 3 October 2005).

8   Priplata AA, Niemi JB, Harry JD, *et al*. Vibrating insoles and balance control in elderly people. *Lancet* 2003;**362**:1123–4.

9   *E-Health Insider* Chip in ankle brace may reduce falls in elderly. 2005;**184**. Available at: www.e-health-insider.com/News/Newsletters.cfm?ID=212 (last accessed 3 October 2005).

10 Ebrahim S, Kalache A, eds. *Epidemiology in old age*. London: BMJ Publishing, 1997:361.

11 Fisk MJ. *Social alarms to telecare: older people's services in transition*. Bristol: Policy Press, 2003:210.

12 Miskelly FG. Assistive technology in elderly care. *Age Ageing* 2001;**30**:455–8.

13 Brownsell S, Hawley M. Automatic fall detectors and the fear of falling. *J Telemed Telecare* 2004;**10**:262–7.

14   Mathie MJ, Coster AC, Lovell NH, *et al.* A pilot study of long-term monitoring of human movements in the home using accelerometry. *J Telemed Telecare* 2004;**10**:144–51.

15   Med-e-Tel 2005. *Telemedicine and e-health directory 2005.* Luxembourg: Med-e-Tel, 2005:111. Available at: www.medetel.lu/teldir/tm-dir.html (last accessed 3 October 2005).

16   Sixsmith A, Johnson N. A smart sensor to detect the falls of the elderly. *IEEE Pervasive Comput* 2004;**3**:42–7.

17   Lee T, Mihailidis A. An intelligent emergency response system: preliminary development and testing of automated fall detection. *J Telemed Telecare* 2005;**11**:194–8.

18   Nait-Charif H, McKenna SJ. Activity summarisation and fall detection in a supportive home environment. *Proc 17th Int Conf Pattern Recogn* 2004;**4**:323–6.

19   Kettnaker V, Gahm JK. Closed-loop person tracking and detection. *1st Canadian Conference on Computer and Robot Vision* 2004:314–19.

20   Hauptmann AG, Gao J, Yan R, *et al.* Automated analysis of nursing home observations. *IEEE Pervasive Comput* 2004;**3**:15–21.

21   Doughty K, Lewis R, McIntosh A. The design of a practical and reliable fall detector for community and institutional telecare. *J Telemed Telecare* 2000;**6** (Suppl 1):150–4.

22   Aminzadeh F, Edwards N. Exploring seniors' views on the use of assistive devices in fall prevention. *Public Health Nurs* 2001;**15**:297–304.

23   Brownsell S, Bradley D. *Assistive technology and telecare: forging solutions for independent living.* Bristol: Policy Press, 2003.

24   Brownsell S, Hawley M. Fall detectors: do they work or reduce the fear of falling? *Housing, Care and Support* 2004;**7**:18–24.

25   Ohta S, Nakamoto H, Shinagawa Y, Tanikawa T. A health monitoring system for elderly people living alone. *J Telemed Telecare* 2002;**8**:151–6.

►12

Quarantine and isolation

Susan L. Dimmick and Kunka D. Ignatova

Introduction

During a widespread health crisis, such as an epidemic, authorities attempt to contain the spread of disease. In the US, the Public Health Service Act authorizes the Department of Health and Human Services to make and enforce regulations to prevent the introduction, transmission and spread of communicable disease from foreign countries into the US and from one state or possession into another.[1] Under its authority, people suspected of carrying a communicable disease can be detained, medically examined or conditionally released. Individuals or groups can be quarantined for nine infectious diseases:

- cholera and suspected cholera
- diphtheria
- infectious tuberculosis
- plague
- smallpox
- yellow fever
- viral haemorrhagic fevers (Lassa, Marburg, Ebola, Crimean-Congo, South American and others not yet isolated or named)
- severe acute respiratory syndrome (SARS)
- influenza caused by novel or re-emergent influenza viruses that are causing, or have the potential to cause, a pandemic.

Local and state governments also have the authority to impose quarantine. If a health crisis affects only a single community, the local authority exercises the quarantine option. If the pattern of communicable disease affects more than one community or has the potential to spread across different jurisdictions, the state government assumes quarantine authority. The federal government steps in when a communicable disease incident crosses state lines.[2]

Containment strategies

The three common methods of disease containment used are:

- **quarantine** – the separation and restriction of movement of people who are not yet ill but have been exposed to a person with a specific communicable disease

- **shelter in place (SIP)** – a method for accomplishing quarantine in which individuals are usually confined to their homes
- **isolation** – the separation of people who have a specific communicable illness from healthy people.

In the US, voluntary separation of those exposed is preferred.[3] Generally, people who are quarantined are either directed to their homes or to some kind of large, non-medical facility, such as a sports arena or a hotel.

Shelter in place is one method of quarantining people. Most of the time, SIP orders confine individuals to their homes; however, SIP could relate to other locations, such as the workplace. The intention of SIP is to make a shelter out of the place a person is in when a community-wide health crisis occurs. It is a way to make a building or home as safe as possible.[4] In practice, SIP has often been used in the US as a method of protecting people from chemical spills or radiation emergencies. Mannan and Kilpatrick chronicled the effective use of SIP in a number of chemical release emergencies.[5] This approach has also been used frequently in countries such as Hong Kong, Singapore, China and Canada, where cases of SARS occurred.

Isolation is intended to restrict the movement of people with a communicable illness to stop the spread of the disease.[6] People who need to be isolated are usually confined in a medical facility, where negative pressure rooms are available.

Obviously quarantine, isolation and SIP involve some curtailment of civil liberties, such as privacy and liberty of movement. According to Gostin *et al*, 'contemporary public health practice favours 'sheltering in place', preferably in a person's home'.[3] They also noted that public health staff should resort to isolation or quarantine only if it is the least restrictive or intrusive alternative.[3]

Experience with SARS

Experience in the SARS outbreak in 2003 showed that blocking the transmission of communicable diseases was the key to controlling epidemics. Bloom noted that 'voluntary isolation and quarantine are a great inconvenience for a lot of people, but they are currently our best tools to save lives'.[7]

Shelter in place was the method of choice for the Nassau County Health Department in New York, which used a videophone to deliver care to an individual who was isolated because of potential exposure to SARS. The Health Department initiated video monitoring in January 2004, after it received a report from an emergency department about a patient with upper respiratory tract symptoms. The man had been in Quangdong Province, China, during the SARS outbreak there. The patient did not require hospitalization but agreed to voluntary home isolation. Health Department staff monitored him at least twice daily for fever and symptoms until they had resolved, in accordance with the Centers for Disease Control and Prevention guidelines. The use of a videophone seemed to be an effective and efficient method of closely observing and monitoring the patient during voluntary home isolation and quarantine.[8]

Home telehealth

Whatever method of quarantine is used, the government has an obligation to provide adequate healthcare, food and water, and a means of communication with family and friends. In the US, the Model State Emergency Health Powers Act, passed after the events of 11 September 2001, specifies what the government must do during quarantine and protects individuals from undue government intrusion. The public health authority must maintain places of isolation or quarantine in a safe and hygienic manner, regularly monitoring the health of residents. There must also be due process of appeal for individuals who believe that the government is overstepping its authority during isolation and/or quarantine incidents.[9]

During an epidemic, large numbers of people would probably be ordered into quarantine. People who are ordered into quarantine will require medical care and health monitoring. Home telehealth is a method by which it could be delivered.

Home telehealth technologies

A wide range of home telehealth technologies exist – from asynchronous individual emergency alerts to synchronous televideo systems. Table 12.1 shows a categorization scheme. This framework[10] may be helpful in assessing the types of applications that would be useful in home quarantine or isolation situations:

- Emergency alerting – these kinds of devices could be used for elderly or disabled individuals affected by SIP quarantine orders to enable them to summon assistance in an emergency.
- Medication monitoring and dispensing – this kind of device would be useful in SIP situations in which individuals are required to take medications, either as part of their own pre-existing daily disease management or when medications must be taken to manage the disease for which quarantine was imposed.
- Medical device monitoring – these kinds of devices could be used to deliver a level of care that would include the monitoring and treatment of subacute conditions when individuals are quarantined.
- Therapy telemanagement – these kinds of devices would be useful for quarantined individuals who had therapies that required healthcare providers to make continuous adjustments.
- Telemonitoring – these types of devices would be useful in the care of quarantined or isolated individuals who are not acutely ill but require more than simple vital signs monitoring (Fig. 12.1).
- Televideo patient management – this type of equipment would be useful for caregivers and other family members who need help and support to describe the situation, and would allow providers themselves to see what the patient is experiencing.

Video monitoring was the technology most often used during the SARS crisis. Two-way sound and image transmission make real-time medical assessments possible.

Table 12.1. Classification scheme for home telehealth technologies (from Ref. 10)

System	Description
Personal emergency response	• Automated dialling system (that is, a base unit) that can transmit a coded message to a remote monitoring station when activated by the user or by a sensor (such as air temperature, smoke or fire sensor) • User activation is by means of a small, battery-powered transmitter that may be worn around the neck or on the wrist • Transmitter can send discrete signals to the base unit, which initiates a toll-free call to the monitoring station, which in turn attempts to verify the emergency with the user and then contacts the appropriate emergency service (such as the police or ambulance service) in the user's community • Some base units are speaker phones and allow staff at the monitoring station to stay in contact with the user until local help arrives • Personal emergency response system is an in-home emergency service that enables elderly people and those with disabilities to stay in their homes without caregivers and reduces hospitalization by facilitating early emergency treatment and transport
Monitored medication dispensing	• Programmable device for scheduled dispensing of medications • Alerts a remote monitoring station about patient non-compliance by means of a coded telephone message • Consists of a medication storage compartment that holds a one-week or one-month supply of tablets or capsules and a lock-out feature to prevent access • User's daily regimen is programmed by the provider • Dispensing device may simply release designated scheduled dosage or may display patient instructions on a small LCD screen (for example, a reminder to a patient with diabetes to 'take your insulin'). • Common feature is visual message and/or audio signal that alerts the user that it is time to take the required medication(s). If the patient does not take the medication, the system notifies a monitoring station, which may call to remind the patient. Alternatively, an on-call nurse may contact the patient.
Medical device monitoring	• Permits off-site monitoring of in-home medical devices such as oxygen concentrators and drug delivery systems by a telephone connection that periodically transmits reports about device functioning and patient usage • Teleinfusion is an example of this type of system, in which an infusion device is linked to a telephone line. Solution administration and device operation can be monitored at a remote location. Troubleshooting can be done online. • Minimizes in-home interventions and increases patients' involvement in care and therapy • In other applications, the monitoring device can be attached to a concentrator or ventilator, which may be free-standing in terms of telecommunications capability or may have a wired or wireless connection to a base unit of the personal emergency response system, which provides telecommunications capability
Therapy telemanagement	• Dedicated configuration involving real-time continuous monitoring of in-home therapy administration, automatically tracking the patient's signs and adjusting volumes and flows as indicated • One in-home oxygen conservation device can monitor a patient's blood oximetry in real-time. If the system measures a rise in the patient's blood gas concentration above a predetermined level, it can reduce the flow of oxygen. When the patient's levels drop, the system will increase the oxygen flow accordingly • Systems of this nature need a telecommunications link, which is usually the ordinary telephone network

Table 12.1. Classification scheme for home telehealth technologies (from Ref. 10) *continued*

System	Description
Patient telemonitoring	<ul><li>Involves input of patient data at scheduled intervals to a device that has telecommunications capability or attaches to a standard telephone</li><li>Common application is monitoring patients with asthma and other respiratory conditions. Spirometry is performed by the patient at home to measure peak expiratory flow and forced expiratory volume for one second (FEV_1)</li><li>Typical unit provides digital display of results for the patient and transmits data to a monitoring station, which transmits the results to the provider or allows the results to be viewed via a web interface</li><li>Other applications involve remote sphygmomanometers for monitoring blood pressure and electronic stethoscopes to transmit heart, lung and bowel sounds</li></ul>
Televideo patient management	<ul><li>Videophone configuration that allows voice communication and exchange of low-resolution video images of patient and provider staff</li><li>Images usually displayed on a standard television set</li><li>Video camera and telephone connection also required in the home</li><li>May also incorporate a range of instruments for measuring clinical variables online</li></ul>

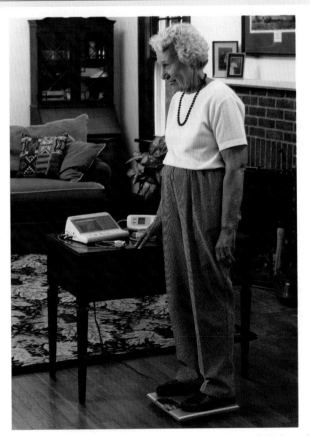

Fig. 12.1. An example of store-and-forward technology to transmit vital signs data to a remote server and provide personalized questions or advice (Viterion 100, Viterion TeleHealthcare LLC)

They permit a visual check of certain types of medication usage. For example, use of diuretics can be determined by inspecting the subject for fluid retention, which is often visible in the face, under the eyes or by looking at the feet. Health education and symptom management can progress at a more rapid rate because two senses (vision and hearing) rather than one sense (hearing alone) are involved. Caregivers and other family members receive help and support because providers can see for themselves what the person is experiencing. Finally, mental healthcare is likely to be a sought-after service during home quarantine or isolation, as occurred during the SARS outbreaks in Toronto. Mental health assessments and counselling can be conducted via home videoconferencing.

Future technology

Advances in wireless technologies make it possible for individuals to provide feedback to public health professionals who may be trying to determine when and where there will be outbreaks of communicable disease. For example, an early warning system for epidemics based on data transmission via mobile phones has been developed (MedDay AB, Sweden). The data are stored on a central server: for example, in a public health department. Communication between the server and the mobile phones can be encrypted.

If there is suspicion that an outbreak of a communicable disease could be imminent, the health department tells users what symptoms to look for. Using their mobile phones, people can report suspicious symptoms to the monitoring server. If the health department concludes that there is community transmission of the disease, the locations of those who are ill and using the monitoring software are known, so the epidemiologists can develop a containment strategy. If individuals are quarantined,

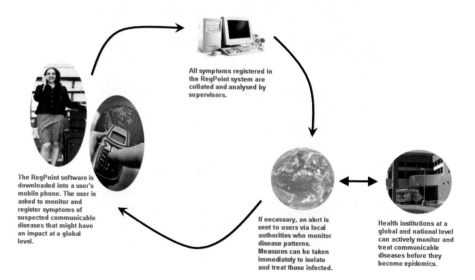

All symptoms registered in the RegPoint system are collated and analysed by supervisors.

The RegPoint software is downloaded into a user's mobile phone. The user is asked to monitor and register symptoms of suspected communicable diseases that might have an impact at a global level.

If necessary, an alert is sent to users via local authorities who monitor disease patterns. Measures can be taken immediately to isolate and treat those infected.

Health institutions at a global and national level can actively monitor and treat communicable diseases before they become epidemics.

Fig. 12.2. Early warning system for epidemics (RegPoint, MedDay AB)

their conditions can also be monitored by using the same wireless mechanism to transmit disease information (Fig. 12.2).

Home telehealth usage during SARS

The SARS episodes of 2003 triggered the widest use of quarantine since the influenza epidemic of 1918. In Canada alone, 20 000 individuals went into voluntary quarantine for 10 days.[11] The quarantine experience may be helpful in predicting what home telehealth technology would be useful in future emergencies.

Because of the voluntary nature of SIP, it is necessary to monitor the level of compliance. During the SARS period, different countries took different approaches to surveillance. Some used police or private guards, some had neighbours report a quarantine violation by calling health officials on a telephone hotline, and some used web cameras or videophones; when violations occurred, electronic bracelets were used to track movement.

In Singapore, quarantined people were required to allow a web camera in their homes. They were monitored for compliance through random calls and directed to turn on their web cameras.[12]

In Singapore and Hong Kong, remote monitoring was used to monitor fever and compliance with SIP and quarantine orders. In Singapore, service workers, such as taxi drivers and bank tellers, checked their temperatures twice a day. If they did not have a raised temperature, they wore 'fever-free' stickers. Thousands of people were quarantined in Singapore. The government, through its security agency, used scanners, web cameras and electronic bracelets to monitor compliance with the quarantine order.[13] Also in Singapore, hospital emergency rooms struggled to contain spread from infectious individuals because the symptoms of SARS were varied and non-specific. After two physicians in a particular hospital became ill with SARS, clinicians became convinced that previous contact with a SARS patient was a critical factor. As a result, a national computerized database of SARS patients and their contacts was established.[13]

In Taiwan, 131 000 citizens were ordered into quarantine. There were two levels of quarantine: Level B quarantine was for 10 days and was for arriving passengers from World Health Organization-designated SARS areas, and Level A quarantine was for 14 days and involved those who were not travellers but who met the criteria for quarantine. Compliance was monitored either by daily visits or telephone calls, but as the epidemic persisted, video monitoring was used to check on compliance.[14]

In an analysis after the event, Eysenbach described information and communication technologies, such as the Internet, wireless devices, mobile phones, smart appliances, smart homes and web cameras, as 'population health technologies'.[15] He said that they could be used to improve the health of populations and not just individuals. He noted that such technologies could make healthcare accessible during disease outbreaks. He summarized a number of technologies that were used during the SARS crisis:[15]

- Singapore General Hospital introduced an online physiotherapy programme that allowed physical therapists to remotely monitor patients with web cameras in their homes.

- Also in Singapore, health officials tested electronic tracking systems that could monitor the movements of every person who entered a public hospital. Staff and visitors wore credit card-sized radiofrequency identification (RFID) tags around their necks to communicate their location to sensors hidden in the hospital ceilings, thereby enabling officials to track all encounters with others. Hospitals saved movement records for 20 days – twice the incubation period for SARS. If one person was infected, the database allowed rapid identification of all encounters. Health officials said it was 10 times faster than traditional methods of asking infected people with whom they had contact.
- In Hong Kong, a company launched a mobile phone service that promised to alert subscribers if they were near 'infected' buildings. Those opting for the service had their phones tracked and would be warned by text messages whenever they came within one kilometre of a building which had had instances of SARS infections.
- Two companies produced technologies that allowed people to enter their vital signs into their personal digital assistants or smart phones and transmit that information to a central monitoring clinic. Both companies claimed that their product could serve as an early warning system for detecting outbreaks.

Health Canada developed an Internet-based public health information system (i-PHIS). This allowed public health staff to enter data on individuals, which could be linked to their laboratory data and quarantine case reports.[16] Most cases of SARS occurred in the greater Toronto area. Most identified SARS cases were in healthcare facilities and were not spread widely in the general population. A sample of quarantined people was asked about problems related to being quarantined. The two most commonly cited problems were emotional difficulties related to confinement and loss of income for the quarantine period.[17] In another survey of people quarantined in Toronto (n=129), mostly healthcare workers, 100% of respondents described a sense of isolation, particularly citing the lack of physical contact with family members. A number of respondents reported symptoms consistent with post-traumatic stress disorder and depression, as measured by validated scales.[18]

To combat SARS-related stress, Canada's Center for Addiction and Mental Health used the Internet to create a website for physicians and patients to chat about SARS. It also created telephone support groups and intranets for quarantined healthcare workers.[19]

Opportunities and challenges

Level of concern is high about a widespread communicable disease epidemic, such as a pandemic of avian flu, occurring some time in the first decade of the twenty-first century. This provides an important opportunity to educate policy-makers and public health professionals about the advantages of using home telehealth to provide healthcare – whether that healthcare be remote monitoring, videoconferencing or other e-health solutions.

The potential of home telehealth for communicable disease containment was noted in a 2004 technology report from the US Department of Commerce. During the same year as the SARS outbreak (2003), the American army's Telemedicine and Advanced Technology Research Center (TATRC) convened a needs assessment workshop, gathering more than 40 experts in healthcare and technology. The goal was to identify how healthcare technologies could best serve homeland security and biodefence. Telehealth was identified as having a number of roles to play by:[20]

- augmenting first responders' capabilities by providing video and telemedicine services at the site of an emergency
- making it possible to concentrate clinical care resources where they are most in demand
- using telehealth to diagnose, monitor and treat patients in quarantine for infectious disease.

Current home telehealth technologies can be used to deliver medical care, monitor chronic disease, reduce social isolation and educate patients for better self-management. Generally, the technologies are simple, and many require only the use of the ordinary telephone network (public switched telephone network, PSTN) to deliver care from provider to isolated or quarantined people, and to transmit data from isolated or quarantined people to a healthcare provider. The implications are that the vital signs of people in isolation can be assessed without entry into the home. Any of the remote monitoring devices or video equipment described in the technology section above could be quickly distributed to SIP homes, as part of a ready pack for emergency response – similar to ready-to-go packages, like CHEMPACK, which are stockpiled in the US for chemical emergencies. Ready-to-go home telehealth packages could be stockpiled as part of the Strategic National Stockpile programme.

In addition, people sheltered in the home and healthcare providers can be seen and heard via video equipment. Dermatological conditions and wounds can be visualized and directions given for care. If quarantine is prolonged, people under SIP orders who have chronic diseases could routinely transmit information such as data on blood glucose levels for diabetes management, for example. Although the telephone network is the most simple transmission medium, more and more devices can be used with wireless technologies and cable or web-based systems (Fig. 12. 3).

The benefits of using these technologies in the home include:

- providing adequate healthcare when SIP is the least restrictive quarantine option in a healthcare crisis
- making the most of scarce resources, such as physicians, nurses and other allied health professionals, by making telehealth visits available
- reducing the risk of transmission by reducing the number of contacts between those who have and those who have not been exposed to a particular infectious agent, thus maintaining strict quarantine and isolation
- reducing the psychological sense of isolation reported by many who were quarantined during the SARS crisis in 2003
- beginning mental health counselling during isolation and quarantine, instead of waiting for problems to develop, as evidenced in the SARS experience in Toronto.

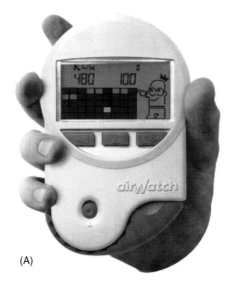

(A)

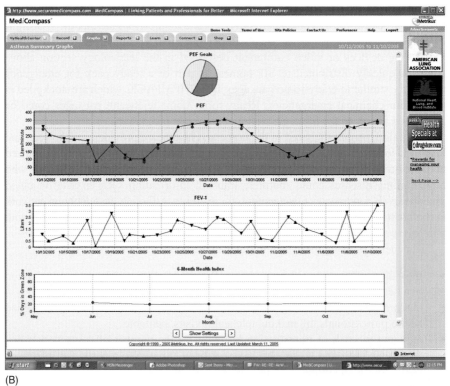

(B)

Fig. 12.3. Asthma monitoring system (iMetrikus, Inc): spirometer transmits data on FEV$_1$ and PEFR via a telephone line (A), and web page shows patient's electronic record in graphical form (B)

Conclusion

During the SARS outbreaks in 2003, home telehealth technologies were used to monitor compliance with quarantine orders in several parts of the world. However, home telehealth could be used for much more than monitoring, including the delivery of healthcare. Experiences with using quarantine, particularly SIP, to contain SARS made it clear that adequate physical and psychological medical care was important to those who were confined to their homes. A number of simple-to-use devices connected via the telephone network allow medical assessments, psychological counselling and ongoing monitoring of chronic conditions. It seems particularly important to provide high-quality care, given the findings from the Toronto study on the psychological effects of SIP, which indicated that the longer quarantine lasted, the greater the incidence of symptoms of post-traumatic stress disorder.[18] There is considerable experience of using telemedicine in mental health (Fig. 12.4).[21]

The same Toronto study found that more than one-third of those quarantined did not monitor their temperatures as recommended, and only 58% remained in their home for the entire quarantine period. Similarly, more than half of the residents of a housing complex that had been quarantined in Hong Kong did not stay in quarantine for the entire 10-day period.[12] One way to make SIP more acceptable might be to use home telehealth to deliver clinical and psychological care during quarantine. Because home

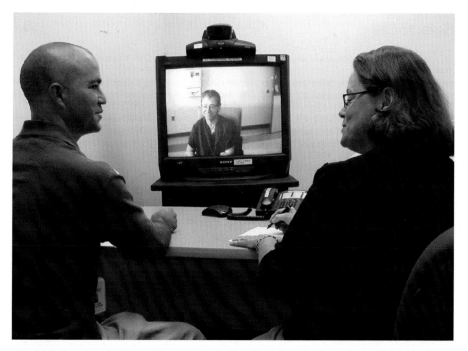

Fig. 12.4. Staff from Ridgeview Psychiatric Hospital (Oak Ridge, TN) using videoconferencing for patients who present in a rural hospital's emergency room in a psychiatric crisis

telehealth technologies generally are simple and use familiar electronic equipment, such as television monitors and telephones, the learning period for providers and those quarantined would probably be short.

During a health crisis, authorities need to perform surveillance, assessment, monitoring, treatment, follow-up and health education. Home telehealth could support all of these needs and would also allow the government to fulfil its healthcare obligations under the Model State Emergency Health Powers Act. Serious consideration should be given to prepacking suitable equipment as part of the national emergency preparations.

Further information

Barrett MJ. *Patient self-management tools: an overview*. Oakland, CA: California HealthCare Foundation, 2005. Available at: www.chcf.org/documents/chronic disease/PatientSelfManagementToolsOverview.pdf (last accessed 15 November 2005).

Bauer JC, Bushnell PG. *The future of home telehealth: unprecedented opportunities in a growing market*. Marriottsville, MD: Bon Secours Health System, 2001. Available at: bshsi.com/tews/docs/TEWS.FutureHomeTelehealth.pdf (last accessed 16 January 2006).

References

1   Misrahi J, Foster J, Shaw F, Cetron M. HHS/CDC legal response to SARS outbreak. *Emerg Infect Dis* 2004;**10**:353–5.
2   Barbera J, Macintyre A, Gostin L, *et al*. Large-scale quarantine following biological terrorism in the United States: scientific examination, logistic and legal limits, and possible consequences. *JAMA* 2001;**286**:2711–17.
3   Gostin L, Bayer R, Fairchild A. Ethical and legal challenges posed by severe acute respiratory syndrome: implications for the control of severe infectious disease threats. *JAMA* 2003;**290**:3229–37.
4   Department of Health and Human Services. *Chemical agents: facts about sheltering in place*. Atlanta, GA: Centers for Disease Control and Prevention, 2004. Available at: www.bt.cdc.gov/planning/shelteringfacts.pdf (last accessed 15 November 2005).
5   Mannan M, Kilpatrick D. The pros and cons of shelter-in-place. *Process Saf Prog* 2000;**19**:210–18.
6   Department of Health and Human Services. *Isolation and quarantine*. Atlanta, GA: Centers for Disease Control and Prevention, 2004. Available at: www.cdc.gov/ncidod/dq/sars_facts/isolationquarantine.pdf (last accessed 15 November 2005).
7   Bloom B. Lessons from SARS. *Science* 2003;**300**:701.
8   Greenberg AJ, Sherman M, Maniscalco J, *et al*. Videophone monitoring of SARS patients and contacts under non-hospital voluntary quarantine and isolation: a novel management approach. Presented at the 132nd annual meeting of APHA, Washington DC, US, 6–10 November 2004. Available at: apha.confex.com/apha/132am/techprogram/paper_77963.htm (last accessed 15 November 2005).
9   Gostin L, Sapsin J, Teret S, *et al*. The Model State Emergency Health Powers Act: planning for and response to bioterrorism and naturally occurring infectious diseases. *JAMA* 2002;**288**:622–8.
10 Home Care Management Associates. *Home telehealth systems: a guide for home care providers*. Springfield, PA: Home Care Management Associates, 1998. Available at: members.tripod.com/%7EProviderHelper/index-4.html#PRIMER (last accessed 15 November 2005).
11 Centers for Disease Control and Prevention. Postexposure prophylaxis, isolation, and quarantine to control an import-associated measles outbreak – Iowa, 2004. *MMWR Morb Mortal Wkly Rep* 2004;**53**:969–71.

12 Rothstein M, Alcalde M, Elster N, *et al. Quarantine and isolation: lessons learned from SARS.* Louisville, KY: University of Louisville School of Medicine, 2003. Available at: www.louisville.edu/medschool/ibhpl/images/pdf/SARS%20REPORT.pdf (last accessed 15 November 2005).

13 Singh K, Hsu LY, Villacian JS, *et al.* Severe acute respiratory syndrome: lessons from Singapore. *Emerg Infect Dis* 2003;**9**:1294–8.

14 CDC. Use of quarantine to prevent transmission of SARS – Taiwan, 2003. *MMWR Morb Mortal Wkly Rep* 2003;**52**:680–3. Available at: www.cdc.gov/mmwr/preview/mmwrhtml/mm5229a2.htm (last accessed 15 November 2005).

15 Eysenbach G. SARS and population health technology. *J Med Internet Res* 2003;**5**:e14.

16 Health Canada. *Health Canada's preparedness for and response to respiratory infectious season and the possible re-emergence of SARS.* Ottowa: Health Canada, 2003. Available at: www.phac-aspc.gc.ca/sars-sras/ris-sir/ (last accessed 15 November 2005).

17 Blendon RJ, Benson JM, DesRoches CM, *et al.* The public's response to severe acute respiratory syndrome in Toronto and the United States. *Clin Infect Dis* 2004;**38**:925–31.

18 Hawryluck L, Gold WL, Robinson S, *et al.* SARS control and psychological effects of quarantine, Toronto, Canada. *Emerg Infect Dis* 2004;**10**:1206–12.

19 DiGiovanni C, Conley J, Chiu D, Zaborski J. Factors influencing compliance with quarantine in Toronto during the 2003 SARS outbreak. *Biosecur Bioterror* 2004;**2**:265–72.

20 Brantley D, Laney-Cummings K, Spivack R. *Innovation, demand and investment in telehealth.* Washington, DC: US Department of Commerce, 2004. Available at: www.technology.gov/reports/TechPolicy/Telehealth/2004Report.pdf (last accessed 15 November 2005).

21 Hilty DM, Marks SL, Urness D, *et al.* Clinical and educational telepsychiatry applications: a review. *Can J Psychiatry* 2004;**49**:12–23.

Section 3: Application areas

13. **HIV/AIDS**
    César Cáceres, Enrique J. Gómez, M. Elena Hernando, Felipe García and Francisco Del-Pozo

14. **Home dialysis**
    Veli N. Stroetmann, Michael Nebel, Simon Robinson and Karl A. Stroetmann

15. **Quality of care**
    Barbara Johnston and Sam G. Burgiss

16. **Diabetes**
    Justin Starren, Ruth S. Weinstock, Walter Palmas, Roberto E. Izquierdo, Philip C. Morin and David Kaufman

17. **Congestive heart failure**
    Penny Ford-Carleton, Nancy Lugn, Nhedti Colquitt, Marcia Reissig, Irene Higginson and Joseph C. Kvedar

18. **Home health monitoring**
    Shigeru Ohta, Hiroshi Nakamoto, Yoshimitsu Shinagawa and Toshio Kishimoto

19. **Home-based telecardiology**
    Simonetta Scalvini, Emanuela Zanelli and Amerigo Giordano

20. **Child monitoring**
    Andrea Tura and Luca Quareni

21. **Palliative care**
    Marilynne A. Hebert, J.J. Jansen and Lynn Whitten

22. **Remote asthma monitoring**
    Vedran Ostojić

►13

HIV/AIDS

César Cáceres, Enrique J. Gómez, M. Elena Hernando, Felipe García and Francisco Del-Pozo

Introduction

As other chapters in this book demonstrate, telemedicine can be used successfully in caring for chronically ill patients at home. Patients with human immunodeficiency virus (HIV)/acquired immunodeficiency syndrome (AIDS) can also be managed by home telehealth, although little work has been reported to date. This chapter describes our experience with a home telecare project in Spain.

HIV spread unnoticed during the 1970s, and general awareness of the disease began in the early 1980s.[1] Although the disease can be treated, there is still no definitive cure for HIV infection. Furthermore, the potent combination of drugs called highly active antiretroviral therapy (HAART), which is used to prevent virus replication, has a cost for the patient. First of all, antiretroviral drugs have numerous and some quite serious side-effects,[2] which means that not every patient will tolerate the treatment. It also is important to note that a very high compliance is required – more than 95% – and if it is not achieved, the virus may become drug-resistant.[3] Compliance is also affected by the large number of pills the patient has to take. Highly active antiretroviral therapy consists of three or more antiretroviral drugs, and each could be offered in the form of one to eight pills that have to be taken several times per day. Simplifying the treatment is another aspect that healthcare professionals have to take into account in order to improve compliance, reduce toxicity and save costs.[4] An important aspect of treatment for HIV is its high cost – €1000–2000 per month depending on the particular treatment – and not every country or patient can afford it.[5]

The combination of new antiretroviral drugs (such as protease inhibitors) with existing treatment has reduced the progression to the AIDS terminal phase (Fig. 13.1). Now that the infection is beginning to be better controlled, clinical priorities are giving way to psychological and social aspects.[6] A patient with HIV goes through different psychological stages: shock when the infection becomes known, negation of their own disease state, acceptance of the situation and finally preparation for death. Fortunately, this last phase is now being replaced by learning to live with a chronic disease,[7] which implies new hopes but also new problems for patients. Stress, depression, irritability and anguish are common in patients with HIV.[8] Even today, people living with HIV/AIDS have to face stigmatization and social discrimination.[9] Their quality of life is affected by families' and friends' refusals to accept them, sexual problems, work problems and even financial problems.

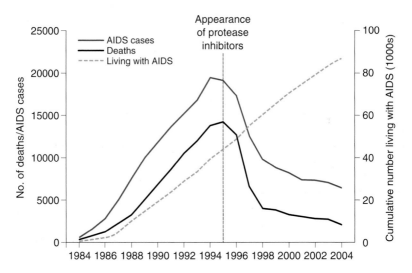

Fig. 13.1. Annual number of AIDS cases and deaths in western Europe. The cumulative number of people living with AIDS is also shown (right-hand axis). Source: EuroHIV

New chronic care models in HIV

The process of HIV/AIDS becoming a chronic disease in industrialized countries involves a dramatic change in the illness paradigm.[10] Patients who previously would have been terminally ill become chronically ill, and palliative care becomes chronic care. The objectives change from prolonging life before entering the terminal phase[11] to improving the quality of life of patients who may delay their entrance to that phase indefinitely.

This situation needs a completely new approach to care of patients with HIV/AIDS. We therefore could learn about how to deal with this new situation from the management of other chronic diseases – such as diabetes, chronic obstructive pulmonary disease and congestive heart failure. Coordination of the care team and involvement of patients in their own care[12] seem to be factors of great importance for good management of chronic diseases.[13] A multidisciplinary care team is also desirable for patients with a disease like HIV/AIDS, where psychological and social factors have an increasing influence on a patient's health status. Chronic care requires a new home-care model that should be holistic – integrating doctors, psychologists, nurses, social workers and pharmacists into the same team, with the patient as a member as well.[14] This is the basis for the telecare model we have developed.

Telecare

Telecare involves the delivery of health and social care to individuals in the home or wider community, with the support of systems enabled by information technology.[15] Telecare introduces new modes of assessment to improve the quality and variety of information about a patient's health status to the clinician. Measures of functional status and quality of life, in addition to physiological monitoring, can be translated into accurate predictors of health risk and can be combined with electronic alarm systems to initiate an appropriate course of action. This allows problems to be identified, sometimes at an earlier stage. Small improvements can also dramatically affect the outcome, function and overall well-being of a patient with a chronic disease.[16]

Telecare can provide a means of coordinating multidisciplinary care inside and outside hospitals – for example, scheduling visits with allied health staff and community health workers, automating the collection of clinical findings and test results, and liaising with hospital and staff specialists. As an example of this concept, home telecare is a means of providing care, monitoring and information sources to patients in their homes.[17] It can also contribute to the process of care team coordination and patient empowerment.[18,19] In particular, the Internet can be used to improve the quality and reduce the cost of caring for chronic complex illnesses such as diabetes and chronic obstructive pulmonary disease.[20,21] In the field of HIV/AIDS, research is still at an early stage,[22,23] but this seems to be one of the most promising fields for home telehealth.

Broadband access

Home telecare obviously requires appropriate network bandwidth. A home telecare system may offer several services to its users. For example:

- Cooperative working space – Both patients and professionals share their experiences and exchange information.
- Coordination centre – Usually a call centre that provides immediate response to any demands made by patients or professionals by managing, routing and filtering incoming calls or messages.
- Telemonitoring of variables such as glucose, heart rate, body temperature, body weight and body position – The patient's unit is usually provided with special devices that monitor physiological signals and communicate with the system.
- Improved communication – Between professionals for collaborative working, between patients to empower themselves or between patients and healthcare professionals for consultations.
- Information repository – Provides validated information about the disease.
- Intelligent data management – Automatic analysis of patient data and any other relevant information to detect specific patient status or deviations from the care plan whenever the recorded data/signal features deviate from pre-established normal ranges and generation of the appropriate action.
- Access to the electronic health record (EHR) – This is the core of any telemedicine system, and efficient and secure access must be provided to the whole care team.
- Other home services – Maintenance of the equipment, catering, house cleaning, receiving the drugs at home or a visit from any member of the care team. These are complementary services that the patient could need and that could improve his or her quality of life.

- Multi-access connectivity – Allows users to decide the terminal they want to use to interact with the system.[24]
- Interoperability – To exchange information with any user of the common shared space, the existing electronic health records that the system must deal with and the patient's monitoring devices.

In a web-based system, some of these services are available with no need for broadband access. Nevertheless, some – such as videoconference consultation, medical image transmission or real-time telemonitoring – certainly need broadband communication. Nowadays, with the expansion of digital subscriber line (DSL) services, broadband communication is much cheaper and more readily available. In general, therefore, telecommunications bandwidth is no longer a critical issue in the industrialized world.[25]

VIHrtual Hospital

To support the new chronic care model for HIV/AIDS described above, we have developed the so-called 'VIHrtual Hospital'. This covers the care process of the chronically ill patient as a whole: visits; clinical, psychological and social follow-up; pharmacology and quality of life. The main goals are the definition, development, clinical routine installation and evaluation of a telemedicine service that complements standard care with telecare follow-up for stable HIV-infected patients during the chronic phase of their disease. Potential users of the home telecare system include:

- Patients – In a chronic care model, the patient should be part of the care team. The patients may be homebound or mobile, and, depending on the disease, they will need different health-related services. The advantages of working with patients with HIV/AIDS are that they are relatively young (average age 40 years), their follow-up does not need complex monitoring (just a blood analysis and some questionnaires) and they have routine visits every three months.
- Patient's caregivers – The patient is usually not alone when making his or her health decisions. The partner, parents, children or other relatives may be involved in the patient's care. Home telecare systems could also be aimed at these caregivers.
- Healthcare professionals – A multidisciplinary care team is always desirable, but it is even more desirable when managing a patient with a chronic illness. Depending on the field of application of the telecare system, different disciplines will participate in its use. In the case of a patient with HIV/AIDS, an interdisciplinary care team usually interacts with the patient. Collaboration among members of the care team normally takes place for some specific reason and is not done routinely. In the VIHrtual Hospital project, the care team comprises an HIV/AIDS specialist doctor, a psychologist, a nurse, a pharmacist and a social worker.
- Technical staff – Other professionals, such as the user's administrator and the development and maintenance technical teams, need to interact with the system.

In the VIHrtual Hospital, a user's administrator signs in both professionals and patients and manages the timetables for visits. The development team provides new versions of the system during the clinical trial. An important aspect of the project was that installation and maintenance of the patient's units were subcontracted to a company that trains the patient during installation.

Main services

The VIHrtual Hospital has four main services (Fig. 13.2). These services are:

- virtual community
- virtual library
- virtual consultations
- telepharmacy.

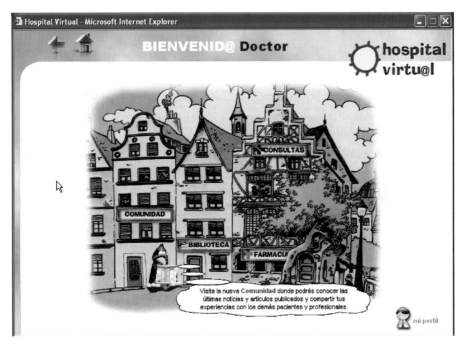

Fig. 13.2. Main menu of the VIHrtual Hospital website

Virtual community

The virtual community creates spaces to exchange information about the disease and the project, to share opinions and to comment about articles and news (Fig. 13.3). This tool offers different information depending on the user: for example, healthcare professionals and patients receive different information. The clinical session option is exclusive for professionals and allows them to share opinions about the cases they are currently covering.

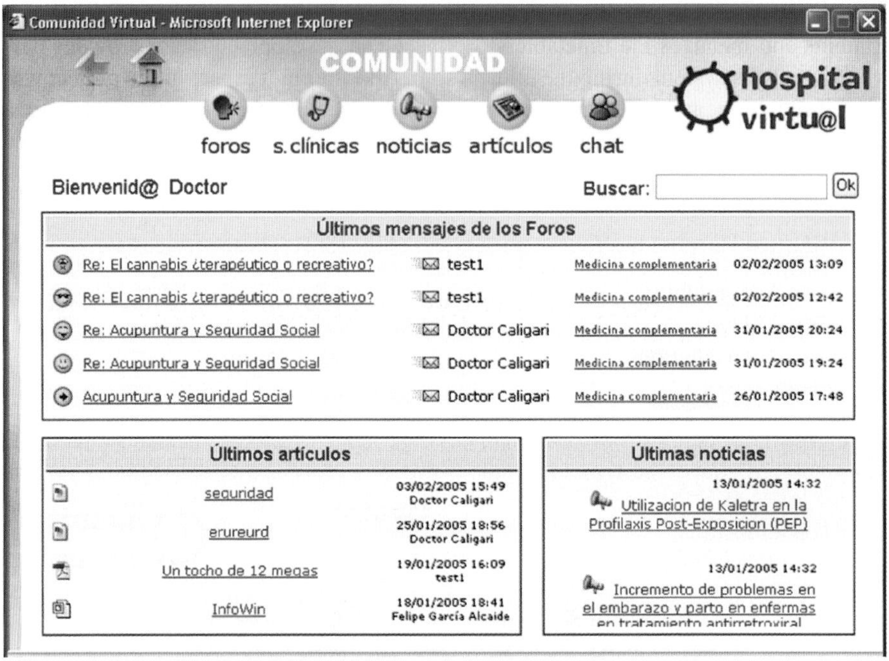

Fig. 13.3. Main menu of the virtual community of the VIHrtual Hospital

Virtual library

The virtual library stores validated basic information about HIV/AIDS as links to other web pages for both patients and professionals. Different sections are included for validated links (links inserted by professionals) and non-validated links (links inserted by patients), although the latter can be upgraded after validation by a professional. All links are categorized by the type of source and are included in different groups according to the subject to which they refer.

Virtual consultations

Virtual consultations can be delivered using videoconferencing, chat sessions or through the exchange of messages. During any of these sessions, both the participating professional and the patient have access to the EHR (Fig. 13.4). Psychological and social data are recorded in the EHR, as the care is holistic. An agenda also is available so that patient and professional can make the next appointment at the end of the 'visit'.

Telepharmacy

With telepharmacy, the pharmacist receives electronic prescriptions and consults with the patient about compliance, adverse effects and interactions with other drugs. The drugs are sent to the patient's home by courier. Follow-up of the treatment is done by the doctors, pharmacists and patient. Before sending the drugs to the patient's home by

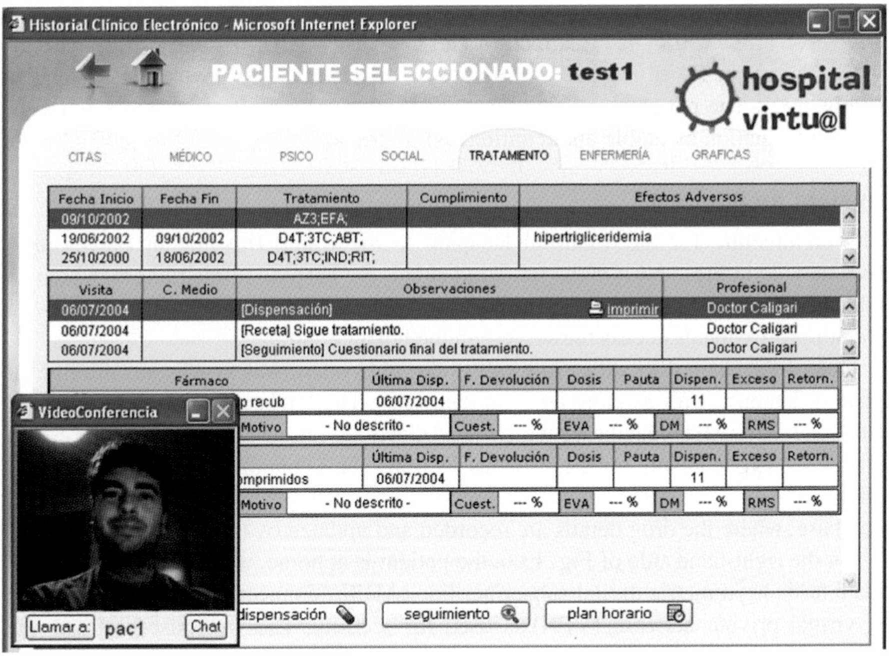

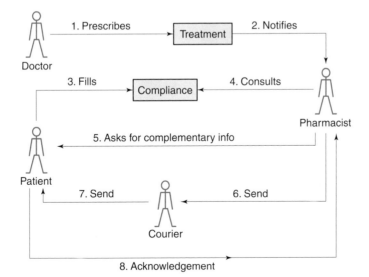

Fig. 13.4. Example of a videoconference with simultaneous access to the electronic health record of the VIHrtual Hospital

Fig. 13.5. Collaboration process in telepharmacy as part of the VIHrtual Hospital

courier, the pharmacist usually wants to visit the patient and check whether there are any problems with the treatment. This is also done virtually, through the videoconference facility of the VIHrtual Hospital system. This new process is shown in Fig. 13.5. The patients can also visualize their own treatment on charts and view basic information available about antiretroviral drugs.

System architecture

The architecture for the VIHrtual Hospital in the Clinic Hospital in Barcelona is summarized in Fig. 13.6. On the left-hand side is the hospital infrastructure, where we added our server to the existing hospital intranet, which is protected by a firewall. Health professionals access the server via the hospital intranet.

One of the main difficulties in establishing the system was synchronization of the project database with existing hospital databases. The VIHrtual database was loaded from the HIV/AIDS database, which the Infectious Diseases Service of the Clinic Hospital had been using for the previous 15 years. This contained details of more than 3000 patients with HIV/AIDS. The server was also connected to the pharmacy database, where the drug details are recorded and updated by the pharmacists.

On the right-hand side of Fig. 13.6, the patient is at home, with access to the server via a basic asymmetric digital subscriber line (ADSL) connection (at 512/128 kbit/s). A virtual private network (VPN) is used for security. The web-based system was developed with equipment that integrated well in the home environment. The graphical interface was also designed carefully to make it easy to use for professionals and patients (see Figs 13.2–13.4).

Another main goal was developing a low-cost system to increase the number of patients for the clinical trial. Therefore, low-price home web cameras and ADSL connections were chosen.

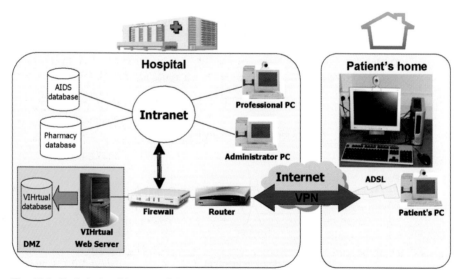

Fig. 13.6. Technical architecture of the VIHrtual Hospital

Security issues

Security is an important aspect of any telecare system. Four security services are usually associated with telemedicine systems: access control, authentication, confidentiality and data integrity. In the case of the VIHrtual Hospital, the experimental nature of the project and the disease characteristics dictated the need for strict security measures. Data on patients were encrypted, and all personal identifiers were removed. Fingerprint recognition could also be used to access the system.

Preliminary results

A randomized, crossover, open clinical trial is being conducted. One hundred HIV/AIDS patients were randomized into two groups: 50 patients with the new telecare model and 50 with the usual care model. The project will last for two years, with crossover after 12 months. The evaluation is being carried out by infectious disease, mental health, pharmacy and social services staff of the Clinic Hospital, Barcelona, and involves 20 healthcare professionals (11 HIV/AIDS specialist doctors, a psychologist, a psychiatrist, two nurses, four pharmacists and a social worker). The evaluation is also being monitored by an independent expert on quality of life.

Initial results – as yet unpublished – show better coordination between members of the care team, tighter control by healthcare professionals and better patient self-control. It is still too soon to determine cost-effectiveness, but some cost reductions have occurred. Preliminary experience includes various problems and some benefits.

Problems

Firstly, integration of the system with the hospital infrastructure took too long. Although some hospital databases were connected to the project network quickly, other databases, such as those from the pathology laboratories, still need to be added. The process for this integration is too laborious.

Working with a group of 20 professionals was another handicap. Coordination of the care team was sometimes difficult, because they had to convert from an individual, face-to-face care mode to a collaborative telecare mode. Some instances occurred in which virtual appointments were forgotten or messages were unanswered after 48 hours. This was solved with an alert system that was integrated into the VIHrtual Hospital. Both professionals and patients were then able to configure the alerts to be sent to them by email or text-messaging (SMS) to their mobile phones.

Consultations via chat were also disappointing. This kind of consultation was supposed to be an extra resource for patients in case they wanted to ask a relatively urgent question. Professionals were to be available to answer questions from patients. In practice, however, professionals would not wait in the chat room in anticipation of patient questions, claiming that they were wasting time. The solution was to use an instant messaging tool to allow professionals to work at other tasks until patients had questions. However, integration of the instant messaging tool into the system is incomplete.

Benefits

The preliminary results suggest significant benefits to both patients and the healthcare system. These include:

- Patients – Patients prefer to be visited at home (as indicated in preliminary questionnaires). They feel better and more comfortable there, and they can do other things while they wait. Using home telehealth, patients have better access to their clinicians.
- Healthcare system – Coordination of the care team is enhanced thanks to the sharing of data and the virtual community. This is the major contribution of the system to the chronic model of care and improves the quality of care. In addition, professionals do not need to leave their working room to attend these virtual patients. Professionals obtain first-hand, instant and accurate information from the patient and other professionals. Although some staff may think that virtual consultations or messages may result in a heavier workload, other studies have shown the benefits of using these new methods of communication.[26]

Although the cost-effectiveness analysis has yet to be completed, the relatively modest costs of investing in home telehealth should be small compared to the advantages described above. In addition, the interest of the hospital in conducting research in a promising field, such as home telehealth for chronically ill patients, should not be overlooked. The VIHrtual Hospital is now being offered as a routine protocol for any patient with HIV/AIDS who asks to be attended virtually. In the first two months, 18 new patients have joined the service. This, together with the fact that the project was originally proposed by the clinicians, shows that experts in HIV/AIDS are keenly interested in this kind of home telehealth system.

Conclusion

Home telehealth can contribute to the redesign of health services. Virtual environments that allow cooperation and information sharing between health professionals and their patients can now be constructed. Integrated systems make seamless care possible, creating a continuum from health promotion through to clinical care. The main challenge is to facilitate the move from provider-centred to patient-centred healthcare delivery models.

Our newly developed system of virtual care for chronically ill patients with HIV/AIDS seems promising. The care model involves more frequent medical oversight – for example, by permitting doctor visits via telehealth. These medical visits are being supplemented by psychological, social and educational visits, which are also accomplished through telehealth. Although the results of the randomized, clinical trial are not yet available, preliminary results are encouraging. Home telehealth may allow professionals, and patients themselves, to care for illness in a more efficient, cost-effective and comfortable way.

Further reading

AIDS Education Global Information System website. Available at: www.aegis.com/ (last accessed 2 January 2006).

AIDSinfo website. Available at: www.aidsinfo.nih.gov/ (last accessed 2 January 2006).

Whitten P, Cook D, eds. *Understanding health communication technologies*. San Francisco, CA: Jossey-Bass, 2004.

References

1   Centers for Disease Control and Prevention. Kaposi's sarcoma and pneumocystis pneumonia among homosexual men – New York City and California. *MMWR Morb Mortal Wkly Rep* 1981;**30**:305–8.
2   Montessori V, Press N, Harris M, *et al.* Adverse effects of antiretroviral therapy for HIV infection. *CMAJ* 2004;**170**:229–38.
3   High antiretroviral drug adherence key in effort to avoid drug resistance. New study highlights its importance. *AIDS Alert* 2005;**20**:25,27–8.
4   Barreiro P, Garcia-Benayas T, Soriano V, Gallant J. Simplification of antiretroviral treatment – how to sustain success, reduce toxicity and ensure adherence avoiding PI use. *AIDS Rev* 2002;**4**:233–41.
5   Cost imposes barrier to HIV treatment in Missouri. *AIDS Policy Law* 2005;**20**:2.
6   Ruiz Perez I, Rodriguez Bano J, Lopez Ruz MA, *et al.* Health-related quality of life of patients with HIV: impact of sociodemographic, clinical and psychosocial factors. *Qual Life Res* 2005;**14**:1301–10.
7   Morlat P. [The chronicity of HIV infection]. *Rev Prat* 1999;**49**:1781–5 (in French).
8   Leserman J. HIV disease progression: depression, stress, and possible mechanisms. *Biol Psychiatry* 2003;**54**:295–306.
9   Varas-Diaz N, Serrano-Garcia I, Toro-Alfonso J. AIDS-related stigma and social interaction: Puerto Ricans living with HIV/AIDS. *Qual Health Res* 2005;**15**:169–87.
10 Martin DK, Thiel EC, Singer PA. A new model of advance care planning: observations from people with HIV. *Arch Intern Med* 1999;**159**:86–92.
11 Bascunana Morejon de Giron J, Sanz de Barros R, de la Pena Gonzalez M, Candel Monserrate I. Home care for the terminally ill HIV patient. *An Med Interna* 1997;**14**:93–7.
12 Holman HR, Lorig KR. Patients as partners in managing chronic disease. Partnership is a prerequisite for effective and efficient health care. *BMJ* 2000;**320**:526–7.
13 Cretin S, Shortell SM, Keeler EB. An evaluation of collaborative interventions to improve chronic illness care. Framework and study design. *Eval Rev* 2004;**28**:28–51.
14 Wiecha J, Pollard T. The interdisciplinary eHealth team: chronic care for the future. *J Med Internet Res* 2004;**6**:e22.
15 Barlow J, Bayer S, Curry R. The design of pilot telecare projects and their integration into mainstream service delivery. *J Telemed Telecare* 2003;**9** (Suppl 1):1–3.
16 Celler BG, Lovell NH, Basilakis J. Using information technology to improve the management of chronic disease. *Med J Aust* 2003;**179**:242–6.
17 Kinsella A. Home telecare in the United States. *J Telemed Telecare* 1998;**4**:195–200.
18 Weerakkody G, Ray P. CSCW-based system development methodology for health-care information systems. *Telemed J E Health* 2003;**9**:273–82.
19 Graspemo G, Ludvigsson J, Sam N. [Information technology gives opportunity for genuine patient empowerment. Next generation patients with type 1 diabetes can surf to empowerment.] *Lakartidningen* 2005;**102**:2316–18 (in Swedish).
20 Hernando ME, Gomez EJ, Gili A, Gomez M, Garcia G, del Pozo F. New trends in diabetes management: mobile telemedicine closed-loop system. *Stud Health Technol Inform* 2004;**105**:70–9.
21 de Toledo P, Jimenez S, Del Pozo F. A telemedicine system to support a new model for care of chronically ill patients. *J Telemed Telecare* 2002;**8** (Suppl 2):17–19.
22 Flatley-Brennan P. Computer network home care demonstration: a randomized trial in persons living with AIDS. *Comput Biol Med* 1998;**28**:489–508.
23 Kinsella A. Telecare for HIV/AIDS patients. *Caring* 1997;**16**:42–5.

24   Hernando ME, Gómez EJ, García A, del Pozo F. A multi-access server for the virtual management of diabetes. *Proceedings of the Fifth Conference of the European Society for Engineering and Medicine, Barcelona, 29 May–2 June 1999*: 309–10.

25   Craignou B, Cordier F, Sejourne D. Broadband telecommunication services – a reality in advanced countries and a challenge for operators in developing economies. *Proceedings of the 18th ITC Workshop for Developing Countries, Berlin, Germany, 31 August–5 September 2003.* Available at: oldwww.com.dtu.dk/teletraffic/papers/2_1_Craignou.pdf (last accessed 5 December 2005).

26   Scherger JE. E-mail 'visits' can save you time. *Med Econ* 2004;**81**:37–8. Available at: www.memag.com/memag/article/articleDetail.jsp?id=123705 (last accessed 3 January 2006).

▶14

Home dialysis

Veli N. Stroetmann, Michael Nebel, Simon Robinson and Karl A. Stroetmann

Introduction

Renal failure is a global issue. More than one million patients with end-stage renal disease (ESRD) receive dialysis treatment worldwide.[1] On a per-capita basis, dialysis is among the most costly of the chronic diseases, with costs of up to €60 000 a year.[2] In 2005, the global market for dialysis services, including clinics, treatments and renal care products, was estimated to be $48 billion.[3]

When the kidneys fail, toxic products build up in the blood. This waste must be removed by artificial means – typically through haemodialysis or peritoneal dialysis (PD). PD is usually undertaken at home, but an exchange of fluid can also be performed at work or during travel. With haemodialysis, patients have to be connected to a dialysis machine – usually located in a hospital or clinic – at least three times a week. The patient's quality of life generally is better with PD than with standard haemodialysis.

Telemedicine and hospital dialysis

Telemedicine has been used successfully to support haemodialysis in small hospitals and clinics. Most physician–patient interactions do not require palpation and therefore are possible by videoconferencing. Some major dialysis centres – such as in the US (Washington DC and Texas) and Australia (Adelaide) – have supported patients undergoing dialysis at satellite units using telemedicine.[4-6] The technique seems to be successful in avoiding unnecessary travel in those satellite centres in which it is used. Indeed, it seems surprising that telemedicine is not used more widely in hospital dialysis to reduce patient and staff travel.

Given the success of teledialysis for patients in small hospitals and clinics, a natural development is to try and support patients being dialysed at home. Encouraging reports exist about the benefits of renal telemedicine to the home from rural areas of countries like Australia, the US and elsewhere.[7,8] The benefits include savings in journeys, time and related financial costs by medical professionals and patients; avoidance of inpatient services; and a sense of increased support and security for patients.

Telemedicine opportunities in home dialysis

In most countries, the percentage of patients who receive haemodialysis at home is very low or negligible, with the exceptions of New Zealand (14%), Australia (10%) and France (5%).[1] PD, which is usually performed at home, also shows wide variations between the countries for which data are available: from 45% of all patients in New Zealand and 19% in Canada, to only 5% in Germany and 4% in Japan.

Home dialysis supported by telemonitoring seems likely to become a major application of home telehealth for three main reasons:

- Home dialysis can produce improved medical perspectives for patients.[9] In addition, more flexibility allows patients better adaptation to a changing work environment and to various leisure activities, which in turn translates into a higher quality of life.
- Although home telemonitoring is still at an early stage of development,[10] the most promising applications are in fields such as chronic illnesses, where it can be used to reduce the number of complications, reduce costly hospital stays and respond to new needs in home care for an aging population. The same advantages can be expected to apply to ESRD.
- Various empirical reports in the literature suggest that home application of both haemodialysis and PD leads to a considerable reduction in overall treatment costs.[11]

Home telemonitoring

Research on home telemonitoring of patients on dialysis – both for haemodialysis[12] and PD[13] – suggests considerable potential to improve the quality of life for some patients with ESRD. A prerequisite is an adequate system approach to the clinically and technically complex situation of haemodialysis, and clear criteria for identifying and selecting patients who may benefit most from home dialysis supported by telemonitoring. Integrating telemonitoring with nightly automated peritoneal dialysis (APD) treatment for difficult paediatric patients has been shown to be useful in detecting and solving the clinical and technical problems associated with this form of treatment.[14]

Nocturnal home haemodialysis with telemonitoring has been piloted by the McGill University Health Centre, Montreal. Patients underwent a 4–6-week training session, during which they were taught to operate the dialysis equipment, properly connect and disconnect themselves, and troubleshoot alarms. They also had to undergo a home evaluation to ensure that requirements for storage, quality of electrical power supply, and water and drainage were met. The dialysis machines were linked via the Internet to a monitoring centre, where trained personnel were available throughout the night to deal with problems.[15]

A similar application has been tested at the Toronto General Hospital. A completely automated system monitors dialysis machines and patients' vital signs. Data from physiological sensors are transmitted wirelessly to a computer in the home, which is connected via a high-speed Internet connection to central servers. If any problems occur with patients or equipment, the system automatically alerts the appropriate caregiver or technician by email or pager.[16]

Automated telemonitoring is designed to give patients the confidence they need to conduct dialysis on their own. Home-based nocturnal haemodialysis is more effective than conventional, clinic-based dialysis, for which patients must travel to a hospital or clinic three times a week. Home nocturnal dialysis enables patients to dialyse at night for 40 hours a week as opposed to the 12 hours a week that is standard practice with conventional haemodialysis.[17] An additional advantage of home dialysis is that patients can spend more time at work and with their family.

European dialysis telemonitoring project

The aim of a recent European project was to develop and test a modular telehealth home-care system for chronically ill people.[18] The aim was to improve outcomes for patients with various chronic diseases, such as heart failure.[19] Here we describe the application for supporting ESRD and its results.

Requirements analysis

A small study of user requirements (from the physicians' point of view) was conducted. The survey concerned whether telehealth applications could be expected to improve the treatment of patients with ESRD. We developed a well-structured questionnaire to guide discussions with 15 nephrologists – specialists in private practice as well as in teaching/university hospitals. The small sample means that the data reported should be regarded as indicative in nature. The specialists believed that home monitoring would probably most benefit patients with comorbidities, specifically hypertension, who were undergoing home haemodialysis or PD (other co-morbidities mentioned were cardiac arrhythmia and coronary artery disease). Neither the age nor the home environment of patients was regarded as an important criterion (Table 14.1).

Table 14.1. Groups of patients who might benefit most from monitoring of vital data at home

Type of patient	Approving answers (%)*
Home haemodialysis	85
Home peritoneal dialysis	70
Comorbidities	
Hypertension	85
Diabetes	45
Living alone	30
Older patients: >70 years	30
Pre-dialysis with hypertension	60

*A total of 21 nephrologists (11 in hospitals, nine with private dialysis clinics and one in a foundation) were approached, of whom 15 participated in the survey. Not all responded to all questions.

Table 14.2. Priorities for improving healthcare through telematics by points (maximum of 100) and rank

Telematics components or systems	Points	Rank
Automatic transmission of data on vital signs from patients' homes to the office computer for patients with:		
• chronic renal failure or pre-dialysis	14	3
• home haemodialysis	28	1
• home peritoneal dialysis	28	1
Electronic information on patient's compliance with medication regimen	6	6
Improved communications with patients via:		
• Internet/email	11	4
• videotelephony	4	7
Improved training and education of patients through special Internet/World Wide Web services	9	5
Others	–	–

Experts were asked to identify the telematic applications they thought would best improve medical services to patients. They were asked to distribute a maximum of 100 points on the items shown in Table 14.2. Home monitoring of data on vital signs from patients on dialysis – whether treated by haemodialysis or PD – received the most points, followed by home monitoring in pre-dialysis patients. PD was the only item in the list that received points from all physicians interviewed.

Pilot trial

On the basis of these results, we conducted a pilot trial of home monitoring of patients on PD. Comprehensive material was prepared to inform patients and obtain their written consent. In parallel, we selected about 25 patients who used continuous ambulatory peritoneal dialysis (CAPD) on the basis of criteria identified through our survey. With CAPD, the patient empties a fresh bag of dialysate into his or her abdominal cavity via a catheter implanted into the abdomen. After 4–6 hours of dwell time, the patient returns the dialysate-containing wastes to the bag. The patient then repeats the cycle with a fresh bag of dialysate. This method does not require a machine, as the process uses gravity to fill and empty the abdominal cavity.

From the 25 patients on CAPD, seven patients with hypertension and one with hypotension were selected for inclusion in the trial in order of medical priority. These patients also had other diseases, including diabetes mellitus type 2, congestive heart failure, coronary heart disease and left ventricular hypertrophy. All eight consented to the trial. During the early phase, two patients were lost to the study: one changed to haemodialysis and another died. One new patient joined the trial, so we were able to collect data on seven patients in total. The staff was trained in handling the software before the equipment was installed in the patients' homes. Fifteen minutes of training was given to patients; this was found to be sufficient, with even older patients quickly gaining confidence in handling the equipment. The system architecture is shown in Fig. 14.1.

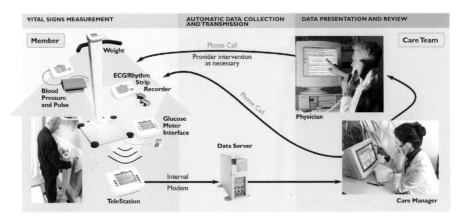

Fig. 14.1. System architecture of the Trans-European Network initiative Home-Care Management System (TENHMS) interactive telemonitoring service

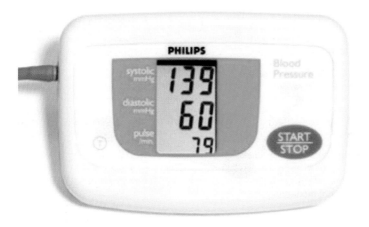

Fig. 14.2. Blood-pressure monitoring device

All patients measured blood pressure and pulse rate four times a day during each exchange of the dialysate (Fig. 14.2). In addition, on the morning before the first exchange, weight was measured (Fig. 14.3) and an electrocardiograph produced (one-lead rhythm strip; Fig. 14.4). One patient with heart failure was also asked to produce an electrocardiograph in the evening. All data were transmitted wirelessly from the measurement devices to a home hub connected to the patient's telephone line. Data were transmitted automatically to the central server at the nephrologist's office in the dialysis clinic. A printer attached to the server allowed printing of charts and reports for filing or for patients who requested their data.

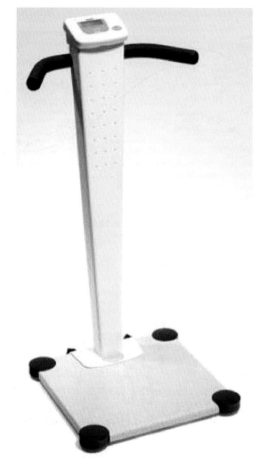

Fig. 14.3. Body-weight monitoring scale

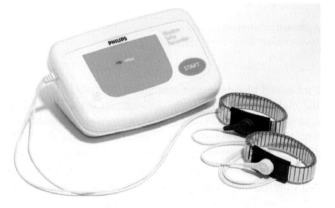

Fig. 14.4. Electrocardiographic monitoring device (one-lead rhythm strip)

General assessment by the nephrologist

The daily transmission of data allowed closer monitoring of patients and enabled more timely reaction to changes in their medical requirements. This became obvious in various instances involving patients whose health deteriorated over a very short time period. The physician was generally satisfied with the home monitoring system and devices. He also made specific suggestions for improving the clinical software, particularly with regard to the user interface.

Integration of the system into the routine processes of daily care did not pose any problems. The physician reported the impression that patients were feeling better looked after and cared for.

Clinical value

A system for differentiating between 'normal' patients on CAPD and 'risky' patients was devised.

- Normal patients – The 'normal' patient on PD has relatively stable physical health and may even go to work daily. They have been selected for treatment via PD, *inter alia*, because of their relatively stable situation. For such patients, the physician in the trial saw no specific medical value in daily home telemonitoring of vital data.
- Risky patients – Not unexpectedly, telemonitoring was particularly useful for patients with blood pressure and body weight concerns. For example, patients who had problems with their fluid balance – either because the filtration was too low or because they tended to drink too much – could be expected to have rapid weight fluctuations in a short time period. It is estimated that for about 10% of all present patients on PD, close telemonitoring would be indicated medically.

When the telemonitoring system becomes available for general introduction, it can be expected that the market potential for PD will expand considerably. Perhaps 10–20% of all new patients who would have required haemodialysis might qualify for treatment with PD. At present, their unstable health requires close monitoring, which requires them to visit the dialysis clinic three times a week. Patients on PD usually visit their physician only once a month or every six weeks.

Thus two types of patients benefited in the trial:

- those who needed only a certain time to determine and stabilize an optimum medication regimen
- those who continually caused considerable problems in establishing a stable medication regimen – that is, those who sometimes, even after only a short period of time, needed some readjustment.

On the basis of this positive initial assessment, four of the seven patients were chosen to continue the trial. Monitoring for two patients who assessed their own health as stable or did not see much benefit was discontinued. Another patient had to be admitted to hospital and could no longer participate.

Assessment by patients

A four-page, easy-to-answer, written questionnaire survey and informal discussions showed that patients responded very positively to the trial, with all reporting high acceptance of the monitoring devices (Fig. 14.5). Three patients reporting on their perception of the system's effect on their health indicated the subjective feeling that they were much better cared for due to the daily monitoring (5 points on a scale from 1 to 5), two patients said that their care was considerably improved (4 points) and two noted 'only somewhat better care' (2 points). As people usually hesitate to vote for extreme values of 5 or 1 on a Likert scale, these results show that most patients had a high acceptance of the monitoring system and a positive assessment of its effect on their health.

In one case, the system supported attainment of longer-term, stable values, such that both the physician and patient saw no need for a continuation of daily monitoring. The study also showed that some patients will resist – or at least not value – telemonitoring.

Patients provided the following comments about the trial:

- 'I expected a better surveillance by my nephrologist – which indeed was the case.'
- 'I obtained much better control of my blood pressure. Before it was sometimes too high, sometimes too low.'
- 'I expected and received improved medical care by my doctor.'
- 'I hoped for an incentive to better monitor and keep track of my daily vital data and to establish my optimum dialysis parameters. I used to measure my blood pressure only once a month.'
- 'It helps me to not forget the daily measurements.'
- 'It provides me with a certain assurance, and it helps me to better control myself. Like when the blood pressure is too high, I take my drugs earlier, or when more fluid has accumulated or the weight has increased, I take a stronger dialysate.'

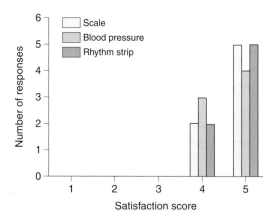

Fig. 14.5. Overall satisfaction of patients with monitoring devices

Technical assessment

In two cases, connection of the monitoring devices caused some problems because of incorrect wiring by the telecommunications provider or an old switchboard in one home. Once it was successfully installed, no significant technical failures of any part of the monitoring system occurred. The high reliability of the whole monitoring system, coupled with very efficient technical support, made it an ideal means of closely monitoring patients at risk, quickly adjusting their therapy in small steps as needed and balancing the medication regimen so that established boundary values were not exceeded.

Summary

The pilot trial showed that daily transmission of vital data – initially planned for six months only but extended for four patients by another six months – resulted in closer monitoring of certain patients on dialysis without interference with their daily routines. The daily collection of data enabled immediate reactions to significant changes in their health status, and adjustments to medication management were accomplished in a few days rather than as a follow-up to their regular 4–6-week visits to their physician. Telemonitoring also reduced patients' fear of performing inadequate dialysis. If additional data, such as temperature and fluid balance, could also be monitored closely, home telehealth could be applicable to an even wider patient population, such as other patient groups currently rated as too unstable.

Future telemonitoring in dialysis

Advances in technology, as well as expected changes in reimbursement systems, will provide important incentives and opportunities for home telehealth services in future. At the same time, they hold the potential to improve the quality of life for quite a few members of this growing patient population. New reimbursement schemes are expected to be implemented soon in Germany and other European countries. These will be based on diagnosis-related groups (DRGs) or, for the treatment of patients on dialysis, on fixed weekly or monthly sums, independent of the specific dialysis regimen. This will also have an effect on the ambulatory sector in general, which is still dominated by fee-for-service reimbursement. Such changes can be expected to provide new stimuli for expanding home dialysis by providing an economic incentive to reduce the costs per case.

Pierratos *et al* observed that, 'There is increasing evidence confirming that quotidian [daily] haemodialysis improves clinical outcomes in a cost-efficient manner. Provided that the reimbursement issues are resolved, these modalities may be used extensively at home as well as at the in-centre facilities. The revitalization of home haemodialysis will compensate for the decline in the use of continuous ambulatory peritoneal dialysis and the nursing shortage encountered in most countries.'[17]

In addition to the medical and direct cost benefits of home-based haemodialysis and PD, there will also be wider economic benefits. Because of the rigours of conventional haemodialysis – with trips to clinics usually three times a week – most patients on haemodialysis do not work. Instead, they are on various forms of disability and income supports. Another option is the combination of home telemonitoring with visits to local/regional satellite centres connected via telemedical equipment to a central hub with specialist nephrologists on duty. Finally, patients on dialysis who value the added security and safety of being telemonitored by their physician might make private payments. Here, too, is a potential for expanding home telehealth.

Acknowledgements

We are grateful to our patients, the staff of the dialysis clinic, and various medical and other colleagues for their involvement in this research project. Financial support was provided by the European Commission in the context of the European Union TEN Telecom (now eTEN) Programme. Philips Healthcare Services Europe, Böblingen, Germany, provided the hardware and software used, as well as technical and financial support.

Further information

Home Dialysis Central website. Available at: www.homedialysis.org (last accessed 3 January 2006).

NephrOnline website. Available at: www.nephronline.com/ (last accessed 3 January 2005).

Royal Infirmary of Edinburgh Renal Unit website. Available at: renux.dmed.ed.ac.uk/ EdREN/index.html (last accessed 3 January 2006).

References

1   US Renal Data System. *USRDS 2005 annual data report: atlas of end-stage renal disease in the United States.* Bethesda, MD: National Institutes of Health, National Institute of Diabetes and Digestive and Kidney Diseases, 2005.
2   Statistisches Bundesamt. *Gesundheitsbericht fuer Deutschland. [Health report for Germany].* Wiesbaden: Statistisches Bundesamt, 1998:257. Available at: www.destatis.de/presse/deutsch/pm1998/ p3610090.htm (last accessed 6 January 2006).
3   Gambro. *Market details.* Stockholm: Gambro, 2005. Available at: www.gambro.com/Pages/ InfoPage.aspx?id=756 (last accessed on 2 January 2006).
4   Winchester JF, Tohme WG, Schulman KA, *et al.* Hemodialysis patient management by telemedicine: design and implementation. *ASAIO J* 1997;**43**:M763–6.
5   Moncrief JW. Teledialysis: desktop based video monitoring for hemodialysis patients and delivery of primary care to dialysis patients. *Telemed J* 1998;**4**:85.
6   Mitchell JG, Disney AP. Clinical applications of renal telemedicine. *J Telemed Telecare* 1997;**3**:158–62.
7   Mitchell JG, Disney APS, Roberts M. Renal telemedicine to the home. *J Telemed Telecare* 2000;**6**:59–62.
8   Jennett P, Scott R, Hailey D, *et al. Socio-economic impact of telehealth: evidence now for health care in the future. Volume two: policy report. Appendix K: critique of renal telehealth.* Calgary: University of Calgary, 2003. Available at: www.fp.ucalgary.ca/telehealth/Appendix%20K.pdf (last accessed 3 January 2006).

9   Mackenzie P, Mactier RA. Home haemodialysis in the 1990s. *Nephrol Dial Transplant* 1998;**13**:1944–8.

10   Meystre S. The current state of telemonitoring: a comment on the literature. *Telemed J E Health* 2005;**11**:63–9.

11   Mignon F, Michel C, Viron B. Why so much disparity of PD in Europe? *Nephrol Dial Transplant* 1998;**13**:1114-17.

12   Skiadas M, Agroyiannis B, Carson E, *et al*. Design, implementation and preliminary evaluation of a telemedicine system for haemodialysis. *J Telemed Telecare* 2002;**8**:157–64.

13   Stroetmann KA, Gruetzmacher P, Stroetmann VN. Improving quality of life for dialysis patients through telecare. *J Telemed Telecare* 2000;**6** (Suppl 1):80–3.

14   Edefonti A, Boccola S, Picca M, *et al*. Treatment data during pediatric home peritoneal teledialysis. *Pediatr Nephrol* 2003;**18**:560–4.

15   Popple I. MUHC patients reap the benefits of sleep with nocturnal home hemodialysis. *Med News Today* 23 June 2005. Available at: www.medicalnewstoday.com/medicalnews.php?newsid=26522 (last accessed 3 January 2006).

16   Zeidenberg J. Toronto General rolls out innovative tele-dialysis service. *Can Healthc Technol* October 2005. Available at: www.canhealth.com/oct05.html#05octstory1 (last accessed 30 October 2005).

17   Pierratos A, McFarlane P, Chan CT. Quotidian dialysis – update 2005. *Curr Opin Nephrol Hypertens* 2005;**14**:119–24.

18   Disease Management Purchasing Consortium. *Philips Medical Systems: interactive remote patient management and personalized education delivered through a patient's home television.* Wellesley, MA: Disease Management Purchasing Consortium, 2005. Available at: dismgmt.com/docs/bestideas05.doc (last accessed 3 January 2006).

19   Cleland JG, Louis AA, Rigby AS, *et al*. Noninvasive home telemonitoring for patients with heart failure at high risk of recurrent admission and death: the Trans-European Network-Home-Care Management System (TEN-HMS) study. *J Am Coll Cardiol* 2005;**45**:1654–64.

▶15

Quality of care

Barbara Johnston and Sam G. Burgiss

Introduction

Home telehealth programmes have been expanding since the mid-1990s, partly in response to the rapidly aging population that requires increasing levels of healthcare. This trend has been fuelled by increased public funding for home care, shortened hospital stays that often result in the need for follow-up care, advances in medical technology that facilitate home-care treatment and the desire of individuals to continue living in their homes rather than moving to obtain services.[1] The growing need for home-care services is expected to continue. The main recipients of home-care services are elderly people.

These factors mean there is an imperative to incorporate telehealth into a health organization's strategies to ensure that high-quality healthcare services can be provided for the aging population. Some studies have shown that telehealth can help keep people well and out of the hospital, as well as allowing scarce medical resources to be stretched.[2] However, only a small number of rigorous research studies have examined home telehealth. Nonetheless, home telehealth clearly has the potential to make a major contribution to solving the present problems of healthcare in America and elsewhere. In one of the earliest randomized controlled trials of home telehealth, published in January 2000, investigators showed that patients who were seen in person received the same quality of care as those who received care by real-time home video systems.[3]

In general, published work shows that home telehealth allows care to be provided in the home effectively, efficiently and clinically appropriately. Telehealth is normally used as part of a home-care programme that continues to include face-to-face traditional care – not as a replacement for all face-to-face care. However, adoption of home telehealth is far from widespread. In the US, fewer than 200 home health programmes (about 2% of home health agencies) existed in 2002.[4] Considerably more research is needed, especially on the best ways of integrating home telehealth into traditional care systems and the changes in management processes required in home-care agencies. Nonetheless, the research conducted to date shows clearly that patients are well satisfied with home telehealth and are delighted when such services can be provided remotely.

Various approaches can be taken in evaluating the quality of health care, including the Donabedian model, which measures structure (qualifications of staff), process (services delivered) and outcomes (results for the clients such as improvements in

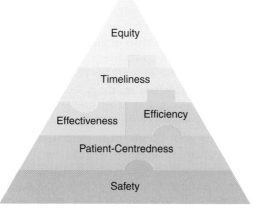

Fig. 15.1. The American Institute of Medicine's six quality aims

quality of life or rehospitalization).[1] In 2001, an authoritative report by the American Institute of Medicine (IOM) called for the healthcare delivery system to be redesigned fundamentally to improve the quality of care and become more consumer centred.[5] The IOM identified six categories to improve quality (Fig. 15.1). These 'quality categories' require health to be:

- safe
- timely
- effective
- efficient
- equitable
- patient centred.

The six categories are relevant to the approaches being taken by various organizations that are using telehealth to provide healthcare to patients in their home. They are considered in more detail below.

Safe

Safety is defined by the IOM as freedom from accidental injury. This means that to improve patient safety in the home telehealth environment, healthcare organizations and professionals must establish and improve systems that minimize the likelihood of error, make visible the errors that do occur, and prevent or mitigate harm from errors that reach the patient.

One of the main reasons for developing telehealth programmes has been to improve access to high-quality healthcare services for the rapidly growing numbers of patients being referred for service, who are being referred in an increasingly acutely unwell state of health because of pressure on hospitals. The level of illness of many patients referred to home care has risen over the past decade. It is not uncommon for patients with complicated treatment plans, including a variety of complex medical devices, to be sent home under the care and supervision of visiting nurses. These nurses must prioritize their visit frequency on the basis of their caseload and the complications of driving between individual patients. Intuitively, it makes sense that more closely monitored patients will be safer, but no study has been done to verify this.

Patients with congestive heart failure are the patients most commonly referred for home care. They require close monitoring of vital signs, body weight and adherence to complex treatment plans to minimize the likelihood of errors due to the lack of information. As is true with other chronic diseases, congestive heart failure requires rigorous disease management to improve quality and longevity of life. When telehealth is used for patients with congestive heart failure, it offers independence to patients and the ability to perform sophisticated clinical measurements, such as blood oxygen saturation, heart and lung sounds, and electrocardiogram recordings. Telehealth systems allow practitioners to treat, evaluate and educate patients in the comfort and safety of their own homes.

Developing and implementing telehealth programmes that provide safe and high-quality care can be facilitated by following the recommendations and techniques described in detail in the American Telemedicine Association's Home Telehealth Toolkit.[6] This toolkit includes information about policies and procedures, vendor-selection processes, accreditation and document requirements, performance improvement and evaluations.

Box 15.1 shows a case study of the safety of telehealth.

Box 15.1. Case study – safety and telehealth

Telehealth is used as a component of a disease management programme for patients with congestive heart failure at the Mercy Hospital, Sacramento, California. Telehealth is used to monitor the patients and provide education and behavioural modification programmes to improve health outcomes. It also improves the safety of the patient by early detection of adverse conditions before the patient's situation worsens. The Mercy telehealth programme allows one clinician to oversee many patients using remote monitoring, which alerts the clinician if and when a patient may need an intervention. The telehealth programme has shown a 73% reduction in hospitalizations.

Comment
The programme allows more efficient use of the organization's resources and, at the same time, encourages staff to make in-person visits when necessary. Using telehealth in a disease management programme helps to deliver more proactive care, education and support. This empowers patients and improves the quality of their lives by allowing them to control their symptoms.[7]

Timely

Timely healthcare can be defined as the process of care being free of undesired delays for those who receive care and those who deliver it. The process of care needs to flow smoothly. and waiting times should be minimized. Several studies have shown that home telehealth can improve client outcomes through timely intervention and health crisis prevention, thereby reducing the frequency of return visits to hospitals and physicians' offices.[8] The US Office of the National Coordinator for Health Information has developed a strategic framework to utilize technology to improve the quality of healthcare. In this strategic framework, telehealth has been identified as a method of providing access to high-quality healthcare, especially in rural communities where delays in access to health services are the result of geographical barriers.[9]

The provision of daily services to patients in a timely manner is equally important. Here, the provision of home telehealth can help by allowing more occasions of service per nurse per week – with some services delivered face to face and some via telehealth, with videoconferencing for direct interaction or home monitoring of vital signs. Telehealth detects when a patient needs care and allows a timely response to that patient rather than depending only on visits with a pre-arranged schedule.

Measurement of outcomes is critical to the use of telehealth in home and hospice care. Outcome measurement allows a programme to evaluate its own performance and to share its experience with other organizations. One of the earliest studies was done by the Kaiser Permanente organization in 1996 and 1997.[3] The patients studied had been diagnosed with chronic obstructive pulmonary disease, congestive heart failure, diabetes, cancer, anxiety, cerebral vascular accident and need for wound care. A control group comprised 110 patients. Patients in the intervention group (n=102) were provided with an interactive video system, electronic stethoscope and sphygmomanometer. The study focused on quality, patient satisfaction, utilization of services and cost of care. The results showed improvements in the flow of timely care and reduced waiting times for patients. Nurse visits in the home required an average of 45 minutes, while telehealth visits required 18 minutes. The time saved in telehealth visits, including travel, indicated that a nurse could see 15–20 patients a day; this compared with 5–6 patients a day for in-person visits. The cost of health care was $2674 for the control group and $1948 for the intervention group.

Effective

In order to prove that effective service delivery is occurring, the IOM recommended the disciplined use of systemically acquired knowledge during the provision of services. This knowledge can be used to identify, and increase, the services that are likely to benefit patients and refrain from providing services not likely to benefit patients.

Home telehealth has the potential to more appropriately allocate high-quality healthcare services. The technologies should be chosen on the basis of the need of the patient population to be served. Patients recently discharged from acute care may need to be seen, evaluated and have their vital signs monitored frequently. Such patients may best be served by real-time, home video systems, which allow home health nurses to see and talk with the patient, obtain vital signs, listen to heart and lung sounds, and, when necessary, obtain blood glucose levels (Fig. 15.2).

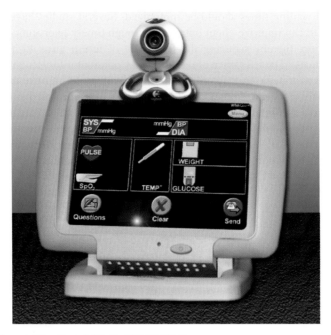

Fig. 15.2. Home telehealth unit (Turtle 800, VitelNet)

Box 15.2. Case study: effectiveness and telehealth (Slater S, personal communication, 2005)

In an early home telehealth project, interactive video equipment was placed in the home of a 56-year-old man in 1998. He was a widower and did not have any other family members at home. He had been in a coronary care unit for many days. He was on a ventilator and suffered several cardiac arrests while being repositioned to prevent skin ulcers, which are common in bed-bound patients. Turning this patient became a high-risk treatment, and he unfortunately developed a large sacral decubitus ulcer. When he was discharged from hospital, he needed very complex dressing changes twice a day to treat the ulcer. His insurance company authorized the use of telehealth so that he could go home to recover. They initially approved home nursing visits twice a day to perform the complex dressing changes. Cost savings from not having to place him in a skilled nursing facility for months were expected to be significant. The patient would also have the comfort of recovering at home.

While the visiting nurse was in the home, the agency telehealth nurse connected via the interactive video equipment using the ordinary telephone network. The nurse on the home visit used a digital camera to document wound healing for the insurance company, and the pictures were transmitted to the telehealth system located in the home-care agency. During the week, remote, interactive video-visits were also made to support the patient. Vital signs were taken with blood pressure/pulse meters, a pulse oximeter and a body-weight scale. An electronic stethoscope was used to listen to his heart and lung sounds. These services benefited the patient and he recovered over a six-month period.

Comment
The use of telehealth allowed this man to obtain the care he needed in his own home and provided beneficial care required for a positive outcome.

In other cases where patients are more stable, the best technology may be remote monitoring systems that do not require the interactive video components. Such telehealth systems can provide disease management through remote monitoring of vital signs, daily reminders about required healthy behaviour and/or health education regarding specific disease categories.

Box 15.2 shows a case study of the effectiveness of telehealth.

Efficient

Efficiency in healthcare is defined as a process of continual reduction of waste, especially waste stemming from overuse of ineffective tests, medications, procedures, technologies and other interventions. Waste also includes any use of a resource that fails to help meet patients' needs, including materials, supplies, time, forms, measurements, reports, motion, duplicated efforts, ideas not used and information that is lost.

Telehealth programmes have the capacity to improve staff productivity and prevent waste by eliminating unnecessary travel time for nurses driving to and from patient's homes. Use of telehealth allows the nurse to use 'windshield time' for the provision of home care. Telehealth represents a form of consumer-centred healthcare that offers opportunities to empower patients with knowledge, improve overall health, deliver services more efficiently and save money. It allows homecare staff to reallocate resources and promote a safe and efficient homecare environment for the consumer by increasing the time available for visits.

At present, the healthcare industry is in the midst of a revolution, with a focus on improving quality of care and encouraging patients to be more directly involved with their own healthcare. In response to increasing healthcare costs and the well-documented need to improve healthcare quality, the American government and leaders from the private sector have set the stage for transforming healthcare through widespread adoption of health information technology.[10] Although telehealth technologies account for a small segment of all healthcare technologies in the US – an estimated $380 million out of $71 billion nationwide – innovation in this area could bring significant improvements in healthcare productivity and quality of life.[11]

Over the past decade, growth has been seen in new products designed to provide health information technology solutions for patients who require varying levels of care in their homes, including real-time video systems and several levels of remote monitoring systems that target the chronically ill. Telemonitoring will be successful only if the service delivery model reflects national health system idiosyncrasies, takes into account established organizational boundaries and adapts to patient quality of life and health professional preferences. Patient-centred care will be required if a seamless and efficient health system is to be achieved.

Equitable

Access to healthcare should be equitable. Access should not differ solely because of characteristics such as sex, race, ethnicity, income, education, disability, sexual orientation or location of residence. Rural communities have experienced a significant growth in population, especially as older people move out of major cities to retire in a less congested and less expensive environment. People who have moved to these rural communities are the most likely to need home health services, because they are the most likely to have developed a variety of chronic conditions. Telehealth systems that monitor conditions such as asthma, diabetes, heart disease and mental illness are effective and can be provided irrespective of the location of the patient.[12] Telehealth allows patients to be seen in their own home, which is important for rural residents. Even if nurse visits can be arranged, nurses may not be able to visit as frequently as needed. Many rural communities also have problems with inclement weather, which can prevent access by home-care staff.

The high costs of care to the patient have the potential to prohibit healthcare for some rural residents. Although many previous studies have examined the cost savings for healthcare organizations, a group of researchers in Arkansas focused their attention on the patient's perspective.[13] They found a significantly positive financial outcome for patients involved with telehealth. Telehealth made healthcare more equitable to rural and remote populations in Arkansas, because healthcare was accessible in the patient's own community without the cost of travel. Thus, 94% of patients would have travelled more than 110 km for medical care, 84% would have missed one day of work and 74% would have incurred $75–150 in additional family expenses. With telemedicine, however, 92% of patients saved $32 in fuel costs, 84% saved $100 in wages and 74% saved $75–150 in family expenses.[13]

The ideal is to keep people in their own communities as long as possible with support from healthcare services. A study conducted in Italy of home-based telecardiology provided to patients with congestive heart failure showed that telehealth was able to detect and prevent clinical instability, reduce rehospitalization and reduce the cost of managing the patients.[14]

The IOM's recommendation about equity is probably the recommendation that has had the most effect on traditional telemedicine systems of care – that is, those focusing on providing care to rural and remote populations. However, it is equally important in the home telehealth environment. Telehealth has been shown to promote equitable access to healthcare and should be incorporated into mainstream healthcare services throughout health organizations, especially in rural communities.

Patient centred

The final IOM category underlines the importance of patient-centred healthcare, that is, healthcare that respects and honours the patient's individual wants, needs and preferences and ensures that the individual patient's values guide all decisions. Telehealth programmes have the capacity to be patient centred by providing access to the patient in the convenience of their own home. Elderly people are the most likely consumers of healthcare services and referrals to home health. In the US, 30 million people were older than 60 years in 2000; this figure is likely to be 60 million by 2025.

Telehealth programmes must be designed to meet the needs of the consumers. Technology must be designed for the needs of the providers, caregivers and patients in order to improve the quality of healthcare. Box 15.3 describes a real example of how telehealth provided patient-centred care at home and also improved the quality of life for the patient and his family.

Many studies have shown high levels of patient satisfaction from those who have participated in telehealth programmes, which confirms that the patient's wants, needs and preferences are being met.[12,13,15] A study at the University of Minnesota involved 53 elderly patients with chronic cardiac, pulmonary and wound-care needs.[16] Interactive videoconferencing and physiological monitoring were used in the homes of the patients who received the telehealth intervention. A total of 576 telehealth and 1057 in-person visits were provided to the patients. The patients' perceptions of home telehealth and their satisfaction with their nurse were evaluated during the project. The virtual telehealth visits were considered to be as useful as the actual in-person visits in 91% of cases.

Box 15.3. Case study – patient-centred and telehealth

Mr Oberheim, a 79-year-old gentleman in Pennsylvania, found himself in a situation that seemed increasingly hopeless. Numerous complications with congestive heart failure and pneumonia had left him with only 25% of his heart functioning properly. Although Mr Oberheim was assigned to self-monitoring and a twice-weekly visiting nurse rotation, undetected changes in his health status had led to frequent emergency interventions. As a result, this once-active deep-sea fisherman had grown increasingly despondent and had become either homebound or hospitalized. 'I asked myself why I should bother taking medications, limit my activities and stay on a diet that I did not enjoy if the outcome was always the same – that I was still being admitted to the hospital quite often,' he said, 'What kind of life is that?' Fortunately, Mr Oberheim was referred to a home-care agency that used telehealth, which provided him with an easy-to-use system to measure and transmit clinical data, including heart rate, blood pressure, oxygen saturation, glucose levels, lung function, body weight and temperature. Mr Oberheim's health-related information was sent directly to the clinical team from the comfort of his home.

The telehealth system enabled Mr Oberheim's medical team to identify changes in his oxygen saturation, which were the precursor to his frequent exacerbations. This was vital information that previous self-reporting had not been able to capture. The telehealth system allowed the nurses who monitored him to detect even subtle changes early enough to begin treatment before the problems escalated or became life threatening.

Comment
Telehealth had a positive effect on Mr Oberheim and his family. In his first year using the system, Mr Oberheim was admitted to the hospital on only two occasions. Each time, the telehealth system detected slight but critical changes to his health well in advance of a major exacerbation. His health improved to the point where he could spend the winters in Florida, and he is even back to deep-sea fishing with friends – one thing he values highly. 'You cannot believe the security my husband and I feel with telehealth,' said Mrs Oberheim. 'I just cannot imagine not knowing that someone is watching over him every day.'

Conclusion

Good evidence shows that the use of home telehealth can improve access to high-quality healthcare for patients. The growing need for health services and the limited human resources to provide high-quality home care have stimulated the development of telehealth programmes. Despite certain challenges, the US Department of Commerce recommended widespread adoption of telehealth. Their report provided a framework for advancing the adoption and application of telehealth, and recommended a strong commitment among all healthcare stakeholders to ensure success.[11] 'If we seize this opportunity and act, the national benefits can be great. Increased adoption of telehealth technologies offers increased access to quality healthcare at lower costs, while simultaneously increasing our nation's security.'[11] The main focus of telehealth programmes must remain on improving access to high-quality healthcare.

Patients need healthcare in their homes, and they want to remain in their homes for as long as possible. Telehealth enables patients to receive, at home, services that were only available previously in care facilities such as nursing homes and hospitals, such as daily and hourly physiological monitoring. The cost of this care typically is lower in the home than in the other settings. Research has shown that home telehealth is an efficacious tool. Widespread adoption of information technology is now regarded as a path to improving healthcare and to achieving the IOM's six quality aims for redesigning care.[17] If telehealth programmes are focused on the IOM's six quality indicators, they will have the potential to improve the quality of care for the communities they serve.

Further information

Institute of Medicine's healthcare and quality website. Available at: www.iom.edu/CMS/3718.aspx (last accessed 24 December 2005).
National Rural Health Association. *Quality through collaboration: the NRHA quality initiative*. Kansas City, MO: National Rural Health Association. Available at: www.nrharural.org/quality/ (last accessed 24 December 2005).
Tracy JA, ed. *A guide to getting started in telemedicine*. Available at: www2.muhealth.org/~telehealth/geninfo/TAD.html (last accessed 24 December 2005).

References

1 Coleman B. Assuring the quality of homecare: the challenge of involving the consumer. Washington, DC: AARP Public Policy Institute, 2000. Available at: www.aarp.org/research/housing-mobility/homecare/aresearch-import-719-IB43.html (last accessed 14 December 2005).
2 Fishman J. House calls: remote monitors can be lifesavers for chronic disease patients. *Most Wired* 10 August 2005. Available at: www.usnews.com/usnews/health/articles/050801/1home.htm (last accessed 14 December 2005).
3 Johnston B, Wheeler L, Deuser J, Sousa KH. Outcomes of the Kaiser Permanente Tele-Home Health Research Project. *Arch Fam Med* 2000;9:40–5.

4   Institute of Medicine. *Quality through collaboration: the future of rural health.* Washington, DC: *National Academy Press,* 2005:153.

5   Institute of Medicine. *Crossing the quality chasm: a new health system for the 21st century.* Washington, DC: National Academy Press, 2001:147–81.

6   American Telemed Association. *Home telehealth toolkit.* Available at: www.americantelemed.org/ ICOT/icot.htm. (last accessed 15 December 2005).

7   Utterback K. Supporting a new model of care with telehealth technology. *Telehealth Pract Rep* 2005;**9**(6):11.

8   Hebert M, Korabek B. Stakeholder readiness for telehomecare: implications for implementation. *Telemed J E Health* 2004;**10**:85–92.

9   Thompson T. *The decade of health information technology: delivering consumer-centric and information-rich health care: framework for strategic action.* Washington, DC: Department of Health and Human Services, National Coordinator for Health Information Technology, 2004. Available at: www.hhs.gov/healthit/documents/hitframework.pdf (last accessed 15 December 2005).

10   Lewin Group. *Health Information Technology Leadership Panel. Final report.* Falls Church, VA: Lewin Group, 2005. Available at: www.lewin.com/Lewin_Publications/Uncategorised/HITLeadershipPanel FnlRpt.htm (last accessed 15 December 2005).

11   Brantley D, Laney-Cummings K, Spivack R. *Innovation, demand, and investment in telehealth,* Washington, DC: US Department of Commerce, 2004. Available at: www.technology.gov/reports/ TechPolicy/Telehealth/2004Report.pdf (last accessed 15 December 2005).

12   Kobb R, Hoffman N, Lodge R, Kline S. Enhancing elder chronic care through technology and care coordination: report from pilot. *Telemed J E Health* 2003;**9**:189–95.

13   Bynum A, Irwin C, Cranford C, Denny G. The impact of telemedicine on patients' cost savings: some preliminary findings. *Telemed J E Health* 2003;**9**:361–7.

14   Scalvini S, Capamolla S, Zanelli E, *et al.* Effect of home-based telecardiology on chronic heart failure: costs and outcomes. *J Telemed Telecare* 2005;**11** (Suppl 1):16–18.

15   Cheitlan Cherry J, Dryden K, Kobb R, *et al.* Opening a window of opportunity through technology and coordination: a multisite case study. *Telemed J E Health* 2003;**9**:265–71.

16   Finkelstein SM, Speedie SM, Demiris G, *et al.* Telehomecare: quality, perception, satisfaction. *Telemed J E Health* 2004;**10**:122–8.

17   Tang PC, Lansky D. The missing link: bridging the patient–provider health information gap. Electronic personal health records could transform the patient–provider relationship in the twenty-first century. *Health Aff (Millwood)* 2005;**24**:1290–5.

►16

Diabetes

Justin Starren, Ruth S. Weinstock, Walter Palmas, Roberto E. Izquierdo, Philip C. Morin and David Kaufman

Introduction

Diabetes mellitus is a worldwide problem, and its prevalence is increasing. It is estimated that in 2000, the number of people with diabetes was 171 million, resulting in 2.9 million excess deaths; this is estimated to increase to 366 million affected individuals in 2030.[1] In the US, it is estimated that more than 18 million people have some form of diabetes. For children born in the year 2000, the lifetime risk of developing diabetes has been estimated to be 33% for males and 39% for females. The rate is higher in ethnic minority groups.[2] In 2002, the estimated direct and indirect costs for diabetes care were more than $132 billion.[3]

Poorly controlled diabetes is associated with the development of microvascular and macrovascular complications, including retinopathy, neuropathy, foot ulcers, nephropathy, heart disease, peripheral vascular disease and stroke – all of which are associated with significant morbidity and mortality. Diabetes remains the leading cause of blindness in adults aged 20–74 years. This makes it the leading cause of end-stage renal disease and non-traumatic amputations in adults. All these complications can be prevented or delayed with improved care. A multifactorial intervention aimed at improving glycaemia, hypertension, dyslipidaemia and microalbuminuria, as well as instituting aspirin therapy, in patients with type 2 diabetes has been shown to reduce microvascular and cardiovascular events by more than 50%.[4]

Prior studies in home telehealth

Almost every home telehealth technology has been used to treat patients with diabetes. The following discussion focuses on the use of home telehealth specifically for the treatment of diabetes – rather than for patients in whom diabetes is an incidental diagnosis.

To date, there have been eight randomized, controlled trials of telemedicine case management for patients with type 1 diabetes mellitus (Table 16.1);[5–12] these were included in a systematic review and meta-analysis.[10] There have been two studies in patients with type 2 diabetes (Table 16.1).[13,14] In the studies in patients with type 1 diabetes, the telemedicine case management intervention consisted of modem transmission of glucometer data and telephone contact by clinicians to adjust therapy.

Participants had inadequate or poor glycaemic control at baseline, and required intensive insulin therapy in five of the eight studies. In one study, the population was composed of pregnant women.[6] Follow-up duration varied from 3 to 12 months in the studies. Only one study involving type 1 diabetes showed a significant improvement in glycaemic management by telemedicine case management: the mean HbA_{1c} changed from 9.1% to 7.8% after six months in the intervention group and from 8.8% to 8.2% in the control group (p=0.03).[10] In the meta-analysis, pooled data showed no significant difference in glycaemic control between telemedicine case management and usual care.

In patients with type 2 diabetes, two controlled trials – both combining remote monitoring with videoconferencing – showed significant results. One showed improvement after three months.[13] A 16% reduction was seen in mean HbA_{1c} (from 9.5% at baseline to 8.2% at three months) in the telemedicine group; this compared with a 9% reduction (from 9.5% to 8.6%) in the control group (p<0.05). The other study (the Informatics for Diabetes Education and Telemedicine Project (IDEATel) described below[14-16]) showed improvement at one year, by which time the mean HbA_{1c} had improved from 7.4% to 7.0% in the telemedicine group and from 7.4% to 7.2% in

Table 16.1. Summary of controlled studies in diabetes home telehealth

Study	Year	Population	Participants		Duration (months)	Result
			Enrolled	Lost to follow-up		
Remote monitoring only						
Ahring *et al*[1]	1992	Adult, type 1	42	4	3	Not significant
Marrero *et al*[5]	1995	Paediatric, type 1	106	0	12	Not significant
Biermann *et al*[8]	2000	Adult, type 1	48	27	8	Not significant
Wojcicki *et al*[6]	2001	Pregnant, type 1	32	2	6	Not significant
Gómez *et al*[7]	2002	Adult, type 1	10	N/A	6	Not significant
Chase *et al*[9]	2003	Adult, type 1	70	7	6	Not significant
Welch *et al*[12]	2003	Adult, type 1	52	28	12	Not significant
Montori *et al*[10]	2004	Adult, type 1	31	3	6	Mean HbA_{1c} in telemedicine group reduced from 9.1% to 7.8% (8.8% to 8.2% in control group; p=0.03)
Remote monitoring and videoconferencing						
Whitlock *et al*[13]	2000	Adult, type 2	28	0	3	Mean HbA_{1c} in telemedicine group reduced from 9.5% to 8.2% (p<0.05)
Shea *et al*[14]	2005	Adult, mostly type 2 (IDEATel)	1665	248	12	Mean HbA_{1c} in telemedicine group was reduced from 7.4% to 7.0% (7.4% to 7.2% in control group; p=0.006)

the control group (p=0.006). Systolic blood pressure improved by 4.7 mmHg in the telemedicine group and 0.9 mmHg in the control (p=0.001). Diastolic blood pressure improved by 3.0 mmHg and 0.9 mmHg (p<0.001) and low-density lipoprotein (LDL) cholesterol improved by 10.7 mg/dl and 2.1 mg/dl (p<0.001) in the groups respectively.

There is still a general lack of controlled studies that compare different types of interventions or compare the effects of telehealth interventions in different populations.

Current approaches

As diabetes is a chronic disease that requires daily self-management, care in the home is critical for maintaining metabolic control and preventing complications. This includes achieving satisfactory blood glucose, blood pressure and lipid levels; being physically active; understanding appropriate meal planning; and following preventive health practices such as wearing proper footwear, regularly inspecting feet, and obtaining dilated eye examinations and influenza vaccinations. An overview of the breadth of telemedicine approaches applied to diabetes has been reviewed in a previous book in this series.[17] This chapter focuses specifically on home telehealth.

Current applications of diabetes home telehealth focus on three broad areas: monitoring, education and management. Home blood glucose monitoring provides data that help direct the use of hypoglycaemic drugs. Without telemedicine, these

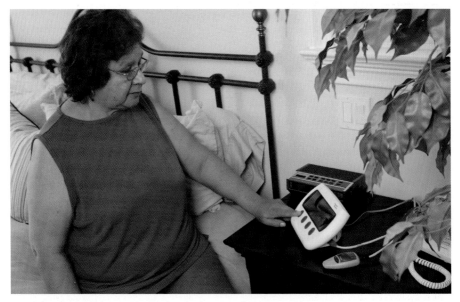

Fig. 16.1. Remote monitoring. The patient is using a remote monitoring device to send glucose results. The patient also answers symptomatic questions using buttons on the device. Image courtesy of Health Hero Network

values are reviewed only by the healthcare provider at routinely scheduled medical visits (for example, every 3–6 months), which results in long intervals between adjustments of the doses of hypoglycaemic medications. Telemedicine allows frequent transmission of blood glucose values, which means that healthcare providers can better change the medical regimen and/or diet. This improves metabolic control.

Virtually all remote monitoring technologies have been applied to diabetes. Interactive telephone systems have been used to allow patients to report glucose values through voice or touchpad. Many interactive video systems support the capture of glucose values from glucometers. Several web-based applications allow patients to enter values into a web-based form.[18] At present, the most common approach to monitoring in the home environment is the use of data collection devices that transmit information from glucometers over telephone lines (Fig. 16.1). The monitoring data, along with symptomatic questionnaire responses, are transmitted to a server. Nurse case managers typically access the server to review the results from multiple patients (Fig. 16.2). The server may include data interfaces that export the monitoring data to an electronic medical record (EMR).[15] More recently, other transmission paths, including broadband, mobile phone-based messaging and proprietary radio networks, have been employed.

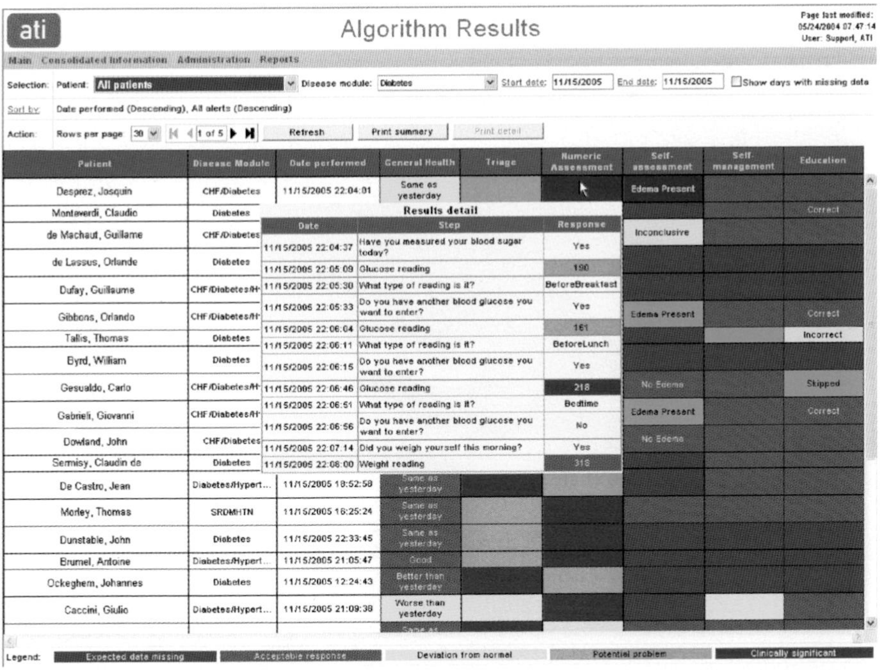

Fig. 16.2. Example of a nurse case manager's summary screen. The screen provides an example of a system for review of remote monitoring data. (Patient names are fictitious.) Note that the screen includes information about physiological measurements, symptomatic questionnaires and compliance with educational modules. The nurse can also view a chronological summary of a single patient. Image courtesy of American Telecare

In addition to monitoring blood glucose levels, other diabetes-related conditions can be monitored with telemedicine in the home. Foot ulcerations and other diabetes foot-related problems can be monitored using telemedicine (see Chapter 8), including the use of videoconferencing equipment and, more recently, mobile phone cameras.[19]

A critical component of diabetes care in any venue is patient education. This education is essential so that patients with diabetes can take the best possible care of themselves.[20] In most diabetes centres, self-management education is provided primarily by specialist nurses or dietician educators. Most people with diabetes are not seen in these centres and are followed by their primary care providers, who may not have access to specialist educators. Many primary care providers do not have enough time or resources to provide extensive education and behaviour modification programmes. In addition, many people with diabetes have poor access to care because of geography, weather, transportation difficulties, lack of insurance coverage, and/or social and cultural barriers.

Diabetes education can be delivered by diabetes educators via telemedicine directly to the patient in their home – bypassing many barriers to care. Such education is provided in two ways. The first is the use of conventional videoconferencing –

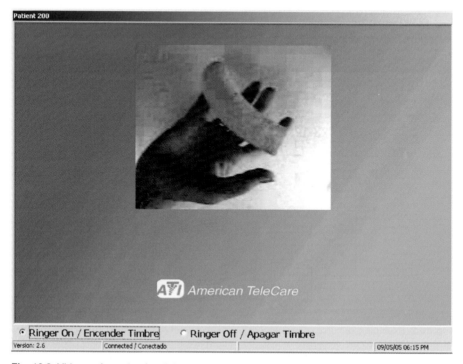

Fig. 16.3. Videoconferencing for diabetes education. The image shows a dietician demonstrating food portion size to a patient via a videophone connection

frequently with video telephones that operate over the ordinary telephone network (public switched telephone network, PSTN) (Fig. 16.3). In addition to face-to-face interactions between the educator and the patient, such systems can provide high-resolution still images of educational aids, such as food portions. The second form of education is through the use of web-based resources, such as those provided by the American Diabetes Association (www.diabetes.org) (Fig. 16.4).

Finally, home telehealth technologies can be used directly in the management of diabetes and its complications. Diabetic retinopathy can limit a patient's ability to provide appropriate self-care. Insulin doses can be monitored through the use of video connections. Fig. 16.5 shows an image of an insulin syringe that has been transmitted over a PSTN video connection. Video can also be used to guide dressing changes for diabetes-related wound care. In all these ways, home telehealth has the potential to decrease diabetes-related morbidity, mortality and costs and improve quality of life.

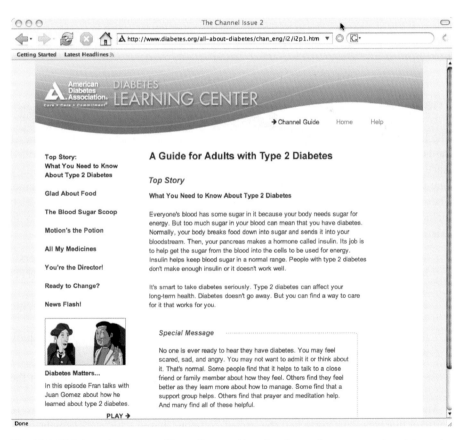

Fig. 16.4. Web-based resources. Many sites provide education and management assistance for patients with diabetes

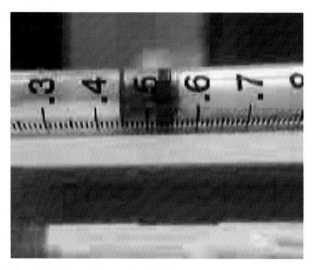

Fig. 16.5. Video-based diabetes management. Close-up image of an insulin syringe being transmitted to a case manager to support the adjustment of insulin dosing in visually impaired patients

The IDEATel project

The Informatics for Diabetes Education and Telemedicine Project (IDEATel) is one of the largest telemedicine studies in the US, with more than 2100 participants enrolled since late 2000.[14–16] The participants were randomized to usual care by their primary care provider or an intervention of case management and education by telemedicine. The intervention participants received a home telemedicine unit (HTU), which included a web-enabled personal computer with a dial-up modem connection to an existing telephone line (Fig. 16.6). The HTU has four other components:

- video camera and microphone for videoconferencing with nurse case managers
- home glucose monitoring device and blood pressure cuff connected to the HTU for transmission of readings
- ability to access patients' own clinical data and post messages at a project-specific web portal
- the capability to access educational websites, including one created for the study participants by the American Diabetes Association.

As part of the installation process, participants received in-person training on the use of the HTU.

The nurse case managers were trained in management of diabetes (most were certified diabetes educators) and the use of computer-based case management tools that facilitated interactions through videoconferencing with patients. Case managers interacted with patients using the home telemedicine unit and followed the tenets of

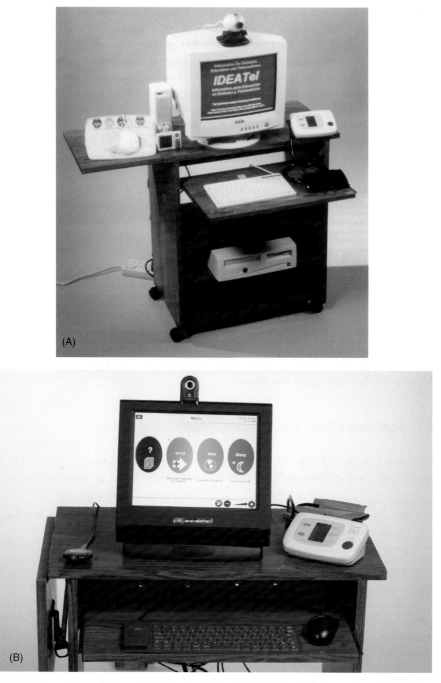

Fig. 16.6. Home telemedicine units: first-generation unit (A) and second-generation unit (B). In the second-generation unit, all computer hardware is behind the touch screen, which makes the unit suitable for countertop placement

the Veterans Health Administration (VHA) *Clinical practice guidelines for the management of diabetes mellitus in the primary care setting.*[21] Video-visits, during which participants met with the diabetes nurse educator and a dietician, were scheduled every 4–6 weeks. During a routine visit, the nurse educator reviewed the recent medical history and current medications. Glucose and blood pressure readings were transmitted to the server. Individualized goals for diabetes management were set, and specific recommendations were made about therapy (whether to change or adjust medications or continue the present antidiabetic therapy). The goals followed the published diabetes standard of care to achieve the targets recommended by the American Diabetes Association: that is, HbA_{1c} <7%, LDL cholesterol <100 mg/dl (<5.5 mmol/l), triglycerides <150 mg/dl (< 8.25 mmol/l) and blood pressure <130/80 mmHg. The dietician discussed the patient's diet and developed an individualized meal plan. The dieticians were able to project images of portion sizes using food models and a document camera. An endocrinologist met daily with the diabetes nurse educators and the dietician to discuss the management plan of these patients and to review the written medical notes, which were then submitted to the primary care provider. The primary care providers who sponsored the participating patients from their practice retained full responsibility and control over their patients' care in both the intervention and control (usual care) groups.

The IDEATel study intervention is scheduled to continue until 2007. The project has already shown that home telehealth can be delivered to patients with diabetes on a large scale and can bridge both geographic and socio-economic divides. As described above, analysis of the first year's results showed significant improvements in HbA_{1c}, blood pressure, cholesterol and lipids.[14]

Clinical workflow and communication issues

The concept for IDEATel was to provide underserved patients with access to specialized diabetes education and care. The strategies were:

- more intensive self-management education of patients with diabetes
- more frequent and more easily accessed results of blood glucose and blood pressure measurements by patients and health providers
- more frequent intervention by the primary care provider than is usual in the US.

All strategies involve enhanced communication between the diabetes support team, the patient and the primary care provider.

In diabetes home telehealth, adjustments to medications are common, and good communication is important. Because telehealth is able to accelerate the normal interaction cycle, it also requires acceleration of the communication cycle. Fig. 16.7 shows the flow of information in the IDEATel project. In the urban arm, physicians were able to review results and televisit reports using the electronic medical records (EMR). In the rural arm, physicians and case managers interacted primarily by telephone and fax. All physicians were offered direct web-based access to the telehealth application, but most preferred paper- or fax-based communication.

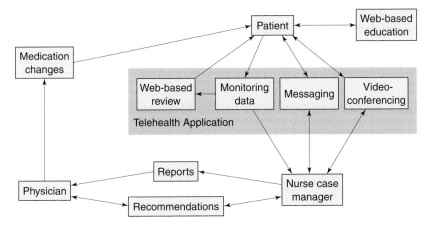

Fig. 16.7. Flow of information in the IDEATel project. Interaction between primary physician and case manager occurred outside the telehealth application. All physicians were offered direct, web-based access to the telehealth application, but most preferred paper- or fax-based methods of communication

A comparison between the urban and rural arms is informative. The urban patients live in the boroughs of New York City, they are often beneficiaries of two federal health insurance programmes (Medicare and Medicaid) and nearly all are patients of providers affiliated to the New York Presbyterian Hospital (NYP) and Columbia University. Communication between the urban case management diabetes support team and the primary care providers is facilitated via the institutional EMR, which contains monitoring data, routine laboratory results, records of televisits, web messages, alerts and notes from case managers' visits.

The rural component of the project shows the challenges of coordinating care with a large number of paper-based primary care practices. More than 500 elderly patients with diabetes live in the 30 000 square miles of New York State that lies west of the Hudson River and north of the Pennsylvanian border. These patients are served by more than 200 different primary care providers. For the rural patients, case manager recommendations were sent to the primary care provider by mail, fax or telephone. About 50% of providers in the rural arm gave written permission for the endocrinologist to adjust diabetes-related medications, such as oral hypoglycaemic agents or insulin.

Although the rural physicians were offered direct web access to the IDEATel telehealth application, few took advantage, because it constituted a significant disruption of their existing workflow. Nationally, the economics of the fee-for-service system means that compensation for self-employed primary care providers is driven by productivity. Any interaction with a home telehealth application must take this into account. In the US, physicians in sole or small-group practice have been the least adoptive of information technology, such as EMRs, electronic access to diagnostic test results and the use of clinical decision support systems to improve practice and patient outcomes.[22]

In the meantime, according to one survey, most American physicians have difficulty assembling basic profile data on a single patient or generating a list of patients whose laboratory results or medications need scrutiny.[22] Telehealth projects thus need to use a variety of methods to communicate with both 'paper' and 'digital' doctors.

Human factors in diabetes home telehealth

In home telehealth, the patient with diabetes interacts directly with at least one medical device – the glucometer. Often the patient must interact with several devices – such as a blood pressure monitor and data-transmission device. Patients are also presumed to be tracking their own blood glucose values, which usually means reviewing the values on a web portal. Systems thus must be usable by a population that traditionally does not use computers.

Older adults are more likely to be novice computer users, less literate and subject to the physical and cognitive effects of aging. These factors all contribute to the difficulties that elderly people experience in using computers and the Internet.[23] We have developed a framework for understanding the barriers to elderly people using web-based systems for disease management. The framework was developed in the context of the IDEATel project, which targeted elderly people without computers.[24] We had observed that, in spite of an initial training session, a substantial proportion of our patients were underutilizing the computer-based resources (for example, they were not using web-based EMRs to monitor blood glucose levels).

We conducted usability testing in the laboratory and patients' homes. The analyses revealed aspects of the system that were suboptimal. These included characteristics of the displays such as font size, text spacing, size of buttons and certain 'widgets' (for example, links, scrollbars, buttons and menus). In addition, certain tasks were unnecessarily complex – requiring too many steps and screen transitions. The problems pertaining to patients' skills and knowledge were of three types (Table 16.2):

- perceptual-motor skills, especially in relation to the use of the mouse
- mental models, which refer to a basic understanding of a system (for example, navigation problems are common among novice web users)
- literacy and numeracy.

Perceptual and motor skills presented significant difficulties for many of the participants. The ability to use a mouse constitutes a significant impediment to computer use. The range of problems include proper grip, halting movements, clicking latency, spatial orientation and coordinating mouse movement with screen coordinates. Previous studies have shown that the mouse is not the best device for elderly people.[25]

The mental models of novice users also interfered with their ability to use the system effectively. Several patients lacked an understanding of how devices such as their glucometer functioned, which led to errors. In order to be able to navigate the web, users need to be able to initiate actions, anticipate consequences, interpret system

Table 16.2. Problems pertaining to patient skills and knowledge

Perceptual/motor skill	Mental model of system	Literacy and numeracy
• Mouse grip	• Blood pressure measuring	• Reading ability
• Fluid movements	devices, glucometers and	• Text comprehension
• Mouse or cursor coordination	other devices	• Understanding graphical user
• Spatial orientation	• Mouse button functions	interface conventions
• Latency or sensitivity of clicks	• Connecting to Internet	• Relations between cells and
• Precision of click on link	• Attending to modem sounds	rows in a table
• Keyboard orientation	• Perceiving cues (screens)	• Correspondence between
• Ability to scan keyboard	• Initiating actions	monitoring device display and
• Locating cursor on screen	• Perceiving system feedback	tabular presentation
	• Anticipating screen transitions	• Recognizing anomalous or
	• Function of widgets: links,	abnormal results
	scrollbars, menus, navigation	• Representations of bounded
	buttons and dialogue box	periods of time
		• Discerning patterns of change
		over time
		• Drawing appropriate inferences

feedback and respond accordingly. Problems that related to basic and health literacy were also observed among patients. Individuals need to have a basic ability to understand relevant materials to participate successfully in a self-management regimen. This involves monitoring one's glucose and blood pressure values, and making the necessary adjustments in one's lifestyle (for example, diet and exercise). In addition, users of home telehealth need to understand the basic properties of a tabular representation and how values may change with time. These problems also served to diminish users' sense of self-efficacy, which affects the willingness to persevere when frustrated or when a task seems daunting. Low self-efficacy was evident in a number of ways. For example, individuals would comment on their lack of experience and reduced ability to learn new things as they became older.

The usability evaluation allowed hardware and software changes. For example, we now employ a touch screen interface (Fig. 16.6), which reduces users' dependence on a mouse and enhances the ease of interaction. We also modified the training programme to provide additional help to patients most likely to benefit.

Conclusion

Telehealth allows diabetes specialists to interact with patients and their primary care providers from hundreds or thousands of miles away. This can eliminate the need for the patient to travel long distances to the specialist and brings specialist care to many who could not otherwise receive it. At the same time, this creates new challenges for the coordination and communication of care. Although progress is being made in the electronic coordination of care across multiple providers, much remains to be done.

The rising incidence of diabetes means that most home telehealth programmes will need to address the needs of patients with diabetes. A wide variety of technological approaches have been deployed successfully; however, many of these technologies remain difficult for elderly patients to use. Although evidence is still sparse, several recent studies have shown the value of home telehealth for the management of diabetes. Demographic and technological trends seem likely to lead to continued growth in diabetes home telehealth. This growth, in turn, will create a need for new methods for the management of these greatly increased volumes of data.

Further information

American Diabetes Association website. Available at: www.diabetes.org (last accessed 22 November 2005).

IDEATel Project website. Available at: www.ideatel.org (last accessed 22 November 2005).

Joslin Diabetes Center website. Available at: www.joslin.org (last accessed 22 November 2005).

References

1   Roglic G, Unwin N, Bennett PH, *et al*. The burden of mortality attributable to diabetes: realistic estimates for the year 2000. *Diabetes Care* 2005;**28**:2130–5.

2   Narayan KM, Boyle JP, Thompson TJ, *et al*. Lifetime risk for diabetes mellitus in the United States. *JAMA* 2003;**290**:1884–90.

3   Hogan P, Dall T, Nikolov P. *Economic costs of diabetes in the US in 2002. Diabetes Care* 2003;**26**:917–32.

4   Gaede P, Vedel P, Larsen N, *et al*. Multifactorial intervention and cardiovascular disease in patients with type 2 diabetes. *N Engl J Med* 2003;**348**:383–93.

5   Marrero DG, Vandagriff JL, Kronz K, *et al*. Using telecommunication technology to manage children with diabetes: the Computer-Linked Outpatient Clinic (CLOC) Study. *Diabetes Educ* 1995;**21**:313–19.

6   Wojcicki JM, Ladyzynski P, Krzymien J, *et al*. What we can really expect from telemedicine in intensive diabetes treatment: results from 3-year study on type 1 pregnant diabetic women. *Diabetes Technol Ther* 2001;**3**:581–9.

7   Gómez EJ, Hernando ME, Garcia A, *et al*. Telemedicine as a tool for intensive management of diabetes: the DIABTel experience. *Comput Methods Programs Biomed* 2002;**69**:163–77.

8   Biermann E, Dietrich W, Standl E. Telecare of diabetic patients with intensified insulin therapy. A randomized clinical trial. *Stud Health Technol Inform* 2000;**77**:327–32.

9   Chase HP, Pearson JA, Wightman C, *et al*. Modem transmission of glucose values reduces the costs and need for clinic visits. *Diabetes Care* 2003;**26**:1475–9.

10 Montori VM, Helgemoe PK, Guyatt GH, *et al*. Telecare for patients with type 1 diabetes and inadequate glycemic control: a randomized controlled trial and meta-analysis. *Diabetes Care* 2004;**27**:1088–94.

11 Ahring KK, Ahring JP, Joyce C, Farid NR. Telephone modem access improves diabetes control in those with insulin-requiring diabetes. *Diabetes Care* 1992;**15**:971–5.

12 Welch G, Sokolove M, Mullin C, *et al*. Use of a modem-equipped blood glucose meter augmented with bi-weekly educator telephone support lowers HbA1c in type 1 diabetes. *Diabetes* 2003;**52** (Suppl 1):A100.

13 Whitlock WL, Brown A, Moore K, *et al*. Telemedicine improved diabetic management. *Mil Med* 2000;**165**:579–84.

14 Shea S, Weinstock RS, Starren J, *et al*. A randomized trial comparing telemedicine case management with usual care in older, ethnically diverse, medically underserved patients with diabetes mellitus. *J Am Med Inform Assoc* 2006:**13**:40–51.

15   Starren J, Hripcsak G, Sengupta S, *et al.* Columbia University's Informatics for Diabetes Education and Telemedicine (IDEATel) project: technical implementation. *J Am Med Inform Assoc* 2002;**9**:25–36.

16   Shea S, Starren J, Weinstock RS, *et al.* Columbia University's Informatics for Diabetes Education and Telemedicine (IDEATel) Project: rationale and design. *J Am Med Inform Assoc* 2002;**9**:46–92.

17   Batch J, Smith AC. Diabetes and telemedicine. In: Wootton R, Batch J, eds. *Telepediatrics: telemedicine and child health.* London: Royal Society of Medicine Press, 2005:89–104.

18   McMahon GT, Gomes HE, Hickson Hohne S, *et al.* Web-based care management in patients with poorly controlled diabetes. *Diabetes Care* 2005;**28**:1624–9.

19   Braun RP, Vecchietti JL, Thomas L, *et al.* Telemedical wound care using a new generation of mobile telephones: a feasibility study. *Arch Dermatol* 2005;**141**:254–8.

20   Strine TW, Okoro CA, Chapman DP, *et al.* The impact of formal diabetes education on the preventive health practices and behaviors of persons with type 2 diabetes. *Prev Med* 2005;**41**:79–84.

21   Veterans Health Administration. *Clinical practice guidelines for the management of diabetes mellitus in the primary care setting.* Washington, DC: Veterans Health Administration, 1999. Available at: www.humanitas.com/vha/download.htm (last accessed 6 January 2006).

22   Audet AJ, Doty MM, Shamasdin J, Schoenbaum SC. *Physicians' views on quality of care: findings from the Commonwealth Fund national survey of physicians and quality of care.* New York, NY: Commonwealth Fund, 2005. Available at: www.cmwf.org/usr_doc/823_Audet_physicians_views_quality_survey.pdf (last accessed 6 January 2006).

23   Fisk AD, Rogers W, Czaja SJ, *et al. Designing for older adults: principles and creative human factors approaches.* Boca Raton, FL: CRC Press, 2004.

24   Kaufman DR, Patel VL, Hilliman C, *et al.* Usability in the real world: assessing medical information technologies in patients' homes. *J Biomed Inform* 2003;**36**:45–60.

25   Czaja SJ. Computer technology and the older adult. In: Helander M, Landauer TK, Prablu P, eds. *Handbook of human–computer interaction.* Amsterdam: Elsevier Science, 1997:797–812.

▶17

Congestive heart failure

Penny Ford-Carleton, Nancy Lugn, Nhedti Colquitt, Marcia Reissig, Irene Higginson and Joseph C. Kvedar

Introduction

A major increase has been seen in the number of cases of congestive heart failure in the industrialized countries of the world. Over the last decade, treatment has improved the survivability of acute events, thus prolonging the course of chronic cardiovascular disease. As the population continues to age, both the prevalence and incidence of congestive heart failure will increase dramatically.

Prevalence and incidence

Many studies in Europe and the US have addressed the epidemiology of heart failure. The lack of a universal definition and differences in methods have complicated international comparisons and confounded the accurate estimation of overall prevalence and incidence. In industrialized countries, however, the prevalence of heart failure is known to range from 3 to 20 cases per 1000 of the population; this increases to more than 100 cases per 1000 in people older than 65 years.[1] Currently, the US has about 4.9 million cases of congestive heart failure, which represents 2.3% of the population.[2] Europe has about 10 million cases.[3] These estimates include only symptomatic heart failure. The prevalence of asymptomatic heart failure is similar and would double the estimated prevalence.[3]

The incidence of heart failure in middle age is about 1–2 cases per 1000 per year, but it rises to 20–30 cases in people older than 85 years.[1] The relative incidence doubles for each decade of life after the age of 45 years.[4] The lifetime risk of developing congestive heart failure after the age of 40 years is one in five.[2] The US has about 550 000 new cases per year.[2]

Cost

The cost of managing heart failure in the early 1990s was estimated to be 1–2% of total healthcare expenditure in many industrialized countries.[1] The most recent estimates of the total cost of heart failure are $27.6 billion in the US and £905 million in the UK.[2,5] About 60% of costs in the US and 70% of costs in the UK are for hospital care.[4,5] In 1991, the hospitalization cost for heart failure exceeded that for cancer and myocardial infarction combined.[6]

Disease trajectory

Despite the financial resources devoted to heart failure, patient prognosis remains poor;[7] indeed, the prognosis and quality of life in congestive heart failure is as poor as in common types of cancer.[7] In the Framingham Study, the median survival time was 1.7 years for men and 3.2 years for women, and the one-year survival rate was 57% for men and 64% for women.[4] The one-year survival rate for those who required hospitalization for an acute heart failure exacerbation was even lower – 39%.[8] In 2001, there were 52 828 deaths in the US; the overall death rate was 18.7 per 1000.[2]

In the US and UK, congestive heart failure is the most common diagnosis that leads to hospital admission.[9] About three million patients per year are admitted to hospitals in the US with a primary or secondary diagnosis of heart failure.[2] Admission rates in the US and many European countries have doubled over the past 10–15 years.[10] The dramatic increase in hospital discharges for heart failure – more than fourfold over 20 years in the US – is illustrated in Fig. 17.1.[11] The in-hospital mortality rate for heart failure is decreasing due to improved therapy for acute events. However, more patients are being discharged to long-term care facilities and home-care follow-up.[12]

Readmission rates are 29–47% within 3–6 months of discharge,[10] and some patients are rehospitalized repeatedly in this period.[13] A number of factors contribute to the need for readmission. These factors extend beyond traditional medical and pharmaceutical control of contributing factors (such as hypertension) to include behavioural factors (such as adherence to medication or diet recommendations), social and economic factors (such as isolation or poverty), and in adequate discharge planning and education.[14]

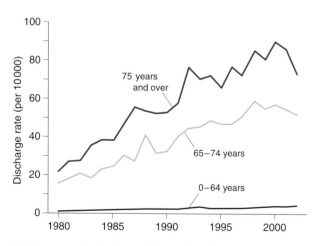

Fig. 17.1. Hospital discharge rates for heart failure as first-listed diagnosis (per 10 000 population in the US, 1980–2002)[11]

Approaches to disease management of congestive heart failure

The Disease Management Association of America (www.dmaa.org) defines disease management as a system of coordinated healthcare interventions and communications for populations with conditions in which there is significant patient self-care. The objective of a disease management programme is to improve healthcare outcomes and the cost-effectiveness of care. Such programmes are designed to address the many factors described above that contribute to the exacerbation and progression of chronic heart disease.

Several different kinds of healthcare delivery models exist. Some disease management programmes are led by physicians (primary care physicians or specialists) and others are led by nurses. The programmes may be based in the hospital, specialty clinic or home healthcare agency. Providers may also contract with disease management services.

Despite the heterogeneity of approaches, emerging evidence supports the positive effects of many of these programmes. In 2004, investigators in Canada, Spain and the US published systematic reviews of randomized, controlled trials that examined the effectiveness of disease management programmes for heart failure.[15–17] Each review examined readmission or hospitalization rates, among other outcomes, and two reported on mortality. All reviews concluded that readmissions were lower with disease management programmes than usual care. One review reported a trend towards reduced mortality,[17] and the other noted reduced mortality risk but only with approaches that included follow-up by a specialized multidisciplinary team.[15] The economic effectiveness of disease management programmes was evaluated by a meta-analysis of 67 studies with published measurements of direct economic outcomes. The results suggest that economic effectiveness is greatest with disease management of the most severely ill patients.[18]

Despite this evidence of positive effects, the resource intensity of these programmes is a challenge that will be magnified as the demand for management of chronic disease increases with the aging of the population. Consequently, technology-enabled disease management is of great interest. Two technology-enabled approaches to disease management in heart failure have been taken:

- telephone interventions
- telemonitoring.

Telephone interventions

Care provided by telephone – such as patient follow-up, education and counselling – is an integral component of many disease management programmes. Specially trained nurses supported by clinical guidelines and/or practice algorithms are usually responsible for these calls. The most extensive evaluation of the effectiveness of telephone intervention in congestive heart failure was conducted in Argentina. The DIAL trial was a multicentre, randomized, controlled study, in which more than 1500 patients with stable heart failure were assigned randomly to telephone intervention or to usual care.[19] A significant reduction in hospital admissions for heart failure exacerbations was seen in the intervention group, with no significant difference in mortality between the groups.[19]

Telephone interventions usually rely on reports by patients about changes in physiological variables, such as blood pressure and body weight. Some investigators have questioned the reliability of self-reporting. In one study of blood pressure monitoring for control of hypertension, patients tended to under-report measurements of blood pressure.[20] Consequently, telemonitoring may be preferable, as it will eliminate reporting inaccuracies and has the potential to reduce the effort required to track changes while providing more continuous information.

Telemonitoring

Telemonitoring has been examined in patients with marked functional compromise: New York Heart Association (NYHA) Class III or IV (see Table 17.1 for definitions).[21] Such patients are at high risk of symptom exacerbation and hospital readmission. In 2002, a team of investigators in the UK published a comprehensive systematic review of international telemonitoring studies for congestive heart failure.[22] They defined telemonitoring as the 'home monitoring of patients using special telecare devices in conjunction with a telecommunication system'.[22] The systematic review included published studies and abstracts presented at international meetings from 1996 to 2002. Most of the studies identified were observational in design; others were trials consisting of non-randomized, control groups, such as historical controls, or comparison with past cost data, and some were randomized trials without adequate power calculations for sample size determination. The authors concluded that although telemonitoring might have a significant role in improving the effectiveness of care for patients with heart failure, as suggested by some studies, more evidence was required. Specifically, large-scale, multicentre, randomized, controlled trials (RCTs) that are adequately powered for clinically relevant outcomes would be required before broader adoption of telemonitoring could be recommended.

Since 2002, the results from four large-scale, randomized, controlled trials have been published.[23-26] Table 17.2 summarizes these studies, including their study designs, results and conclusions. There are differences in population, setting, interventions and outcome measures between these studies. For example, two studies enrolled only participants with NYHA Class III or IV heart failure[23,24], a third study enrolled

Table 17.1. New York Heart Association functional classification system[21]

Functional classification	Degree of symptom intolerance
Level I	No symptoms
Level II	Symptoms with moderate/marked activity
Level III	Symptoms with mild activity
Level IV	Symptoms at rest

Table 17.2. Large-scale, randomized, controlled trials of telemonitoring for congestive heart failure (published from 2003 to 2005). NYHA = New York Heart Association

Study feature	Study			
	Benatar et al, 2003[23]	Goldberg et al, 2003[24]	Galbreath et al, 2004[25]	Cleland et al, 2005[26]
Objective	• To compare heart failure outcomes of two healthcare delivery methods for three months after discharge	• To determine whether daily reporting of body weight and symptoms in patients with advanced heart failure would reduce rehospitalization and mortality	• To determine effectiveness of telephone-based disease management programmes in a large, heterogeneous population of patients with congestive heart failure	• To determine whether home telemonitoring improves outcomes compared with nurse telephone support and usual care for patients with heart failure at high risk of hospitalization or death
Study design	• Prospective, randomized, controlled trial • Single centre in US	• Prospective, randomized, controlled trial • Multicentre in US	• Prospective, randomized, controlled trial • Single centre in US	• Prospective, randomized, controlled trial • Multicentre in UK, Germany and Netherlands
Participants	• 216 participants (NYHA Class III or IV) randomized to: – nurse telephone management (n=108) – home nurse visits (n=108)	• 280 patients (NYHA Class III or IV) from 16 heart failure centres randomized to: – intervention group (n=138) – standard care (n=142)	• 1069 patients (NYHA Class I to IV, stratified for analysis) randomized in a 2:1 ratio to – disease management intervention (n=710) – usual care (n=359) • Additional randomization in intervention group to subgroup that received blood pressure monitor and oximeter	• 426 patients (symptomatically controlled on enrolment, with previous NYHA Class IV episodes) randomized in a 2:2:1 ratio – home telemonitoring (n=168) – nurse telephone support (n=173) – usual care (n=85)
Outcome measures	• Heart failure readmissions and hospital length of stay • Heart failure hospitalization charges • Anxiety, depression, self-efficacy and quality of life	• Hospital readmission rate • Mortality • Heart failure readmission rate • Hospital emergency department visitation rate • Quality of life	• All-cause mortality • Performance on six-minute walk test • Improvement in functional therapeutic class • Total healthcare costs	• Primary endpoint: duration of survival or hospitalized for nurse telephone support or home telemonitoring after 240 days • Other measures: all-cause mortality, symptoms and optimization of medication

Table 17.2. *continued*

Study feature	Study			
	Benatar *et al*, 2003[23]	**Goldberg *et al*, 2003**[24]	**Galbreath *et al*, 2004**[25]	**Cleland *et al*, 2005**[26]
Intervention	• Telephone management consisted of home monitoring of body weight, blood pressure, heart rate and oxygen saturation, transmitted daily to a secure Internet site • Advanced practice nurse working with cardiologist subsequently treated patients via telephone	• Specialist physician-directed daily monitoring of body weight and symptoms, with a monitor linked via a standard telephone line to a computerized database monitored by trained cardiac nurses • Changes outside parameters reported to doctor	• Contract with disease management firm with care directed by physicians • Programme administered telephonically - initially weekly and then monthly • All members of disease management treatment group received scales; half also had blood pressure and oximeter monitoring, activity monitors for 2–6 weeks and thoracic impedance cardiac output measured at six months	• Home telemonitoring consisted of twice-daily patient self-measurement of body weight, blood pressure, heart rate and rhythm, with sensors connected wirelessly to a hub and transmitted to a cardiology centre • Nurse also made a monthly telephone call • Nurse telephone support consisted of specialist nurses who were available to patients by telephone
Control	• Home nurse visit followed heart failure programme clinical pathways • 9–12 visits over five weeks	• Standard care (i.e. outpatient therapy, including recommendation for daily assessment of body weight; most patients in heart failure programme with additional nursing resources)	• Usual care (i.e. managed as usual by physicians)	• Usual care (i.e. patient management plan sent to primary care physician who was asked to implement it)

Table 17.2. *continued*

Study feature	Study			
	Benatar *et al*, 2003[23]	**Goldberg *et al*, 2003**[24]	**Galbreath *et al*, 2004**[25]	**Cleland *et al*, 2005**[26]
Results	• After three months, the telephone management group had highly significant reductions in heart failure readmissions, with shorter lengths of stay • Hospitalization charges were significantly less for telephone management group at three months, as were cumulative readmission charges at 6 and 12 months • Quality-of-life scores significantly improved for both groups	• No observed differences in hospitalization rates • Highly significant reduction in mortality for intervention group	• Significant reduction in mortality rate with telephonic disease management • Total and congestive heart failure-related healthcare utilization – including medications, office or emergency department visits, procedures or hospitalizations – not decreased by disease management	• No significant difference in days lost as a result of death or hospitalization • Number of admissions and mortality similar among patients assigned to nurse telephone support or home telemonitoring, but mean duration of admission and number of home and office visits reduced substantially with home telemonitoring compared with nurse telephone support • Patients receiving usual care had higher one-year mortality than patients assigned to nurse telephone support or home telemonitoring
Conclusions	• Telephone monitoring of patients with heart failure with advanced practice nurse care under the guidance of a cardiologist significantly improves heart failure management while reducing cost of care	• Cardiologist-driven, in-home daily body weight and symptom monitoring system in advanced heart failure has mortality benefits • Survival improved without increasing healthcare resource utilization	• Participation in disease management resulted in significant survival benefit, most notably in symptomatic patients with systolic heart failure; healthcare resource utilization not reduced by disease management • Disease management conferred no cost saving	• Reduction in mortality without an increase in duration of time spent in hospital • Further investigation and refinement of home telemonitoring warranted, as it may be valuable for the management of selected patients with heart failure

symptomatically stable patients with previous NYHA IV episodes[26] and the fourth targeted a more heterogeneous population that included patients with NYHA I to IV classifications.[25]

Two studies were multicentre trials; one was conducted in the US and the other in Europe.[25,26] One study recruited patients from clinical sites with cardiac transplant centres or community-based cardiology practices,[24] and another recruited from hospitals without a comprehensive heart failure management organization.[26] One of the single-centre studies was based in a specialized unit with cardiologists and advanced nurse practitioners,[23] and the other study centred on a disease management service with back-up from primary care physicians.[25]

The telemonitoring interventions varied between the studies, as did the standard care provided to the control groups. One study compared transtelephonic home monitoring of body weight and symptoms to standard outpatient heart failure therapy.[24] The other three studies included transtelephonic physiological monitoring of blood pressure and other physiological variables in addition to body weight.[23–26] Two of these studies included a second intervention arm of nurse telephone support.[25,26] Standard care in the first of these studies was home nurse visits,[23] and in the other two studies, the control group received the usual care provided by the referring physician.[25,26]

The most frequent outcome measures in the studies were hospital readmissions,[23–26] mortality,[24–26] quality of life,[23,24] hospitalization charges[23] and total costs.[25] The study that compared telemonitoring of physiological variables with home nurse visits reported a highly significant reduction in readmissions for heart failure, with a corresponding reduction in hospitalization charges.[23] The other three studies found no significant difference in readmissions; however, all three reported a significant reduction in mortality without an increase in healthcare resource utilization.[24–26]

The findings of the Trans-European Network-Home-Care Management System (TEN-HMS) study are of particular interest. This study compared the value of home telemonitoring with nurse telephone support. Although the number of admissions and mortality were similar among patients randomly assigned to nurse telephone support and home telemonitoring, the mean duration of hospital admissions and the number of home and office visits were substantially reduced with home telemonitoring compared with nurse telephone support.[26] Another finding of note was from the study that enrolled the most heterogeneous patient population, in which the greatest survival benefit was observed in the most symptomatic patients with systolic heart failure.[25]

In summary, evidence is emerging in support of the positive benefits of telemonitoring for congestive heart failure. However, given the heterogeneity of the studies and the multifaceted nature of the interventions, much work remains to be done to establish the incremental value of specific interventions for particular subgroups of patients.

Additional experience

In the US, the Veterans Health Administration has extensive experience with telemonitoring for congestive heart failure and other chronic diseases. Chapter 9 summarizes that experience.

In Boston, the Partners Home Care and Partners Telemedicine organizations have examined the effect of home-based monitoring from the perspective of a home-care nursing agency. Home healthcare traditionally has been a less costly alternative to hospitalization, and many patients prefer the home setting to the hospital. The current manpower shortage in home healthcare, coupled with increasing labour and administrative costs, has motivated care providers to evaluate new technologies for home-based care.

A non-randomized, controlled trial was conducted to assess the effectiveness of home telemonitoring devices in patients with Class III or IV congestive heart failure.[27] The intervention group received home telemonitoring for two months after hospital discharge (n=83). A cohort of historical controls received usual care, which consisted of home nurse visits (n=83). Patients in the telemonitoring group transmitted their body weight, blood pressure and oxygen saturation daily to a telenurse, who evaluated each patient with a follow-up telephone call. The end points included the number of home nursing visits, rehospitalization rate, use of the emergency department and costs. The quality of life of the intervention group at the start and end of the study period was also measured.

Patients in the telemonitoring group required significantly fewer home nursing visits than the usual care group, which resulted in cost savings. No significant differences were seen in hospitalizations or emergency room visits. Patients in the telemonitoring group reported improved quality of life over the course of the study. The study thus suggests that daily home-care telemonitoring can reduce the frequency of home nursing visits required and provide cost savings with improvement in patient-perceived quality of life. These findings are preliminary, however, given the non-randomized study design and the potential for bias due to confounding variables. In addition, the study did not distinguish the effect of telemonitoring from the daily nurse telephone call in the reduced need for home nursing visits.

The American government-funded health insurance scheme for people aged over 64 years and those with disabilities, Medicare, recently began a pilot programme to improve chronic care. One element of this pilot work is that improvement plans for chronic care must include, where possible, monitoring technologies that enable patient guidance through the exchange of pertinent clinical information, such as vital signs, symptomatic information and health self-assessment. The experience gained from the demonstration projects under way should improve our understanding of the effectiveness of disease management and telemonitoring interventions for congestive heart failure.

Technologies for telemonitoring

Several systems for remote monitoring of patients with congestive heart failure are commercially available. Fig. 17.2 illustrates the basic components. In general, a number of patient devices are connected by telecommunications links to clinician information systems. Patients typically use the system once each day, usually at a scheduled time, to collect and transmit health information.

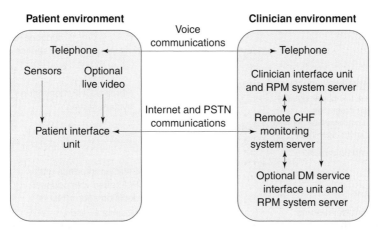

Fig. 17.2. Generalized design of commercial remote systems for monitoring patients with congestive heart failure. PSTN is the ordinary telephone network

Current approaches

Although all commercially available remote monitoring solutions for congestive heart failure are designed to meet the same clinical needs, variations in technological approaches exist (Fig. 17.3). In the patient's environment, the equipment typically includes a number of sensors for measuring variables such as body weight and blood

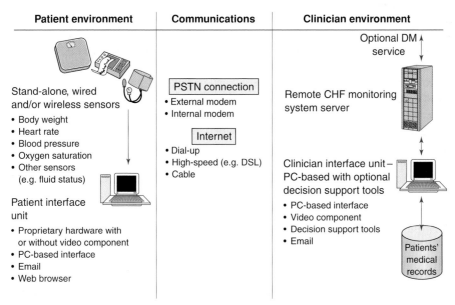

Fig. 17.3. Design variations in current remote systems for monitoring patients with congestive heart failure

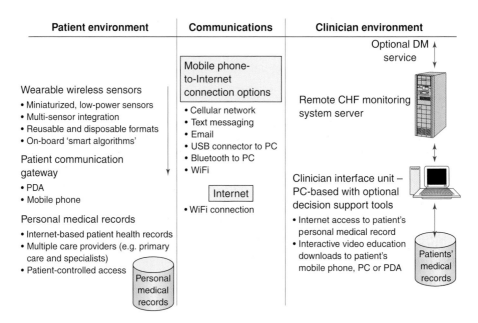

Patient environment

Communications

Clinician environment

Wearable wireless sensors
• Miniaturized, low-power sensors
• Multi-sensor integration
• Reusable and disposable formats
• On-board 'smart algorithms'

Patient communication gateway
• PDA
• Mobile phone

Personal medical records
• Internet-based patient health records
• Multiple care providers (e.g. primary care and specialists)
• Patient-controlled access

Personal medical records

Mobile phone-to-Internet connection options
• Cellular network
• Text messaging
• Email
• USB connector to PC
• Bluetooth to PC
• WiFi

Internet
• WiFi connection

Optional DM service

Remote CHF monitoring system server

Clinician interface unit – PC-based with optional decision support tools
• Internet access to patient's personal medical record
• Interactive video education downloads to patient's mobile phone, PC or PDA

Patients' medical records

Fig. 17.4. Technology options for future remote systems for monitoring patients with congestive heart failure

pressure (including pulse rate). These sensors can be wired or connected wirelessly to a patient interface unit in the home. Symptoms can also be monitored at the patient interface unit through keyboard entry of patient responses to individualized questions. The physiological and symptom data are then transmitted to a central server for storage and subsequent review by clinicians.

In addition to physiological sensors and symptom monitoring, some patient interface units include a videoconferencing unit to enable a clinician to conduct teleconsultations. During teleconsultations, the patient performs measurements of vital signs, which are immediately transmitted to the clinician. The information can also be stored automatically in the patient's electronic medical record (EMR).

Two other important technologies in systems for remote monitoring of patients with congestive heart failure are email and 'smart' systems design. Email has made it possible to efficiently manage part of the non-critical communication between patients and clinicians. Smart systems design – the use of knowledge-based, optimizing algorithms – allows better management of the patient's information and improved decision-making for clinicians as well as patients. Smart systems design is not new, but the recent availability of more powerful computers has made it possible to move the requisite processing into the communications interfaces and sensor devices themselves. As a result, sensor devices now are designed to capture physiological measurements as well as compute and store data trends. Smart interactive, personalized, health questionnaires have become a common patient interface feature.

In addition, advanced information management and decision-support tools are becoming available.

Future approaches

Wireless technology, mobile devices, the Internet and smart systems design are likely to transform remote monitoring for congestive heart failure (Fig. 17.4). As monitoring moves from the hospital to the home, the simplicity and ease of use of technology becomes particularly important. Most patients and families have no medical training and are under considerable health-related stress. In addition, patients and families are concerned about the 'medicalization' of the home environment when devices are installed there. Therefore, a number of research groups are trying to develop minimally intrusive, 'wear-and-forget' sensors that fit into the lifestyle of patients at home and in the community. The design of one such system, developed by a team of investigators at the Massachusetts General Hospital and the Center for the Integration of Medicine and Innovative Technology (CIMIT), is illustrated in Fig. 17.5.

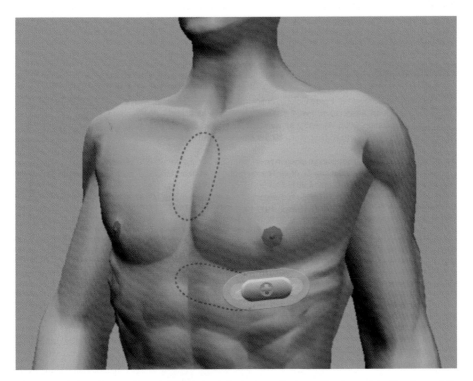

Fig. 17.5. Artists impression of CIMIT physiological monitoring adhesive patch. Courtesy of Dr Nathaniel Sims' laboratory and CIMIT (work supported by USAMRAA)

Conclusion

Home telehealth for congestive heart failure shows promise and its use is growing. The number of well-designed, large-scale, randomized, controlled trials is increasing. Nonetheless, many questions remain. The benefits of telemonitoring compared to telephone intervention and traditional disease management for particular subgroups of patients must be explored further. The question is what should be done and for whom? Technology innovation is likely to continue to drive what can be done, but the evidence already suggests a great opportunity to improve the lives of patients with congestive heart disease and their families.

Further information

Coye MJ. *Remote patient management: the sleeper technology. Most Wired* 2005 24 January. Available at: www.healthtech.org/Common_site/news/docs/Molly_ MostWired_RPM.pdf (last accessed 22 December 2005).

New England Health Care Institute. *Remote physiological monitoring: innovation in the management of heart failure*. Cambridge, MA: New England Health Care Institute, 2005. Available at: www.nehi.net/CMS/viewPage.cfm?pageId=29 (last accessed 14 December 2005).

References

1   McMurray JJ, Stewart S. Epidemiology, aetiology, and prognosis of heart failure. *Heart* 2000;**83**:596–602.
2   American Heart Association. *Heart disease and stroke statistics – 2005 update*. Dallas, TX: American Heart Association, 2005. Available at: www.americanheart.org (last accessed 14 December 2005).
3   Remme WJ, Swedberg K. Guidelines for the diagnosis and treatment of chronic heart failure. *Eur Heart J* 2001;**22**:1527–60.
4   Kannel WB. Vital epidemiologic clues in heart failure. *J Clin Epidemiol* 2000;**53**:229–35.
5   Stewart S, Jenkins A, Buchan S, *et al*. The current cost of heart failure to the National Health Service in the UK. *Eur J Heart Fail* 2002;**4**:361–71.
6   O'Connell JB, Bristow MR. Economic impact of heart failure in the US: time for a different approach. *J Heart Lung Transplant* 1994;**13** (Suppl):107–12.
7   Stewart S, MacIntyre K, Hole DJ, *et al*. More 'malignant' than cancer? Five-year survival following a first admission for heart failure. *Eur J Heart Fail* 2001;**3**:315–22.
8   Jaagosild P, Dawson NV, Thomas C, *et al*. Outcomes of acute exacerbation of severe congestive heart failure: quality of life, resource use, and survival. SUPPORT Investigators. The study to understand prognosis and preferences for outcomes and risks of treatments. *Arch Intern Med* 1998;**158**:1081–9.
9   Davis RC, Hobbs FD, Lip GY. ABC of heart failure: history and epidemiology. *BMJ* 2000;**320**:39–42.
10 Hobbs FD. The scale of heart failure: diagnosis and management issues for primary care. *Heart* 1998;**82** (Suppl IV):8–10.
11 National Center for Chronic Disease Prevention and Health Promotion. *Diabetes surveillance system: hospitalization for heart failure as first-listed diagnosis*. Atlanta, GA: National Center for Chronic Disease Prevention and Health Promotion, 2005. Available at: www.cdc.gov/diabetes/statistics/cvdhosp/hf/table7.htm (last accessed 14 December 2005).
12 Haldeman GA, Croft JB, Giles WH, Rashidee A. Hospitalization of patients with heart failure: National Hospital Discharge Survey, 1985 to 1995. *Am Heart J* 1999;**137**:352–60.
13 Krumholz HM, Amatruda J, Smith GL, *et al*. Randomized trial of an education and support intervention to prevent readmission of patients with heart failure. *J Am Coll Cardiol* 2002;**39**:83–9.

14   Opasich C, Febo O, Riccardi PG, *et al.* Concomitant factors of decompensation in chronic heart failure. *Am J Cardiol* 1996;**78**:354–7.

15   McAlister FA, Stewart S, Ferrua S, McMurray JJ. Multidisciplinary strategies for the management of heart failure patients at high risk for admission: a systematic review of randomized trials. *J Am Coll Cardiol* 2004;**44**:810–19.

16   Gonseth J, Guallar-Castillon P, Banegas JR, Rodriguez-Artalejo F. The effectiveness of disease management programmes in reducing hospital re-admission in older patients with heart failure: a systematic review and meta-analysis of published reports. *Eur Heart J* 2004;**25**:1570–95.

17   Phillips CO, Wright SM, Kern DE, *et al.* Comprehensive discharge planning with post-discharge support for older patients with congestive heart failure: a meta-analysis. *JAMA* 2004;**291**:1358–67.

18   Krause DS. Economic effectiveness of disease management programs: a meta-analysis. *Dis Manage* 2005;**8**:114–34.

19   GESICA Investigators. Randomised trial of telephone intervention in chronic heart failure: DIAL trial. *BMJ* 2005;**331**:425–9.

20   Mengden T, Hernandez Medina RM, Beltran B, *et al.* Reliability of reporting of self-measured blood pressure values by hypertensive patients. *Am J Hypertens* 1998;**11**:1413–17.

21   New York Heart Association. *Nomenclature and criteria for diagnosis of diseases of the heart and great vessels.* New York: New York Heart Association, 1963.

22   Louis AA, Turner T, Gretton M, *et al.* A systematic review of telemonitoring for the management of heart failure. *Eur J Heart Fail* 2003;**5**:583–90.

23   Benatar D, Bondmass M, Ghitelman J, Avitall B. Outcomes of chronic heart failure. *Arch Intern Med* 2003;**163**:347–52.

24   Goldberg LR, Piette JD, Walsh MN, *et al.* Randomized trial of a daily electronic home monitoring system in patients with advanced heart failure: the Weight Monitoring in Heart Failure (WHARF) trial. *Am Heart J* 2003;**146**;705–12.

25   Galbreath AD, Krasuski RA, Smith B, *et al.* Long-term healthcare and cost outcomes of disease management in a large, randomized, community-based population with heart failure. *Circulation* 2004;**110**:3518–26.

26   Cleland JG, Louis AA, Rigby AS, *et al.* Noninvasive home telemonitoring for patients with heart failure at high risk of recurrent admission and death: the Trans-European Network-Home-Care Management System (TEN-HMS) study. *J Am Coll Cardiol* 2005;**45**:1654–64.

27   Myers S, Grant RW, Lugn N, *et al.* Impact of home-based monitoring on the care of patients with congestive heart failure (submitted).

▶18

Home health monitoring

Shigeru Ohta, Hiroshi Nakamoto, Yoshimitsu Shinagawa and Toshio Kishimoto

Introduction

In Japan, one-quarter of the population will soon be older than 65 years as a consequence of the increasing life span and the decreasing birth rate. Consequently, more social services will be needed, such as home helps for elderly people living alone. Japan has been a keen developer of monitoring systems for elderly people. Continuous monitoring may be of physical activities, physiological functions or daily habits in order to estimate a health condition.

Many kinds of techniques for monitoring the elderly exist. For example, satellite navigation (the global positioning system, GPS) and mobile phones can be used to track mentally confused elderly people if they wander outside the house.[1] People being monitored, however, need to carry the necessary devices at all times. Although the equipment can be incorporated into clothing, it may not be worn if it is too heavy. Monitoring that does not require the person to carry a sensor therefore may be preferable.

Monitoring systems can be categorized into four groups, depending on how the monitoring is performed and what is measured (Table 18.1). Wireless monitoring requires a sensor, such as a pedometer, that is carried at all times but does not restrict the movement of the person monitored. Passive monitoring does not require sensors to be attached to the human body; for example, a person's presence in a room can be sensed with a motion detector. Vital signs monitoring deals with variables such as heart rate, blood pressure and body temperature. Motor function monitoring is concerned with posture, walking and position. Examples of the four categories include:

- category A: wireless monitoring of vital signs
- category B: wireless monitoring of motor functions

Table 18.1. Classification system for home monitoring

Method of monitoring	Category	
	Vital signs monitored	Motor functions monitored
Wireless	A	B
Passive	C	D

- category C: passive monitoring of vital signs
- category D: passive monitoring of motor function.

Category A: wireless monitoring of vital signs

A number of groups have demonstrated the wireless monitoring of blood pressure.[2-4] Yang et al monitored pulse waves.[5]

Category B: wireless monitoring of motor functions

Information about posture and walking condition can be derived from the output of an accelerometer worn by a subject, and a GPS device can be used to track elderly people. The combination of an accelerometer and GPS allows detailed information about physical activity and the location of a subject to be obtained.

Category C: passive monitoring of vital signs

Tamura et al monitored distribution of body temperature with sensors installed in a bed and applied this to measure body movement during sleep, which was calculated from the transition of body temperature distribution.[6-8] Acebo et al monitored sleep with pressure sensors and measured the time of falling asleep and wakening.[9] Ishijima et al monitored the electrocardiogram (ECG) during sleep with a specially woven sheet of conductive threads.[10] This method represented the ideal of wireless ECG monitoring during sleep and also enabled monitoring of respiration.[11] The same group showed that it was possible to carry out ECG monitoring while the monitored person was taking a bath.[12] Tamura et al also constructed a system for monitoring pulse wave and respiration.[13] Yamaguchi et al monitored body weight, stool weight and leg blood pressure while the person was in the lavatory.[14] They also measured body weight changes during defecation using ballistocardiography. This technique led to an integrated health-monitoring system.[15,16]

Category D: passive monitoring of motor functions

Celler et al installed infrared, light, temperature and magnetic sensors in various rooms and a refrigerator in the house of an elderly person.[17] The data allowed monitoring of the frequency of use of each room and the refrigerator. Yamaguchi et al extended this idea and tracked the movement of the inhabitant inside a house.[14]

Advantages and disadvantages

The advantages of monitoring using wireless techniques (categories A and B) are that the measurements are precise. This approach, however, is not appropriate for long-term monitoring of elderly people, because carrying a sensor is a burden on the person monitored, and the sensor may not be carried all the time.

Passive monitoring of vital signs (category C) is appropriate for long-term monitoring. Vital signs are useful for health monitoring, although artefacts in category C are larger than those of category A. The space needed for appropriate sensor placement may prevent continuous monitoring. The signal data obtained, such as the ECG, may not be in accordance with the standard format used in medicine. Interpretation of such data therefore needs to be agreed upon in advance.

Category D, passive measurement, also allows long-term monitoring. Infrared sensors can be used in various rooms, but it is difficult to estimate the health condition of people from their location in a house. Togawa pointed out that elderly people had little privacy because of the monitoring system.[18] Privacy should be respected; it is easy to watch elderly people with a video camera inside a house, but such direct monitoring would not be acceptable to everyone.

Conventional emergency call systems do not fall into the categories A–D, as they require active operation of a transmitter that is carried by the user. These systems seem to function well in many countries.[19] One reason may be that the elderly people are allowed to make calls for less important matters. In Japan, however, which at present does not have sufficient numbers of home helpers, many local governments limit the use of emergency call systems to real emergencies.

Health monitoring

Long-term monitoring is valuable because it establishes a baseline against which current data can be evaluated. However, monitoring cannot be carried out in the long term if the system disturbs users' lives or puts them under pressure. Ideally, monitoring should be wholly unobtrusive. We therefore have developed a remote health-monitoring system for elderly people living alone.[20,21] Our health-monitoring system falls into category D. We have monitored the daily health status of elderly people living alone by placing infrared sensors, which sense body temperature, in their homes. The people are monitored without operating any sensor, without wires and without them being aware.

System configuration

The architecture of our system is shown in Fig 18.1. An in-house unit gathered data from the infrared sensors and controlled external communications. The time (to the nearest millisecond) when the sensors detected movement of human bodies was sent to an offsite server via an asymmetric digital subscriber line (ADSL). Information was then stored in the database for subsequent analysis. When the server received a request for information from family members (typically a son or daughter) who were living away from the elderly person, it retrieved the necessary data and automatically converted it into hypertext markup language (HTML) format. Family members thus could view the latest information about their relative via their personal computers.

Data gathering

Many kinds of sensors are used to monitor vital signs,[10,12,14,15,18] but it is hard to select one that can be used for a long time without the person being conscious of it, which restricts movement. The time when electrical appliances are used in the home can be

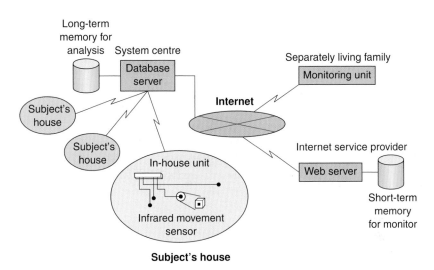

Fig. 18.1. Block diagram of the health-monitoring system. Movement data are sent to a database server via an in-house unit and stored in a database for subsequent analysis. Periodically, new data are converted into HTML format and posted to a web server. Other family members can examine the data from personal computers via the Internet

detected, and the consumption of electricity, gas or water can be measured. Some appliances, however, consume energy at all times – such as a refrigerator. We decided that infrared sensors were the best way to monitor elderly people in their homes.

We continuously monitored clients' in-house movements by placing infrared sensors at various points in each house (Fig. 18.2). The sensors used a passive infrared sensing (PIR) element (AMP2109 and AMN1111-2; Matsushita Electric Works, Japan). The infrared sensors could detect the heat (at a wavelength over 5 μm) radiated from human bodies.[14] Therefore, when a person was in a sensor's field of view, a signal was obtained from the sensor. This signal changed to off when the heat-emitting body moved out of the sensor's field of view. As the sensors could not differentiate more than one heat source, we received contaminated signals when the person had visitors. Although the sensors also reacted to cats and dogs, this effect was negligible in the preliminary trials.

Because the sensors were inexpensive, we were able to place them in every appropriate room of the person's house. The sensors recorded the exact time when someone entered the room. Knowing when and where the previous sensor had been activated, we could calculate the speed and distance moved by the person.

Many medical emergencies occur in bathrooms and lavatories; however, infrared sensors are unsuitable for areas of high temperature or high humidity. We therefore placed the infrared sensor in the changing room next to the bathroom (a common arrangement in Japanese homes), but used a water-resistant emergency call button in the bathroom itself.

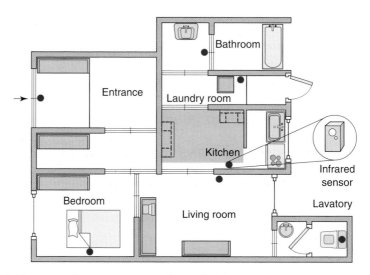

Fig. 18.2. Placement of movement sensors in a typical Japanese house

Classification of behaviour patterns

We monitored eight elderly people who were living in their own houses, and obtained data for more than 155 months in total. The details are shown in Table 18.2. It was difficult to use the raw data obtained from the infrared sensors directly, because the sensors recorded only the time when they detected and lost sight of the person. We therefore analysed the raw data using statistical methods because of the large numbers of data points.

Table 18.2. Participants monitored

Participant	Sex	Age (years)	Date monitoring started	Duration (months)
A	Woman	83	July 1996	5
B	Woman	87	October 1996	8
C	Woman	85	August 1996	19
D	Woman	73	January 2000	20
E	Man	90	April 2000	47
F	Woman	85	April 2001	30
G	Woman	73	May 2001	34
H	Woman	73	July 2001	32

Results

Infrared sensors generate a few erroneous signals as a result of artefacts. To confirm the reliability of the sensors, we checked the miscounts from sensors in a person's house when it was vacant for a week. The one-week average of total recorded counts included true counts and miscounts. The error rate of the sensors was defined as the one-week miscounts divided by the one-week total counts. The error rate was <0.06%, which indicates the reliability of the sensors used in the experiment.

Measurement of in-house movements

The sensors were installed so that they each covered one room. Thus, if the sensor in the living room was activated, it meant that a person was present in that room. Long-term monitoring showed that the pattern of movements of the people in their houses was reasonably constant. The in-house movements can be represented in a transition diagram (Fig. 18.3). The person's location, which is indicated by the sensor number, is plotted against time. The time of meals or sleep can be estimated from this diagram.

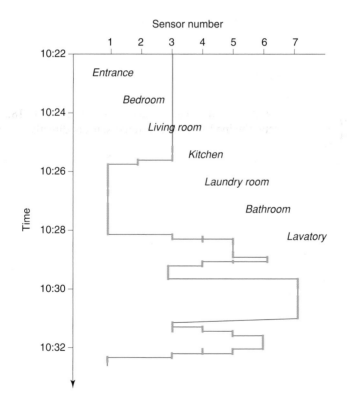

Fig. 18.3. Example of a transition diagram (representation of the person's movements in their house). The location of the elderly person at any time can be checked on this diagram. Thick vertical lines represent periods when the sensors were activated, and thin lines represent the transition to another sensor. The person's location, which is indicated by the sensor number, is plotted against time. The time of meals or sleep can also be estimated from this diagram

Classification of behaviour patterns

Although daily activity patterns did not vary greatly, it was difficult to identify immediately the occurrence of illness or injury. Nevertheless, it was possible to classify the days as usual or unusual based on:

- duration of stay in each room
- no-response time interval
- movement patterns.

When the data were out of the expected range or when the trend deviated from the average, the day was categorized as an unusual day. A relationship between health conditions and movement patterns could be inferred in this way. For example, during the monitoring trials, we detected one case of overstaying in a lavatory, which was caused by the person having severe diarrhoea. When an unusual pattern was found, our monitoring system informed the family members by telephone or email. After an emergency was detected, family members called the person immediately. If necessary, consultation with a doctor was arranged. If a sudden disease or accident was suspected, a home help or ambulance was arranged. Thus, by using human analysis, we increased the credibility of our system's problem detection.

Our unrestricted long-term monitoring has potential for managing the medical problems of the elderly living alone. We found 80 unusual days indicated by overstaying in any room during 20 months of monitoring of four people. At this rate, every family would receive one telephone call (or email message) once a month on average.

The distance between any given two detector-sensing areas can be measured easily. This allows the total moving distance for a day to be estimated. Each sensor covered

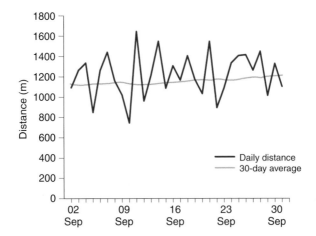

Fig. 18.4. Daily distance moved by the person in the house over the course of a month. The thin line shows the 30-day moving average. Daily moving distance is a rough index of health status, because a decrease is likely to reflect illness

an area of about 2 m in diameter, so the calculated moving distance was approximate. However, we think that it can be used as an index of health condition, because a decrease may reflect illness (as well as absence, for example). Fig. 18.4 shows an example of the fluctuation of these values over one month for one person: the clear upward trend suggests improving health.

Comparison between sensor responses

Histograms of the sensor responses provide information about the person; Fig. 18.5 shows the number of sensor events during each 30-minute period. The infrared sensor we used had a 10-second holding time after it detected a change in its field of view. If another change occurred during the holding time of 10 seconds, the 'on' state would continue. This means few on/off events if a person moved frequently in a room. To solve this problem, when an on period continued for more than one minute, we added to the event total (that is, if the on period was recorded as three minutes, it would be counted as an extra three on/off transitions). The vertical axis of Fig. 18.5 expresses this modified event frequency. Each histogram bar is approximately proportional to the total period for which the person stayed at that time.

We can classify the data as usual or unusual by matching the pattern to previously stored data. However, simple matching may not be appropriate. For example, someone may have a habit of getting up early, although the exact time is not always the same. Matching by time is therefore inapplicable. Instead, we used the dynamic programming matching method.[22–24] This is commonly used in the field of speech recognition, where time variations due to delay have been well studied in human speech analysis.

Maximum duration of stay in a room

We found that the duration of stay in a room that has a specific purpose, such as a lavatory or kitchen, showed a consistent pattern. Fig. 18.6 shows the maximum stay in

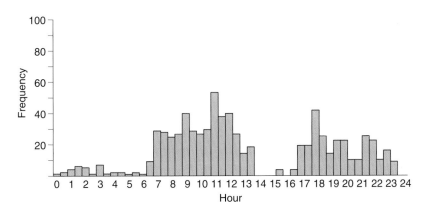

Fig. 18.5. Movement events detected by a sensor over 24 hours (each bar covers 30 minutes). Movement data can be classified as usual or unusual by matching the current pattern to previously stored data

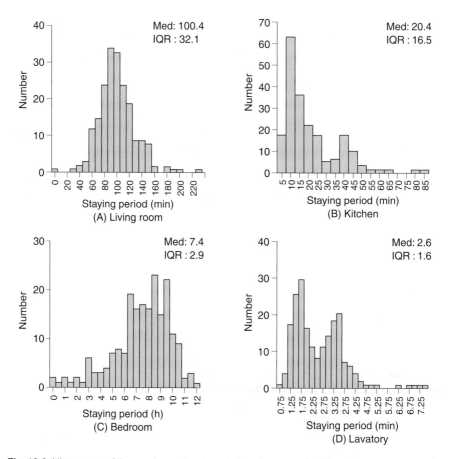

Fig. 18.6. Histograms of the maximum duration of stay of a person in different rooms over one day: living room (A), kitchen (B), bedroom (C) and lavatory (D). Length of stay in a specific room, such as a lavatory or a kitchen, is characteristic of the person. From the values of median (Med) and interquartile range (IQR) shown here, the distribution of maximum length of stay in each room seems fairly predictable

each room for one day for participant C (see Table 18.2), as well as the median and interquartile range for each room. The distribution of maximum duration of stay in each room was reasonably constant. We added an automatic emergency call function to our system by checking the duration of stay in specific places in a house.

Discussion

In our health-monitoring system, measurement was achieved without a person being conscious of it and without restricting their movement with wires. Measurements could therefore be made for a long period – 155 months in total. The use of a video camera would have deprived the people of their privacy. In this sense, a camera is not a desirable monitoring tool. The information obtained from infrared sensors does not reflect a person's health condition directly, but the pattern of the person's movements can still be analysed to determine whether it is usual or unusual. There are some limitations: for example, infrared sensors can detect a person's movements but cannot identify the reason for them. We found that people had their own specific daily pattern of movements and particular personal characteristics, such as how long they stayed in one type of room. We also found that such patterns are influenced by daily environmental conditions, such as weather or temperature. We are able to estimate a person's health condition by checking the duration of stay in specific rooms, such as the lavatory, in comparison with the previous data. If an unusual state is detected after analysis, we can inform the family of the incident. One person was hospitalized after the system identified decreased patterns of activity in their house.

The monitoring system can detect an unusual state by analysing the current information and comparing it with past data. However, it is still difficult to detect immediately an emergency, such as sudden illness or injury. A rapid reaction from family members who live away from their parent is also required. When the system informs them of an unusual state that indicates a possible emergency, the family members must confirm the elderly person's real health condition by, for example, telephoning the person or a neighbour. If a sudden illness or accident is suspected, a home help or ambulance should be arranged. Infrared sensors are suitable for unrestricted monitoring. They are inexpensive, small and need little maintenance.

We asked six of the eight subjects who were still living alone if they wished to continue monitoring after the experiment was over. All six answered in the affirmative. The system reduced anxiety for both the monitored people themselves and their family members by providing family members with information on the monitored person's health condition through the Internet. The system is very valuable for monitoring the health condition of elderly people who live alone.

Other similar systems

In 2002, when we published our research,[20,21] the Japanese company Matsushita Electric Works, who originally provided our infrared sensors, commercialized the basic concept of our system. Their monitoring system informs family members of the current location of a person via a mobile phone, but without any statistical analysis, which is the unique feature of the Japanese system.

In 2004, a commercial monitoring system called Quiet Care was introduced in the American system. This seems to operate in a very similar way to our system. Quiet Care deduces the location of a person in their home and also provides information on the basis of normal patterns of behaviour.

In 2005, a subsidiary of Nippon Telegraph and Telephone Corporation, Marketing Act, released a monitoring system. The system was called 'Mimamori eye' – literally 'a watching eye' in Japanese. The basic concept of the Mimamori system is the same as our monitoring system. With the use of infrared sensors in the house of an elderly person, Mimamori tracks the location of the person in the house, detects a motionless condition that lasts a long time and displays the data on its website. Minor differences are that the call centre for the Mimamori system accepts questions about health from elderly people under its watch, notifies family members of an abnormal incident if anything happens, helps by calling an ambulance for emergencies, sends a message to family members in response to a simple button-push in the house and calls the elderly people to ascertain their health condition periodically. This system is being adopted by many local governments and welfare institutions in Japan.

Conclusion

In our health-monitoring system, measurement was achieved without the person being conscious of it and without restricting their movement. We found that each person had a specific pattern of movements. We estimated their health condition by comparing the duration of stay in specific rooms, such as the lavatory, with previously recorded data. The system can detect an unusual state by analysing the current information and comparing it with past data. When the system detects an unusual state that indicates a possible emergency, the family members must confirm the elderly person's health condition. If a sudden disease or an accident is suspected, a home help or an ambulance should be arranged. In our trial, six of eight people who were still living alone after the experiment finished wished to continue monitoring. The system reduced anxiety for the elderly people and their family members by giving information on health conditions to family members through the Internet. Thus, this system is very valuable for monitoring the health condition of elderly people who live alone.

Further information

Matsushita Electric Works website. Available at: www.naloc.co.jp/setumei/ MIMAMORINET/index.html. Note: this site can be viewed only in Japanese.
Mimamori eye website. Available at: www.mimamori-eye.com/ (last accessed 19 January 2006). Note: this site can be viewed only in Japanese.
Quiet Care website. Available at: www.quietcaresystems.com/how_it_works.htm (last accessed 19 January 2006).
Welfare System Research Association website. Available at: www.wesranet.com/ home_en.html (last accessed 21 November 2005).

References

1   Urakami D, Makikawa M. Ambulatory behavior map, physical activity and biosignal monitoring system. *Methods Inf Med* 1997;**36**:360–3.
2   Yamakoshi K, Rolfe P, Murphy C. Current developments in non-invasive measurement of arterial blood pressure. *J Biomed Eng* 1988;**10**:130–7.
3   Kawarada A, Shimazu H, Ito H, Yamakoshi K. Ambulatory monitoring of indirect beat-to-beat arterial pressure in human fingers by a volume-compensation method. *Med Biol Eng Comput* 1991;**29**:55–62.

4   Tanaka S, Yamakoshi K. Ambulatory instrument for monitoring indirect beat-to-beat blood pressure in superficial temporal artery using volume-compensation method. *Med Biol Eng Comput* 1996;**34**:441–7.

5   Yang BH, Rhee S, Asada H. A twenty-four hour tele-nursing system using a ring sensor. *Proceedings of the 1998 IEEE International Conference on Robotics and Automation, Leuven, Belgium,* May 1998:387–92.

6   Tamura T, Togawa T, Murata M. A bed temperature monitoring system for assessing body movement during sleep. *Clin Phys Physiol Meas* 1988;**9**:139–45.

7   Tamura T, Fujimoto T, Tsuji T, *et al.* Multichannel bed temperature recorder as a monitor of pressure sores. *J Clin Eng* 1990;**15**:315–20.

8   Tamura T, Zhou J, Mizukami H, Togawa T. A system for monitoring temperature distribution in bed and its application to the assessment of body movement. *Physiol Meas* 1993;**14**:33–41.

9   Acebo C, Watson RK, Bakos L, Thoman EB. Sleep and apnea in the elderly: reliability and validity of 24-hour recordings in the home. *Sleep* 1991;**14**:56–64.

10 Ishijima M. Monitoring of electrocardiograms in bed without utilizing body surface electrodes. *IEEE Trans Biomed Eng* 1993;**40**:593–94.

11 Ishijima M. Cardiopulmonary monitoring by textile electrodes without subject-awareness of being monitored. *Med Biol Eng Comput* 1997;**35**:685–90.

12 Ishijima M, Togawa T. Observation of electrocardiograms through tap water. *Clin Phys Physiol Meas* 1989;**10**:171–5.

13 Tamura T, Yoshimura T, Nakajima K, *et al.* Unconstrained heart-rate monitoring during bathing. *Biomed Instrum Technol* 1997;**31**:391–6.

14 Yamaguchi A, Ogawa M, Tamura T, Togawa T. Monitoring behavior in the home using positioning sensors. *Proceedings of the 20th Annual International Conference of the IEEE Engineering in Medical and Biological Society* 1998;**20**:1977–9.

15 Tamura T, Togawa T, Ogawa M, Yoda M. Fully automated health monitoring system in the home. *Med Eng Phys* 1998;**20**:573–9.

16 Ogawa M, Tamura T, Togawa T. Automated acquisition system for routine, noninvasive monitoring of physiological data. *Telemed J* 1998;**4**:177–85.

17 Celler BG, Earnshaw W, Ilsar ED, *et al.* Remote monitoring of health status of the elderly at home. A multidisciplinary project on aging at the University of New South Wales. Remote monitoring of health status of the elderly at home. *Int J Biomed Comput* 1995;**40**:147–55.

18 Togawa T. Home health monitoring. *J Med Dent Sci* 1998;**45**:151–60.

19 Ohguma Y. *Netakiri roujin no iru kuni inai kuni. [Bedridden elderly people: countries where this problem is critical].* Tokyo: Budosha, 1990:32-5 (in Japanese).

20 Ohta S, Nakamoto H, Shinagawa Y, Tanikawa T. A health monitoring system for elderly people living alone. *J Telemed Telecare* 2002;**8**:151–6.

21 Ohta S, Shinagawa Y, Tanikawa T, Nakamoto H. Remote health monitoring system for the elderly living alone. *Biocybern Biomed Eng* 2002;**22**:123–34.

22 Sakoe H, Chiba S. Dynamic programming algorithm optimization for spoken word recognition. *IEEE Trans Acoust* 1978;**ASSP-26**:43–9.

23 White G, Neely R. Speech recognition experiments with linear prediction, bandpass filtering and dynamic programming. *IEEE Trans Acoust* 1976;**ASSP-24**:183–8.

24 Sakoe H. Two-level DP matching algorithm, a dynamic programming based pattern matching algorithm for connected word recognition. *IEEE Trans Acoust* 1979;**ASSP-27**:588–95.

▶19

Home-based telecardiology

Simonetta Scalvini, Emanuela Zanelli and Amerigo Giordano

Introduction

Cardiovascular disease is the major cause of morbidity and mortality in Western countries. Despite progress in early diagnosis and intervention, ischaemic heart disease still is the leading cause of mortality in men older than 45 years and in women older than 65 in Europe. Furthermore, the aging population is contributing to an increase in the number of patients with cardiovascular disease and thus the resources required to manage this pathology. Telemedicine seems to be particularly promising in cardiovascular disease, because early tailored interventions could be life saving. It thus is unsurprising that telecardiology – the transmission of an electrocardiogram (ECG) – has a long history.

Augustus Waller (1865–1922) was the first person to show that the beating heart produces a weak electrical potential, which can be registered by a measuring device connected to electrodes attached to the skin. Willem Einthoven (1860–1927) developed a 'string' galvanometer, which was much faster and more sensitive than the system used by Waller. Einthoven's electrocardiograph was ready for use in 1903. To facilitate investigations of patients, Einthoven connected his instrument to the Academic Hospital in Leyden, by a telephone line. The first successful tele-ECG was transmitted on 22 March 1905. The heart sounds were registered by connecting a specially developed microphone placed on the patient's chest to another string galvanometer. The event therefore was a first for both tele-electrocardiography and telephonocardiography.[1]

Types of telecardiology

Two main types of telecardiology exist:

- continuous or intermittent monitoring – that is, one-way transmission of data, such as an ECG, from a patient to a monitoring centre
- real-time consultation – that is, an ECG, which may have been recorded a few moments beforehand, is transmitted to a specialist who conducts a real-time consultation with the patient.

The two primary types of telemedical interaction therefore are store-and-forward and real time.

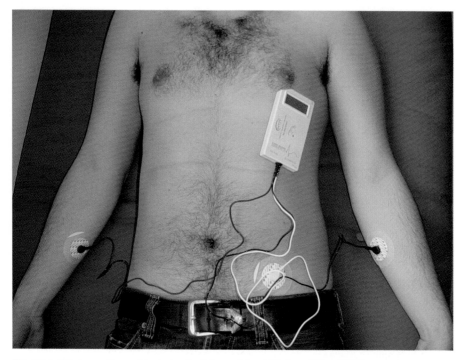

Fig. 19.1. Electrocardiographic device for telemedicine. This is a 12-lead ECG recorder

Electrocardiographic devices for telemedicine generally are small, hand-held and with electrodes, if needed, placed in designated positions on the patient's body (Fig. 19.1). Once activated, the device modulates the acquired ECG signal and acoustically transmits it through the telephone handset to a monitoring centre, where a personal computer-based, ECG-receiving station acquires and displays the transmitted ECG (Fig. 19.2).

The type of connection will affect the speed of data transmission and the quality of any videoconference that may be conducted. Standard telephone lines (public switched telephone network, PSTN) are sufficient for the transmission of a one-lead ECG from a patient's house, and transmission is even possible with a mobile phone. Digital lines (integrated services digital network, ISDN) provide higher bandwidth and may be necessary if good-quality video pictures are to be transmitted in real time.

Telecardiology applications in the home

Home telecardiology may involve the patient, the family, the general practitioner (GP) and a specialized cardiac monitoring centre, so a multidisciplinary approach is required. If implemented successfully, telecardiology can reduce hospitalization rates,

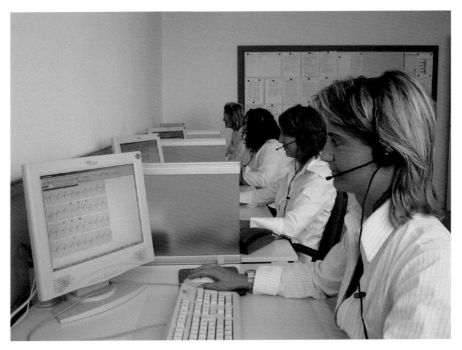

Fig. 19.2. Operator's display at a cardiac monitoring centre

improve patients' quality of life and reduce health service costs. This is particularly true for chronic cardiac diseases, such as congestive heart failure (CHF).[2,3]

Telemonitoring permits patients to stay at home and use special telecare devices connected via standard telephone lines, cable networks or broadband lines to keep in touch with their healthcare providers. Telemonitoring allows evaluation of patients once daily or even continuously, which may help in decisions about patients' management.[4] Interest in home telehealth as an alternative method of providing care has been stimulated by the rising costs of hospital care, rapid advances in telecommunications and diagnostic technology, and wider availability of low-cost, patient-friendly telehealth equipment. There is some evidence that a multidisciplinary management programme and home-based intervention can reduce hospital readmission rates and length of hospital stay in patients with chronic cardiac disease. Several studies have shown significant reductions in hospital readmission rates, but more evidence of efficacy is required before its widespread adoption can be recommended.[3]

Home telecardiology has been used for several different purposes. These include:

- management of chronic cardiac diseases
- telerehabilitation
- diagnosis of arrhythmia
- cardiological second opinions for GPs.

Management of chronic cardiac diseases

Chronic cardiac disease has prompted the development of disease management programmes driven by patient self-assessment or by the nurse. As described in Chapter 17, this approach works especially well in CHF. In a multidisciplinary programme,[5,6] the nurse can identify most patients' problems and answer questions in a few minutes with a telephone call (Fig. 19.3). The use of the one-lead ECG device is important to inform the nurse's decisions about the control of heart rate, in the diagnosis of arrhythmia and in the implementation of β-blocker therapy. The electronic link between the GP and cardiologist permits sharing of the patient's care (Fig. 19.4).

Telephone interventions are not new. Clinical interventions in most previously reported programmes, however, were based solely on subjective information solicited from patients or their family members. Use of transtelephonic transmission of an ECG and other physiological signals creates a real-time connection between the nurse, GP and cardiologist. Telemedicine performed this way allows the choice of the right therapeutic strategy at the right time for patients with chronic cardiac disease. Scheduled consultation and further scheduled telemonitoring are the principal actions taken by the nurses. Commonly, the intervention requires medication adjustments. Physician-supervised, nurse-mediated implementation of pharmacological guidelines has been found to be safe and efficacious.[7]

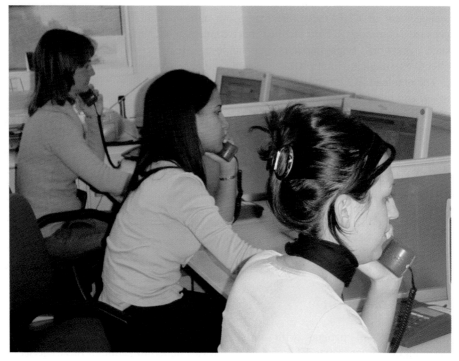

Fig. 19.3. Cardiac monitoring centre

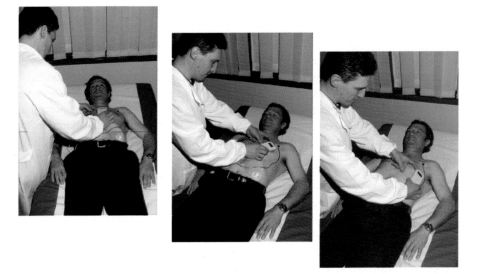

Fig. 19.4. Telehealth link between general practitioner and cardiologist allows the patient's care to be shared

Although different cardiologists, internists and GPs have different practices in the management of CHF, these differences are abolished in a telemedicine network, because a common CHF protocol has been implemented. Nurses play a critical role in such a network. Engaging nurses in home-based interventions has proved to be effective in reducing multiple readmissions and out-of-hospital deaths.[8]

The one-lead ECG recording for a patient with CHF is a simple device that is easy to use and relatively inexpensive. Patients with heart failure can benefit from control of their heart rate, especially during drug titration, and the checks on arrhythmia. Patients are able to use the assigned devices with quite good compliance. No clear data are available at present about which device is the most efficacious and cost-effective in these multidisciplinary programmes. Very few studies have assessed the cost-benefits of telemonitoring, but implementation of a telemonitoring programme decreased annual medical costs compared with the previous year in some cases. This reduction in cost was mainly attributable to lower hospitalization costs.[9,10]

Analysis of existing studies, and new, large, multicentre, randomized, controlled trials are necessary to evaluate the potential benefit and cost-effectiveness of these evolving interventions.

Telerehabilitation

Only 11–20% of patients with coronary artery disease participate in cardiac rehabilitation programmes. This highlights the vast underutilization of these services, especially in older adults and women. Other groups who are underserved include poor, uneducated patients and minorities. The degree of ECG surveillance is linked inversely with the patient's cardiac stability. Self-monitoring of pulse rate, cardiac symptoms and perceived exertion may suffice for many low-risk patients who exercise at home or in community recreation facilities. Continuous or transtelephonic ECG monitoring could be employed for higher-risk patients. Like all contemporary medical strategies, cardiac rehabilitation programmes will require documentation of their efficacy and cost-effectiveness to hospital administrators and health insurers.[10,11] Outcomes analysis is an important part of this process and should include not only clinical variables and quality-of-life measures but also recurrent cardiac events as well as intermediate health outcomes (see Chapter 2). The former are measurable physiological changes, whereas the latter are those experienced or reported by patients.

Home exercise rehabilitation should be promoted, because of its lower cost, increased practicability and convenience, and potential to promote independence and self-responsibility. For low-risk patients, medically directed home-based rehabilitation and supervised group programmes have shown similar safety and efficacy. Treatment of smoking and hyperlipidaemia can also be achieved successfully in a home-based rehabilitation setting. Given its apparent potential, why isn't telerehabilitation flourishing? The reason could be that there is no single best protocol for telerehabilitation. Different problems require different technologies and procedures. Insufficient outcomes research has compared telehealth to conventional approaches and different forms of telehealth with each other. In addition, the limited diffusion of electronic health records and standardized protocols in rehabilitation makes incorporation of telehealth tools more difficult.

Diagnosis of arrhythmia

Palpitation is a common symptom that sometimes results from a substantial cardiac arrhythmia. Establishing the cause of palpitations is difficult, because historical clues are not always accurate. A 24-hour Holter monitor is usually used, but the utility of this instrument is low in patients whose symptoms occur infrequently. Another instrument used to study palpitations is a transtelephonic event recorder. Patients are given this hand-held device to apply to the chest when symptoms occur; the patient presses a button to record about 30 records of cardiac rhythm, which are stored in the device's memory. The recording is later transmitted to a cardiac monitoring centre for printing and interpretation (Fig. 19.5). With this method, patients receive a rapid, accurate diagnosis.

The event recorder is able to create an ECG trace during palpitations in about 70% of patients. This is considerably higher than with Holter monitoring, in which only about 35% of patients successfully record an ECG trace during palpitations. Event recording thus should be used instead of Holter monitoring whenever possible.[12]

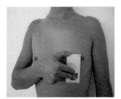

Patient

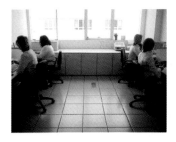

Nurse

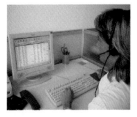

Service centre

Fig. 19.5. Transmission of recordings from patient to nurse

Cardiological second opinions for GPs

General practitioners are faced with an increasing number of patients with cardiac disease. Like so many other patients, those with cardiac disease are often discharged early from hospital. Access to a telecardiology service can support the GP's diagnostic process and therapeutic decisions.[13] Teleconsulting has been applied mainly to the diagnosis of arrhythmia, but it has also been used by GPs as an alternative to ambulatory visits for patients with chronic conditions or systemic hypertension. Preliminary data have confirmed its efficacy in these situations. The advantages of teleconsulting include early diagnosis and tailored therapeutic interventions, home management of chronic conditions, availability of specialist teleconsultation out of the hospital, and improvement in the appropriateness of hospital admissions and referrals to emergency departments.[14–16] The diagnostic accuracy of telecardiology services is high, and it has the potential for cost savings for the National Health Service.[17,18]

Atrial fibrillation in elderly people could be a possible application for GPs.[19] Epidemiological studies have shown that GPs often have to manage patients with atrial fibrillation and experience problems related to therapy and co-morbidity. These patients are often referred to the emergency department at hospital. Telecardiology can help GPs optimize their management of patients with atrial fibrillation, by more closely monitoring their therapy and thus allowing more appropriate referrals to the hospital. Effective teleconsultations depend on an experienced cardiologist and GPs who know their patients well. This kind of telecardiology application supports the goal of mutual reliance between GPs and specialists in managing problems and following common diagnostic and therapeutic protocols.

Benefits and limitations

Despite the diversity of models and the lack of systematic research, successful programmes for telecardiology have been developed (see References for examples). Although some problems remain, they are often the same problems that challenge other telemedicine programmes. In developing a telecardiology programme, therefore, the following aims should be borne in mind:

- a clearly articulated mission that provides direction for the programme as well as specific goals to be achieved
- an accountable governance structure, as well as an effective authority structure for decision-making to facilitate operations and coordinate activities in the organization
- a well-defined service for a well-defined target population, which determines who receives the service and on what basis
- identification of service providers, including the provision of services that match the needs of the target population
- detailed procedures and protocols for activities, which range from appointment scheduling to quality-control procedures
- an appropriate choice of technology that fits the specific clinical needs of the providers and the capabilities of the community
- a well-conceived and well-executed evaluation programme that includes outcomes research
- an economically viable and self-sustaining programme that is based on a sound economic framework that delivers significant value for the investment.

Limitations to the routine implementation of telecardiology include the many different software, hardware and telecommunications options. None of these are designed specifically for cardiology, and no uniform standards for the assessment of health technologies exist, so each component normally functions in isolation. In addition, no clear strategies for promoting wider utilization exist, and dissemination of research results from extant telecardiology programmes is limited. To date, few telemedicine lawsuits have taken place, so legal questions may arise when a tertiary care centre provides equipment or support to a referring hospital or practice. Finally, reimbursement for teleconsultations is limited, and this may discourage many physicians from practising telecardiology.

Conclusion

Telecardiology is a fast-growing field in telemedicine – 38 indexed publications on telecardiology have been published in the last five years. A significant volume of published clinical data already exists, with some randomized, multicentre trials that provide definitive answers to the most important questions. Chronic cardiac diseases such as chronic heart failure benefit from a multidisciplinary approach that can reduce hospitalization and improve the patient's quality of life, while lowering costs for the National Health Service. In addition, GPs gain educationally and hospital follow-up appointments may be reduced in number, because the GPs can handle more advanced medical problems.

The successful contribution of telecardiology to the emergency treatment of patients with cardiac disease, and its application in chronic cardiac care, undoubtedly improves the quality of healthcare and may help to contain rising costs. Nevertheless, stronger study designs are needed, particularly those that are randomized and controlled, as this will permit researchers to determine whether telecardiology is an effective, efficacious and cost-effective way to manage cardiac care. Despite Einthoven's early demonstrations of telecardiology over a hundred years ago, we are still awaiting the full-scale implementation of these achievements.

Further information

OpenECG project. *Interoperability in digital electrocardiography*. Available at: www.openecg.net/ (last accessed 7 January 2006).

References

1   Hjelm NM, Julius HW. Centenary of tele-electrocardiography and telephonocardiography. *J Telemed Telecare* 2005;**11**:336–8.
2   Rich MW, Beckham V, Wittenberg C, *et al.* A multidisciplinary intervention to prevent the readmission of elderly participants with congestive heart failure. *N Engl J Med* 1995;**333**:1190–5.
3   Louis AA, Turner T, Gretton M, *et al.* A systematic review of telemonitoring for the management of heart failure. *Eur J Heart Fail* 2003;**5**:583–90.
4   Wasson J, Gaudette C, Whaley F, *et al.* Telephone care as a substitute for routine clinic follow-up. *JAMA* 1992;**267**:1788–93.
5   Cleland JG, Louis AA, Rigby AS, *et al.* Noninvasive home telemonitoring for patients with heart failure at high risk of recurrent admission and death: the Trans-European Network-Home-Care Management System (TEN-HMS) study. *J Am Coll Cardiol* 2005;**45**:1654–64.
6   Scalvini S, Zanelli E, Volterrani M, *et al.* A pilot study of nurse-led, home-based telecardiology for patients with chronic heart failure. *J Telemed Telecare* 2004;**10**:113–17.
7   West JA, Miller NH, Parker KM, *et al.* A comprehensive management system for heart failure improves clinical outcomes and reduces medical resource utilization. *Am J Cardiol* 1997;**79**:58–63.
8   Stewart S, Pearson S, Luke CG, Horowitz JD. Effects of a home-based intervention on unplanned readmissions and out-of-hospital deaths. *J Am Geriatr Soc* 1998;**46**:174–80.
9   Jerant AF, Azari R, Nesbitt TS. Reducing the cost of frequent hospital admissions for congestive heart failure: a randomized trial of a home telecare intervention. *Med Care* 2001;**39**:1234–45.
10 Franklin BA, Hall L, Timmis GC. Contemporary cardiac rehabilitation services. *Am J Cardiol* 1997;**79**:1075–7.
11 Winters JM, Winters JM. A telehomecare model for optimizing rehabilitation outcomes. *Telemed J E Health* 2004;**10**:200–12.
12 Kinlay S, Leitch JW, Neil A, *et al.* Cardiac event recorders yield more diagnoses and are more cost-effective than 48-hour Holter monitoring in patients with palpitations. A controlled clinical trial. *Ann Intern Med* 1996;**124**:16–20.

13   Shanit D, Cheng A, Greenbaum RA. Telecardiology: supporting the decision-making process in general practice. *J Telemed Telecare* 1996;**2**:7–13.

14   Scalvini S, Zanelli E, Domenighini D, *et al.* Telecardiology community: a new approach to take care of cardiac patients. *Cardiologia* 1999;**44**:921–4.

15   Scalvini S, Zanelli E, Gritti M, *et al.* [Appropriateness of referral to the emergency department through a telecardiology service]. *Ital Heart J Suppl* 2000;**1**:905–9 (in Italian).

16   Scalvini S, Zanelli E, Conti C, *et al.* Assessment of prehospital chest pain using telecardiology. *J Telemed Telecare* 2002;**8**:231–6.

17   Molinari G, Valbusa A, Terrizzano M, *et al.* Nine years' experience of telecardiology in primary care. *J Telemed Telecare* 2004;**10**:249–53.

18   Scalvini S, Zanelli E, Volterrani M, *et al.* [Potential cost reductions for the National Health Service through a telecardiology service dedicated to general practice physicians]. *Ital Heart J Suppl* 2001;**2**:1091–7.

19   Scalvini S, Piepoli M, Zanelli E, *et al.* Incidence of atrial fibrillation in an Italian population followed by their GPs through a telecardiology service. *Int J Cardiol* 2005;**98**:215–20.

►20

Child monitoring

Andrea Tura and Luca Quareni

Introduction

Telepaediatrics is an important application of telemedicine.[1] It includes telemedicine applications related to children and adolescents under 18 years of age. Many applications in telepaediatrics involve connection between two health centres for teleconsultation purposes, but telepaediatrics also includes applications at home. These are important for several reasons. First, the ability to improve illness and recover health is higher in young people than elderly people, so there is more chance of proving the cost-effectiveness of the telemedicine application. Second, interventions performed on young patients are usually more long-lasting than those in elderly people, so the initial investment for the technology involved in the intervention is exploited better. Third, young individuals are usually confident with technology, which increases the possibility of success in the use of the equipment. On the other hand, applications for adolescents (and especially children) require special attention to some aspects, as will be pointed out later.

Applications of home telepaediatrics

Telepaediatrics in the home setting to date has largely been experimental. A number of health conditions have been examined, including:

- diabetes mellitus
- renal failure
- neurological impairment
- palliative care
- asthma
- burns
- cardiology.

Diabetes mellitus

Patients with type 1 diabetes require frequent blood glucose measurement to optimize insulin therapy. In many patients, and especially in young people, compliance is low, and this leads to poor glycaemic control, which often results in hospital admission. Thus, some healthcare programmes have been developed to help patients improve their metabolic control. In a study by Liesenfeld et al,[2] 61 young patients (mean age 13.3 years and mean duration of diabetes 5.5 years) under intensive insulin therapy were admitted to a telemedical programme. These patients had a history of frequent episodes of hypoglycaemia and ketoacidosis (7.8 and 4.2 per 100 patient years, respectively). All patients were provided with a glucometer for domiciliary use and were asked to measure glucose concentrations at least four times each day. Once a week, they transmitted the data to a remote diabetes centre through a telephone line. At the remote centre, diabetologists examined the data and contacted the patients by telephone to provide therapeutic advice. The advice was related to the time schedule for insulin injections, the type of insulin to be used, diet, physical exercise and education about recognition of possible hypoglycaemia or ketoacidosis. On average, the programme required four months to reach optimum glycaemic control. In the 54 patients who completed the programme, mean blood glucose decreased significantly – from 9.3 mmol/l to 8.8 mmol/l. The number of hypoglycaemic events was also reduced.

The glucometer had a local storage capability and recorded time- and date-stamped blood glucose concentrations, insulin doses and carbohydrate levels in the diet. The patients also had a palmtop computer with an integrated modem (connected via an ordinary telephone line) for data transmission. The software for data examination at the remote diabetes centre was Camit Pro (Roche).

In an American study,[3] five patients (mean age 14.2 years) were admitted to an intensive telehealth programme. Four patients had type 1 diabetes and one had type 2 diabetes but with similar need for insulin therapy. The patients reported their blood glucose measurements, details of insulin injections and their food intake every day for three months by telephone contact. After one month, they were also offered videophone contact. At the end of the programme, levels of glycosylated haemoglobin were reduced in all five patients. Few technical details were reported. A low-bandwidth videophone (ViaTV, 8X8) was used.

Renal failure

Renal failure that requires dialysis is a chronic condition, except in the few cases where transplantation is possible. Home telehealth has been used for children undergoing automated peritoneal dialysis.[4] Two children (aged 10 and 12 years) were admitted to the project. The equipment included a teleperitoneal cycler and a videoconference system. The cycler transmitted dialysis data to a personal computer (PC) in the remote dialysis centre via a modem connection. The data were stored and then examined by health professionals, who were able to understand whether the patients were compliant with their dialysis schedule or had manually changed some dialysis parameters. Real-time communication occurred by videoconferencing between the patients and the operators at the remote centre during some treatment sessions. The videoconference system included a high-resolution, colour, digital camera. The camera was placed on the ceiling of the patient's room and could be zoomed and rotated. It was possible, therefore, to focus both on patient and on dialysis cycler, including its display. The camera was controlled from the dialysis centre. Real-time transmission of images and sounds to a PC at the remote centre was via integrated services digital network (ISDN) lines.

At the end of the seven-month study, it was concluded that the patients were highly compliant. Only once in the study did a single patient shorten the treatment, and this was the result of a technical problem with the equipment. The videoconference connection was useful for helping the patients to perform the treatment procedure properly and ensuring correct cleaning and medication. The home telehealth system thus ensured high-quality treatment and excellent compliance, which is not often seen in patients undergoing peritoneal dialysis.

Neurological impairment

Some home telehealth projects have been developed for neurologically impaired children. Guest *et al* established a videoconference link between children's homes and the paediatric neurologists at the hospital. No technical information was provided.[5] The three-year project started at the end of 2003 and involved three children. The system seemed to produce very positive outcomes: as a result of the high quality of the video link, the neurologists were able to make diagnoses and change treatment immediately; in some cases, this prevented admissions to the hospital or emergency unit. All the children had gastrostomies, which were easily controlled through the video link. The system also had positive effects in the patient's and family's moods, reducing the sense of anxiety and isolation. Preliminary results suggest that the system could be extended to other children – even those with very severe neurological impairment.

In the field of home telehealth for children with neurological impairment and mental retardation, another project used telemonitoring of some physiological parameters.[6] This study is described in more detail below.

Palliative care

Telehealth has also been used in palliative care.[7] Again, a video link was used between home and hospital. The link was based on an Internet-based videophone specifically designed for the application. The videophone was a custom-made unit that contained a PC. A web camera was mounted over a flat-screen monitor. The system was designed for ease of use. With the simple press of a button, the PC was configured to start up automatically, connect via the Internet and open the videoconference application (Fig. 20.1). The videoconference software used was NetMeeting (Microsoft). Another advantage of this system was that it used the ordinary telephone network for transmission, in contrast to many videoconference systems that require a broadband connection.

The system was tested on one child supported by palliative care. In the first month of the trial, six video calls were conducted. The calls were initiated by the palliative care nurse at the hospital. The family reported an increased feeling of security.

Asthma

Mantzouranis followed five asthmatic children using a home PC that provided a videoconference connection to the outpatient clinic through a wireless, broadband network.[8] Again, the ease of use of the equipment was important. By pressing the 'call

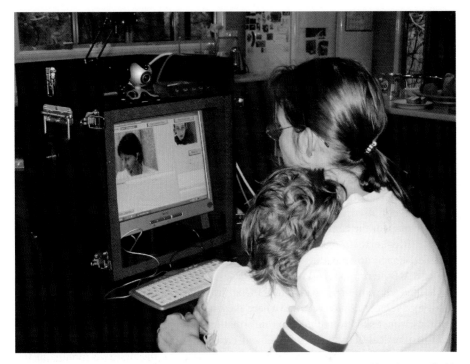

Fig. 20.1. Palliative home-care patient with her mother. They are conducting a videophone call with a palliative care nurse. Photo credit: M Bensink

the doctor' button, all the operations for remote connection were performed automatically. The equipment also included an electronic stethoscope, so the doctor could listen to the patient's chest sounds via the Internet.

Five patients who lived in the neighbourhood were also admitted to the project and obtained a video link that reached the children's homes, where the equipment was installed. During the trial, each patient was examined 12 times. Each televisit lasted for about 30 minutes and was performed by the same specialist who followed the child at the clinic. To complete the televisit, the patients were examined with an electronic stethoscope. During the trial, none of the patients experienced an acute exacerbation or admission to the hospital or emergency room. All the children and 90% of their parents expressed satisfaction with the system.

In a study by Chan *et al*, 10 asthmatic children (mean age 7.6 years) received a digital video camera and a computer with Internet access.[9] The video camera was used to record videos of the patient using a peak flow meter and an inhaler for administration of corticosteroids or other medications. The reading of the peak flow meter was also recorded through the camera. Twice a week, the video recordings were transmitted to the paediatric clinic, with a diary recording the asthma symptoms daily. At the clinic, the project case manager examined the transmitted data and sent email messages in reply to adjust the action plan for asthma care. Furthermore, patients were randomized into two groups that received asthma education through an interactive website or through traditional education during scheduled visits at the clinic. All patients were seen at the clinic at prescribed dates during the six months of the trial. All the patients had very good asthma control during the trial, and unscheduled visits to the clinic occurred rarely. No patients were admitted to the hospital or emergency unit. The web-educated group also showed an increased quality-of-life survey score.

Burns

A recent application for home telepaediatrics is the follow-up care of patients with burns, who may require lengthy follow-up after treatment of the acute injury (sometimes lasting for years). In a study by Johansen et al,[10] four patients' families used a digital camera to obtain images of the child with burns. Three low-cost digital cameras were used (Canon Power Shot, Sony DSC and Nikon Coolpix). The requirements for the cameras were ease of use, acceptable lens quality, resolution of at least 2 Megapixels, macro capability, JPEG image reproduction, rechargeable batteries, image downloading to a PC without the need of special software, memory size of 8 MByte or more and price $400 or less.

The images were downloaded to a PC at the child's home and then transmitted by email to a remote clinical centre, where they were examined by the specialist team. Families were asked to include text information in the email, such as skin condition, level of physical activity and movement capability, possible presence of sores and current treatment. Transmission occurred every week in the first two months of the

Table 20.1. Main features of trials in home telepaediatrics

Pathology/condition	Main equipment and monitoring strategy	Number of patients	Average duration (months)
Type 1 diabetes[2]	• Glucometer • Telephone link	54	4
Type 1 and type 2 diabetes[3]	• Glucometer • Telephone • Video link	5	3
Renal failure[4]	• Teleperitoneal dialysis cycler • Videoconference	2	7
Neurological impairment[5]	• Videoconference	3	36
Physical or mental impairment[6]	• Multivariable monitoring device • Website	9	2
Palliative care[7]	• Internet-based, low-bandwidth videophone	1	1
Asthma[8]	• Electronic stethoscope • Wireless videoconference	10	Not reported
Asthma[9]	• Peak flow meter • Inhaler • Internet-based video link	10	6
Burns injuries[10]	• Low-cost digital camera • Email	4	6
Cardiology[11]	• Videoconference	14	Not completed

trial and every two weeks for the following four months. After each transmission to the clinical centre, the burns team replied to the family. The study showed that most of the received images were of sufficient quality for clinical decision-making despite the use of low-cost, non-professional cameras. The patients and families generally were satisfied with the service, although some improvements were suggested, such as variable frequency of data transmission according to the condition of the child.

Cardiology

A well-established application in telemedicine is telecardiology. At home, this commonly consists of monitoring the heart through an ECG device. Traditionally, the ECG data are transmitted via the ordinary telephone network; however, despite the large number of telecardiology programmes, there seem to be few studies specifically focused on children at home. In Northern Ireland, a group of children discharged with complex congenital heart disease was monitored at home with videoconferencing.[11] For comparison, a control group was monitored by telephone contact only. The preliminary results suggest advantages with videoconferencing. The topic of cardiology in older people is covered in greater detail in Chapter 19.

The main features of the studies described are summarized in Table 20.1.

Equipment for home telehealth

Some aspects of the equipment required for home telehealth need careful consideration. In general, these mainly relate to the safety and comfort of use of the equipment. Some aspects are of special importance when the telehealth application concerns children.

With respect to safety, any devices used by children should be powered with batteries in order to decrease the risk of electric shock. Long battery life is also a requirement, but this sometimes conflicts with another requirement, which is compact size and modest weight. Portability and wearability are also important. Wireless devices tend to increase wearability and comfort. Increasingly, technologies such as Bluetooth or WiFi (short-range wireless transmissions) and general packet radio service, GPRS, or universal mobile telecommunications system, UMTS (long-range network connections) are reliable and available at an affordable price. However, they increase the power requirements and thus are somewhat at odds with the low power requirement mentioned above.

Devices for applications in children and adolescents should be easy to use. Although the patient is completely supported by the adults in the family in most cases, some children may wish to learn how to use the equipment themselves (especially older children). Devices in home telepaediatrics thus should have a few simple functions, which should be accessed through few buttons, possibly of large size and identified by different colours (or, even better, through easily recognized icons). The device display, if any, should be of graphical type and with colours. It should be comfortable to interact with the equipment through a remote control or voice commands – this is especially important for children with reduced physical activity.

In the design of devices for paediatrics, special attention should also be given to cosmetic aspects. Consider, for example, a monitoring device for continuous measurement of respiration rate. Simple and inexpensive sensors, such as thermistors, can be positioned between the nose and mouth using adhesive tape; however, this is not satisfactory from a cosmetic point of view. A more acceptable technique is to use a piezoelectric belt worn on the chest or abdomen. The belt can be hidden under the clothes, which may be important if the child is participating in social activities while measurements are being taken.

Much equipment in home telehealth includes a PC or similar device. Sometimes, the PC is used only as a bridge to transmit information through the Internet from equipment at home to the remote centre. In other cases, the patient uses the PC to receive messages or education from the remote centre.

New devices

A number of devices that can measure physiological variables of interest in home telehealth have been developed recently. To our knowledge, they have not been used in home telehealth trials devoted to children. Some of these new devices are available commercially, whereas others are still prototypes. Commercial devices include:

- Wearable Acquisition Device (WAD) by MS WebCare,[12] which includes sensors able to measure several physiological variables, such as ECG, respiration, body temperature, and body inclination and acceleration. It can also connect to external medical devices. The WAD includes a pocket-sized communication unit able to connect to external media and equipment through different wireless technologies (both short and long distance). For better portability, a special shirt has been developed to house the communication unit and the sensors with their cables.

- SenseWear PRO2 Armband by BodyMedia[13,14] is a body monitor wearable on the back of the upper right arm (in the tricep area). It measures body acceleration, heat flux, skin and near body temperatures, and galvanic skin response. Through these measures, some lifestyle information can be derived, such as energy expenditure, physical activity, and sleep and awake states. This type of information could be important in home telemonitoring of various conditions. Variations in the patient's habits could be an indication of worsening health status. The data measured by the device can be downloaded to a PC wirelessly or through a cable connection.

- Vivago WristCare by International Security Technology Oy[15,16] is a wristwatch-like device able to measure skin temperature and conductivity and the patient's movement. Again, these measures provide information on the patient's activity level and type of actions. If some variations in the normal activity level are detected (such as an unusual period of immobility), an alarm is sent. Alarm data are transmitted wirelessly to a base unit connected to the telephone network. The alarm information thus reaches a call centre and possibly the personal phone of family members. The patient also can send a manual alarm by pressing a button on the device.

- LifeShirt by VivoMetrics[17,18] consists of a garment that includes sensors for monitoring ECG signals and respiratory patterns by patented inductive

plethysmography. Activity and posture are also measured. Data are stored in a recording unit and then downloaded to a PC. External medical devices can be connected to the recording unit. The garment is produced in different sizes, including special sizes for children.

- Smart Shirt by Sensatex is a similar device based on a garment.[19,20] It is able to measure ECG, respiration patterns and body temperature. An interesting feature of this device is that the sensors, as well as the conductive fibres that connect them to a recording unit, are incorporated into the shirt's fabric. The fabric also includes optical fibres and a microphone. The recording unit is the size of a wristwatch and is located at the waist portion of the shirt. Data are transmitted remotely from the unit through a wireless long-distance connection.

Other projects are trying to obtain 'smart' fabrics that incorporate sensors for monitoring physiological variables, but to our knowledge these devices are still prototypes.[21,22] Another interesting device still at the prototype stage is the SILC device.[23] This is a wristwatch-like device that is able to measure ECG, body temperature, and forearm position and acceleration. It generates alarms if a worsening of the health condition is detected. The data are shown on the device display and downloaded to a base unit through a wireless (Bluetooth) connection. The device also includes an infrared remote control module that could be used for domestic applications.

Children with neurological impairment and mental retardation

In a project part-funded by the European Commission, a home telehealth device was developed for the management of children and adolescents with physical and/or mental impairment (Karma2 project). Care of these patients involves many health professionals, including those from medicine, nursing, and social and psychological care, and sometimes other entities such as associations of patients' families and volunteers. The project created a network to coordinate and manage all those involved and the necessary activities. This allowed updated information to be delivered to the participants, making them able to undertake the most pertinent actions.

Equipment

A key element in the project consisted of the home telemonitoring of important physiological variables. For this purpose, a device was developed that could be worn on a belt, thus leaving the patient free to move while measurements are taken.[6] The device measures blood oxygen saturation, heart rate, breath rate and the patient's activity level through accelerometers. The device contains different electronic boards interconnected through sockets inside the device case. This solution allows modularity and flexibility: a board is not mounted if the corresponding function is not required, and this results in a lower cost for the device. Fig. 20.2 shows the device being worn by a 14-year-old patient.

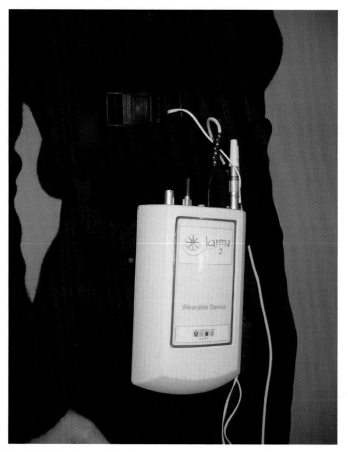

Fig. 20.2. The Karma2 device

The pulse oximetry signal is obtained through a paediatric finger probe. Respiration rate is measured through a piezoelectric sensor encased in a thin box that has a plastic strip connected to it on both sides. A belt allows the sensor to be attached to the patient. During breathing, the piezoelectric sensor undergoes stress as a result of expansion of the chest or abdomen, which provides the respiration rate. A custom-made amplification board was developed to process the piezoelectric signal.

The measured physiological data are stored on a multimedia card (MMC). In contrast to memory components, such as E2PROM chips, the MMC can be removed easily and substituted if necessary. At time intervals, which can be configured properly, the data are read from the MMC and automatically transmitted to a tablet PC through a wireless (Bluetooth) connection. With Bluetooth transmission once per hour, the device can be left on for several days. Data are maintained in the MMC until communication is available for downloading. When the tablet PC receives data from the device, an extensible markup language (XML) file is created and transmitted

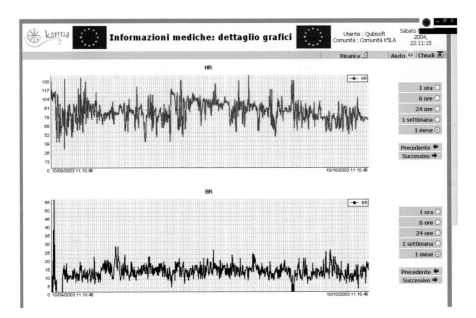

Fig. 20.3. Heart rate and respiratory rate displayed by the web application

through the Internet to a web server located in a service centre. Transmission is made through secure socket layer protocol. The transmitted data can be inspected by the health professionals through a web application running on the server. An example of data display from the web application is shown in Fig. 20.3.

Both the patient's family and other participants in the projects can access the web application. Depending on the user's profile, only specific operations can be performed. The main user types are child/family, general practitioner, paediatrician, speech therapist, rehabilitation therapist, orthopaedic specialist, neurologist, psychologist, municipality (social service), teacher and advocate (the person responsible for the child in the project). An important operation is the management of the weekly planning of patient's activities, which allows all the participants involved in the patient's care to manage the necessary activities, scheduling them at the right day, time and place. Several activities can be scheduled for the patients, each represented by an appropriate icon. Another function of the web application is the use of several communication tools, such as private messages, email and chat lines, which allows all participants to keep in touch easily and effectively.

Results

Nine children were included in the first trial: four with Down's syndrome, three with cerebral palsy and two with mental retardation of unknown aetiology (seven boys, two girls; average age 17 years). The trial lasted for two months. The device gained sufficient acceptance, and all the children provided data, although some of them indicated that reduced dimensions would be appreciated. The web application also

Table 20.2. User satisfaction with the Karma2 device

Satisfaction	No. of patients (%)
Completely satisfied	2 (22)
Sufficiently satisfied	5 (56)
Fairly satisfied	2 (22)
Not satisfied	0 (0)
Total	9 (100)

received good acceptance by the patients and families – thanks to its simple interface and graphical solutions for easy use of the different functions. Some families, however, requested an improved application interface. Improvement of the communication functions seems to be important, as communication was the main reason to access the portal (exchanging messages, reporting a technical or medical problem, arranging appointments) in this first trial. Patients and families were generally satisfied with the system and expressed a desire to continue using it (Table 20.2).

Conclusion

Although home telehealth is increasingly being used, experience with home telehealth for children and adolescents is less common. Furthermore, much of the work is limited to establishing a link between the home and the clinic: trials that include quantitative measurements of the health condition, such as monitoring of the vital signs, are even less common.

One wonders why so few experiences have been reported. It could be the result of the challenges of developing home telehealth systems for children. In our opinion, however, the main obstacles are not technological but organizational in nature. This, of course, holds for any home telehealth application and, more generally, any work in telemedicine. The creation of a new telemedicine application means changing the way that people work – and often there is reluctance for various reasons. Another factor that limits the diffusion of home telehealth is the problem of reimbursement by the public healthcare system. Nonetheless, home telehealth undoubtedly has value for paediatric work, and its increasing adoption seems likely in the coming years.

Further information

Agency for Healthcare Research and Quality. *Telemedicine for the Medicare population: pediatric, obstetric, and clinician-indirect home interventions.* Rockville, MD: Agency for Healthcare Research and Quality, 2001. Available at: www.ahrq.gov/clinic/tp/telemedsuptp.htm (last accessed 23 December 2005).
Gott M. *Telematics for health: the role of telehealth and telemedicine in homes and communities.* Oxford: Radcliffe Medical Press, 1995.

Tang P, Curry R, Gann D, eds. *Telecare: new ideas for care and support at home.* Bristol: Policy Press, 2000.

References

1   Wootton R, Batch J, eds. *Telepediatrics: telemedicine and child health.* London: Royal Society of Medicine Press, 2005.
2   Liesenfeld B, Renner R, Neese M, Hepp KD. Telemedical care reduces hypoglycemias and improves glycemic control in children and adolescents with type 1 diabetes. *Diabetes Technol Ther* 2000;**2**:561–7.
3   Gelfand K, Geffken G, Halsey-Lyda M, *et al.* Intensive telehealth management of five at-risk adolescents with diabetes. *J Telemed Telecare* 2003;**9**:117–21.
4   Ghio L, Boccola S, Andronio L, *et al.* A case study: telemedicine technology and peritoneal dialysis in children. *Telemed J E Health* 2002;**8**:355–9.
5   Guest A, Rittey C, O'Brien K. Telemedicine: helping neurologically-impaired children to stay at home. *Paediatr Nurs* 2005;**17** 20–2.
6   Tura A, Badanai M, Longo D, Quareni L. A multi-functional, portable device with wireless transmission for home monitoring of children with a learning disability. *J Telemed Telecare* 2004;**10**:298–302.
7   Bensink M, Armfield N, Russell TG, *et al.* Paediatric palliative home care with Internet-based videophones: lessons learnt. *J Telemed Telecare* 2004;**10** (Suppl 1):10–13.
8   Mantzouranis EC. User friendliness aspects of home care telematics. *Methods Inf Med* 2002;**41**:370–5.
9   Chan DS, Callahan CW, Sheets SJ, *et al.* An Internet-based store-and-forward video home telehealth system for improving asthma outcomes in children. *Am J Health Syst Pharm* 2003;**60**:1976–81.
10 Johansen MA, Wootton R, Kimble R, *et al.* A feasibility study of email communication between the patient's family and the specialist burns team. *J Telemed Telecare* 2004;**10** (Suppl 1):53–6.
11 Morgan GJ, Grant B, Craig B, *et al.* Supporting families of critically ill children at home using videoconferencing. *J Telemed Telecare* 2005;**11** (Suppl 1): 91–2.
12 MS WebCare. *WAD – wearable acquisition device.* Milan: MS WebCare. Available at: www.mswebcare.it/wad_en.php (last accessed 23 December 2005).
13 BodyMedia. *SenseWear PRO2 Armband.* Pittsburgh, PA: BodyMedia, 2005. Available at: www.bodymedia.com/products/healthwear.jsp#sw (last accessed 23 December 2005).
14 Cole PJ, LeMura LM, Klinger TA, *et al.* Measuring energy expenditure in cardiac patients using the Body Media Armband versus indirect calorimetry. A validation study. *J Sports Med Phys Fitness* 2004;**44**:262–71.
15 IST International Security Technology. *Vivago WristCare.* Helsinki: IST International Security Technology, 2005. Available at: www.istsec.fi (last accessed 23 December 2005).
16 Paavilainen P, Korhonen I, Lotjonen J, *et al.* Circadian activity rhythm in demented and non-demented nursing-home residents measured by telemetric actigraphy. *J Sleep Res* 2005;**14**:61–8.
17 VivoMetrics. *VivoMetrics.* Ventura, CA: VivoMetrics, 2004. Available at: www.vivometrics.com/site/index.html (last accessed 23 December 2005).
18 Grossman P. The LifeShirt: a multi-function ambulatory system monitoring health, disease, and medical intervention in the real world. *Stud Health Technol Inform* 2004;**108**:133–41.
19 Sensatex. *Sensatex.* Bethesda, MD: Sensatex, 2005. Available at: www.sensatex.com (last accessed 23 December 2005).
20 Wolf J. Wearable wireless wonder. Remote monitoring transmits data for patient assessment in the field. *Health Manage Technol* 2000;**21**:30–1.
21 Wealthy. *Wealthy – Wearable Health Care System.* Wealthy, 2002. Available at: www.wealthy-ist.com (last accessed 23 December 2005).
22 Institut de Médecine et de Physiologie Spatiales. *VTAMN PROJECT (RNTS 2000). Vêtement de Téléassistance Médicale Nomade". 'Medical Teleassistance Suit'.* Toulouse: Institut de Médecine et de Physiologie Spatiales, 2004 (in French). Available at: www.medes.fr/VTAMN.html (last accessed 23 December 2005).
23 Information Society Technologies. *Supporting independently living citizens.* Brussels: Information Society Technologies, 2005. Available at: www.fortec.tuwien.ac.at/silcweb/silc_en/SILC.html (last accessed 23 December 2005).

►21

Palliative care

Marilynne A. Hebert, J.J. Jansen and Lynn Whitten

Introduction

It is generally agreed that the hospice is a 'concept of care' designed to provide comfort by alleviating pain or disease symptoms, and giving support to patients and their families in the final stages of a terminal illness. In 2003, more than 885 000 terminally ill people in the US chose to spend their last months in hospice care.[1] Eighty per cent of this care was provided in the patient's home, a family member's home or a nursing home.[2]

Most palliative care is delivered at home, but palliative care is changing. First, societal demographics are shifting, with a growing population of elderly people and a relatively diminishing number of healthcare providers. Patients are also being discharged from hospital sooner, resulting in a heavier home care caseload, with more patients having complex needs.

Hospice provides clinical, emotional and spiritual care for terminally ill patients. The concept originated in England and was first introduced in the US in 1974.

Box 21.1. Early work in telehospice

Gary Doolittle and his colleagues in Kansas and Michigan conducted some of the earliest work in telehospice, starting in the mid-1990s. They established videoconferencing equipment in the patients' homes, connected via the ordinary telephone network. Using this equipment, patients could see and hear the hospice staff. The hospice staff could see and hear the patients. The technology included:

- a wide-angle video camera with high depth of field, enabling focus from about 30 cm to infinity
- a 33-cm off-the-shelf television set
- a codec to compress and digitize the video signal for transmission over conventional telephone lines
- an ordinary telephone handset or a speakerphone.

Their findings showed that, generally, nurses were willing to use telehospice, but many preferred to use it for after-hours calls or to assess whether an in-person visit was necessary. Patients were generally satisfied with care delivered with telecommunications technology. The highest levels of satisfaction were expressed by caregivers.

Doolittle also performed a cost-measurement study comparing traditional hospice service versus a telehospice service over two different study periods.[18] For traditional hospice services, the cost per visit was $126 and $141 for the first and second study periods, respectively. This compares to just $29 for telehospice visits.

Telehospice is the delivery of hospice care through real-time videoconferencing. Telehospice normally uses the public telephone network to deliver care. Nurses visit and treat patients without leaving their homes/offices (Box 21.1).

Palliative home care is an effective strategy for reducing the time spent in hospital during the last three months of life.[3] Many rural and remote areas do not have palliative care experts available locally, however, and if the patient prefers to be at home, the informal caregivers may lack support to deal with the issues of care. This creates a new burden in palliative care, as families and friends sometimes feel pressured to care for their loved ones at home (Box 21.2).

Box 21.2. Case study – Carol

Carol, aged 49 years, suddenly found herself looking after her widowed mother Barbara (aged 69 years) who had metastatic breast cancer. Carol had two teenagers still living at home and worked full-time. Her mother wanted to die at home, and, although Carol respected that wish, she had no experience in caring for someone who was so ill. She felt both frightened and resentful.

The home-care nurse suggested they try 'video-visits', so that Carol could be in touch with her weekly and when needed (Fig. 21.1). Carol felt with this additional support she was willing to try providing her mother's care at home.

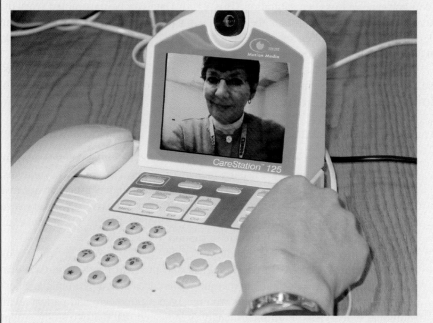

Fig. 21.1. Videophones support communication

Comment
Providing palliative care in the home is a new and often stressful experience for families. Discussing care activities with the nurse represents an opportunity for informal caregivers to obtain support. Although additional home visits may not be possible, video-visits (where the caregiver and nurse each have a videophone) are a cost-effective way for this exchange to occur.

Finally, increased survival rates mean an increased move to provide palliative care in the community. Coyle *et al* observed: 'With advances of medicine, previously lethal diseases like cancer and AIDS have become chronic conditions. There is a growing number of cancer survivors with long life expectancy who are debilitated and dependent on complex medical regimens and equipment. These and other complex palliative care patients are in need of a communication tool that would allow them to be monitored and receive comprehensive care at home.'[4]

Changing societal demographics, complex care requirements in the community and increasing survival rates all strongly suggest that it will be impossible to continue to deliver palliative care services in the traditional manner. These factors will drive the adoption of home telehealth.

Home telehealth

The technology used in palliative homecare is the same as that used in other home telehealth applications. It includes equipment for transmitting digital images of wounds, videophones for real-time consultations and vital signs monitors to measure blood pressure and oxygen saturation (Box 21.3). Data can be transmitted from the patient to the provider through the ordinary telephone network (public switched telephone network, PSTN), special digital lines (integrated services digital network, ISDN) or mobile phone connections (Fig. 21.3).

Roles for home telehealth

In palliative care at home, telehealth can provide support in a number of ways:

- Psychological support – Health problems encountered by dying patients who are receiving palliative home care usually include the control of physical symptoms, especially shortness of breath. However, it is the psychological aspects that cause the most concern to patients, families and healthcare professionals. Wong *et al* pointed out that understanding the needs of palliative home-care patients can assist the healthcare team to plan care to support a 'good' death.[5]
- Symptom management – Technology could play a role in supporting communication to meet both psychological and physical needs. The Canadian video-visits study was designed to measure differences in symptom management and quality of life between patients who received routine care and patients with additional video-visits. Preliminary analysis indicated that the two study groups had similar outcomes, which suggests that patients can maintain appropriate levels of self-management. This supports a care delivery model that integrates technology into routine palliative care.
- Reduced travel – One of the key benefits of home telehealth is reduced travelling times and costs for the nurse, as well as an extension of human resource capacity. The main benefit for the patient is additional visits, which provide assistance in

Box 21.3. Case study – Emma

Emma, a 78-year-old woman, was caring for her 80-year-old husband Carl at home. He had been diagnosed with metastatic lung cancer and was being provided with palliative home care. The home-care nurse visited once a week and was available by telephone for urgent requests. One afternoon Emma called in great distress as she was trying to suction her husband and could not remember the correct way to hold the suction catheter. The nurse tried unsuccessfully to explain the procedure by telephone and then spent two hours driving to and from Emma's house in order to provide assistance.

Shortly after this incident, the home-care nurse suggested that they try two additional ways for Emma and Carl to better manage his shortness of breath. A portable oximeter would enable them to see what Carl's oxygen levels were and start the oxygen before he was in distress. In addition, a videophone would enable Emma to show the nurse what she was having difficulties with (Fig. 21.2). Both the oximeter and videophone would use the existing telephone line to transmit data.

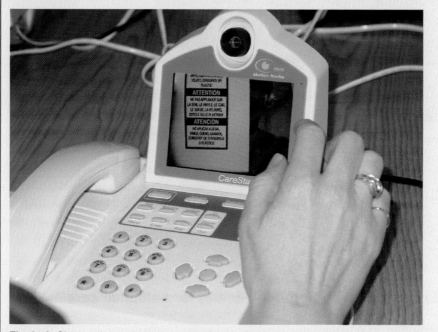

Fig. 21.2. Close-up image provides nurse with details

Comment

Sometimes, reassurance that clinical variables are in the normal range is all the support that carers need. Home monitoring devices can be useful for clients and families to keep track of blood pressure, blood glucose and oxygen levels, for example, and to help clients better manage their symptoms. Practice guidelines for determining whom the technology may be appropriate for can assist the home-care nurse in implementing home telehealth.

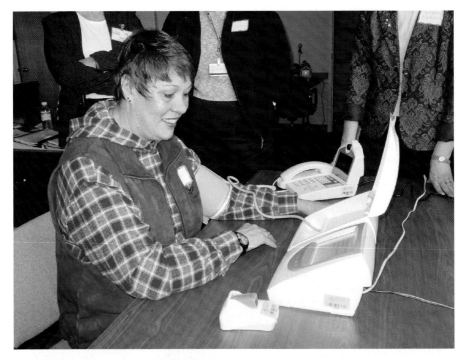

Fig. 21.3. Peripherals demonstrated during training

managing symptoms. Increased contact is possible through video-visits, and, as a result, nurses can help patients to reach more positive outcomes, instil an increased feeling of wellness and support their ability to manage their own health and disease care issues.[6]

Experience with home telehealth for palliative care

More than 3000 hospice programmes exist in the US;[2] however, in 2004, there were only about 15 telehospice programmes.[7]

The limited experience to date shows that telehealth can be used effectively to deliver health care services to the home. However, before the largescale adoption of home telehealth is likely to occur, evidence is required of the clinical and cost-effectiveness at a population level, as well as the readiness of both patients and healthcare professionals to use it.[8] Two projects in hospice palliative care using videophones, one each in the US and Canada, illustrate the differences in how success has been measured and how the use of this technique reflects, in part, differences in healthcare culture and service provision (Table 21.1).

Table 21.1. Comparison of Canadian and American palliative home-care projects

Project feature	Canadian (2003–06)[8]	American (2000–02)[17]
Description	• Three-year multi-method study in province of Alberta • Eligible patients referred to palliative home care randomly assigned for eight weeks to: – routine home care – combination of routine care and video-visits • Nurses have access to technology in 11 rural community offices	• Two-year telehospice project in states of Michigan and Kansas • Telehospice care offered at introductory meeting as an adjunct to care: hospice worker calls at least once a week and patient can use videophone to call anytime • Nurses, social workers, spiritual care counsellors and physicians have access to technology in each rural and urban office
Methods	• Two groups compared in three areas: – patient outcomes (McGill quality of life survey and ESAS symptom assessment tool) • Economic measures (survey of patient preferences for using videophone technology, technology, travel and service utilization costs) • Perceptions of using the technology (nurse focus groups and patient interviews)	• Hospice providers – pre- and post-surveys of perception of using the technology • Hospice patients'/caregivers' perceptions and satisfaction – open-ended telephone interviews • Reasons for patients declining service – survey • Activity logs and patient charts – utilization data
Technology	• Motion Media 125 videophone • Operates over ordinary telephone line (PSTN) • Easy to use with minimal training	• 8x8 ViaTV v160 Teleconferencing Unit • Telephone with separate display screen (e.g. small television) • Operates over ordinary telephone line (PSTN)
Results	• Preliminary analysis suggests no differences between groups with respect to symptom management and quality of life • Less expensive to use videophone if nurse has five or more home visits • Clients prefer face-to-face visits and fewer visits overall • Nurses more reluctant than patients to use the technology	• Hospice providers – cautiously enthusiastic about telehospice; initially sceptical about comparable quality with traditional visits • Patients and caregivers – uniformly positive about service and wished to see increased utilization in own care plans

Implementation factors

Intuitively, it makes sense to use telecommunication to connect healthcare providers with patients when they are in separate locations. However simply adding technology to the current healthcare system will not necessarily produce the expected benefits. Caution should be exercised in promoting the use of technology to enable people to die at home. This is a complex issue, and family choices must play a role – as well as readiness to use the technology.

Patient readiness

Patients may be more or less willing to use home telehealth technology, depending on the stage in their disease trajectory, their mental status and the home support available. In a study of readiness to use home telehealth, patients noted that they were ready and willing to use the technology because it could support their independence.[9] However, the ability of some patients to manage their symptoms will fluctuate according to the daily ups and downs of their disease and treatment. In these cases, telehealth may be only realistic in the early stages of care (Box 21.4).

In the Canadian study, patients stated that they preferred fewer visits of all types, but still preferred in-person nurse visits. Patients also wanted to retain a choice in scheduling and type of visit. Some wanted to use videophones to connect with their family and friends, as well as pastoral and other healthcare providers.

Home telehealth will not be successful under all care conditions or for all patients. Categories of care not suitable for video-visits are those requiring hands-on intervention or assessment, medication preparation or administration, delivery of equipment or supplies, or support for the active phase of dying. On the other hand, patients are willing to receive psychosocial care, caregiver support and teaching through a videophone. However, if the patient's health status worsens, home visits may be more appropriate to provide the human presence and care required.

Nurse readiness

Nurses seem to recognize the value of using video-visits to connect with their patients more often and how it can reduce their travel time. However, palliative care is an area that is traditionally very 'high touch'. Studies of health professionals' responses to the

---

Box 21.4. Case study – Alex

Alex, a 79-year-old man, lives in his own home with his wife. In addition to receiving palliative home care, he suffers from multiple chronic illnesses. With his wife's assistance, he continues to manage at home. The home-care nurse visits every Thursday at 09:00 to check his blood pressure, which he noted 'was never up' at that time. After seeing the home telehealth equipment, he suggested that he check his blood pressure when he did not feel well and send the reading to the nurse using this technology. He could receive guidance on what to do next at the time he needed it.

Alex worked with his home-care nurse to develop a self-management plan, in which he monitored his blood pressure daily using a home-based system. These data were transmitted automatically to the nurse's office via his cable system. Alex followed a number of strategies if his blood pressure was outside the safe range for him. He knew when he was to call the nurse directly. The nurse's visits were reduced to one per month, when she discussed his blood pressure readings and they re-evaluated his management goals.

Comment
Provision of more information for clients and families can empower them to be more in control of symptom management. This also frees up the nurse's time to attend to situations that require nursing expertise. In this case, the nurse was willing to explore alternatives to routine care, which enabled her to find a beneficial solution for the client and herself.

---

introduction of a home telehealth service generally have linked views of the technology to views of professional self-image and status.[10,11]

In the Canadian study, nurses had considerable expertise with home visits, but initially lacked experience of using the home telehealth equipment. This hindered their ability to conduct video-visits. Training to use the equipment and complete the research data collection forms did not adequately prepare many nurses for integrating the videophone into their daily work routine. The nurses taught each other this important information. Once some nurses experienced success, others became less anxious about using the technology. Traditionally, home-care nurses have been older and less experienced in using technology. Given the goals of palliative care to communicate, support and manage symptoms, the nurses' reluctance to accomplish this via technology is understandable. Any changes to care delivery would require consideration of nurse scheduling, available resources, flexibility and ongoing administrative support.

Although home-care nurses often prefer to provide hands-on care, many have not received training in the use of technology to deliver care (Fig. 21.4). Experience shows that their initial perceptions and fears are often not realised.

A patient in the last stages of life anticipates a committed, focused, practical, empathetic interaction with the nurse. The multitasking nurse has to juggle many demands, procedures, priorities and time commitments. When using an analogue videophone, nurses must slow down their movements and speech, as well as attend completely to the patient on the screen. This requires some practice.

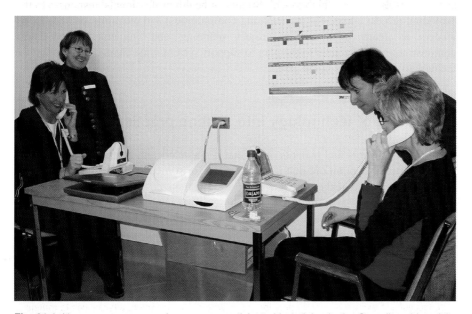

Fig. 21.4. Home-care nurses and managers participated in training in the Canadian video-visits study

Organizational readiness

Use of alternative methods of palliative care delivery requires readiness in the organization as well as readiness among the users. In a study in Missouri, readiness to accept technological innovation was assessed in seven out of 62 hospice organizations. The study found significant differences between disciplines and hospices in relation to the types of devices used and the perceived benefits of videophones.[12] The investigators concluded that introducing videophones for hospice care would require substantial involvement of the users.

The Canadian experience underscores the importance of organizational understanding and support for the required learning – including hands-on training and integration of readiness, attitudes and behaviour into daily practice. A critical factor, often overlooked, is the need to involve all staff in project planning and implementation.

System readiness

The broader political and social environments in which organizations exist must also be ready for change. This 'system readiness' often depends on evidence that the innovation has been successful elsewhere. However, few organizations wish to be the leader in demonstrating success. The American project demonstrated how large-scale, system-wide thinking could result in significant changes in care delivery.[8] Two large hospices in Michigan and Kansas both had a statewide presence, which provided an opportunity to test the introduction of a telehospice service on a large scale.

In the Canadian study, the videophones were demonstrated at every opportunity in an effort to influence system readiness. These included a meeting of the Provincial Deputy Minister of Health with home-care directors, local media attending training, providing project updates in participating communities, and including palliative care leaders as team members in project planning and implementation. These demonstrations contributed to the plan to support system-wide change in adopting the technology in palliative home care.

Integration of technology into routine practice

Healthcare providers and patients agree that home telehealth has potential, although patients frequently point out that it has potential for someone other than themselves.[9] Part of the reason that the potential has not been realized is that attempts are often made to introduce a technology into an existing care system without careful consideration of the changes expected from patients and healthcare professionals. For example, the system may be more effective if patients could contact the nurse when they have a specific concern, rather than the nurse completing a regularly scheduled video or home visit.

Focusing on the definition of 'palliative' may interfere with implementing a home telehealth programme. If disease conditions are used as criteria for participating in a telehealth service, it is important to ensure that providers agree on the definitions so that measurement of outcomes does not become problematic (see Chapter 2).

Box 21.5. Draft nursing guideline recommendations. Adapted from Hebert et al[13]

Nurse–patient relationships
- Nurse initiates therapeutic relationship and performs initial assessment through face-to-face home-care visit before conducting video-visits with palliative patients/families
- When conducting a video-visit, nurse establishes therapeutic nurse–patient/family relationship using the process of providing hospice palliative care, which encompasses patient/family assessment, information sharing, decision-making, care planning, care delivery and confirmation
- To optimize the quality of the therapeutic nurse–patient/family relationship, home-care agency allows flexibility in duration of video-visiting

Competencies
- Nurse must acquire necessary knowledge and clinical experience in hospice palliative care to effectively conduct video-visits
- As in all areas of hospice palliative care nursing practice, nurse conducts video-visits in accordance with national Hospice Palliative Care Nursing Standards of Practice (2002).
- Formal training supports implementation of Nursing Guidelines for Video-Visits in Palliative Home Care for all nurses providing palliative care via video-visits before use of technology with patients and families
- Home-care agency provides educational sessions and resource materials for nurses conducting video-visits and, over time, integrates various of professional development opportunities to support nurses' role in palliative nursing telepractice
- Home-care agency provides, in consultation with vendors and specialized educators in telehome-care, training to patients/families to support them using technology in their home.

Locus of accountability
- When conducting video-visits, nurse provides care consistent with Canadian Nurses Association's Code of Ethics for Registered Nurses (2002) and professional practice standards established by the provincial regulatory body

Security, confidentiality and privacy
- Nurse and home-care agency share responsibility to develop and implement policies ensuring security, confidentiality and privacy of nurse–patient interactions during video-visiting
- Home-care agency develops an appropriate system for documenting video-visit encounters and managing risks
- Home-care agency ensures safety of equipment involved in video-visits and quick access to technical expertise to troubleshoot, maintain or repair equipment quickly

Informed consent and patient choice
- Nurse respects right of patient to be fully informed about choices regarding video-visits, including the right to seek other methods for care
- Nurse determines with general practitioner and patient/family if video-visits are appropriate for meeting the patient's expectations and needs
- Any video-visit in palliative home care would only be done with the full knowledge and informed consent of the patients/families

Professional practice environments
- Before implementation of palliative nursing telepractice programmes, home-care agency develops and adopts related written policies
- When implementing palliative nursing telepractice programmes, home-care agency commits to evaluating outcomes for patients/families and staff
- Home-care agency uses information from systematic evaluation of palliative nursing telepractice programmes to develop and implement strategies for programme improvement

In Alberta, nursing guidelines for video-visits in palliative home care were developed to help integrate the technology into professional practice.[13] The guidelines focus primarily on the expectations and needs of palliative patients and their families rather than the technology. Eighteen recommendations identify the nurse's role and help ensure safety and quality when video-visits are conducted in palliative home care (Box 21.5). The guidelines also highlight recommendations for practice, education, organization and policy.

Telehealth in palliative home care is more concerned with supporting the care than with the technology. Therefore, the tools available for palliative care assessment and nursing care could be adapted when telehealth is implemented. In the Canadian study, a palliative performance scale score (PPSv2) routinely employed in home care was used to determine three levels of general care requirements. Only those patients who required medium-to-low levels of care were recruited into the study. Presumably those with high care needs were too ill to participate or were unable to use the videophones.

Efficiency savings with home telehealth

Video-visits may lower the costs associated with providing home care to chronically ill patients. Fixed costs related to equipment and supplies are relatively easy to calculate. Variable costs, such as nurse travel times and distances, preparation time and long-distance costs require considerable effort to track. In particular, data on travel costs must be collected routinely and meticulously in order to show the economic benefits of video-visits. The Canadian study highlighted some complexity in economic data collection and analysis. For example, some nurses use regional fleet vehicles funded through a global budget, which require no record keeping on mileage or time spent travelling. For others who use their own cars, it is not possible to attribute a specific travel distance to any one patient, because multiple patient visits may be made during a single trip. In most cases, the nurses work part-time and manage caseloads that are a mixture of home care and palliative care, as well as sharing these caseloads with other part-time staff. Initial analysis indicates that there is a threshold at which cost savings are realized if video-visits replace home visits.[8]

Aside from travel costs, other factors to be considered in the economic analysis are: the preference for care, the average time per activity, the cost of equipment/supplies and the health resource utilization (i.e. numbers of doctor, emergency and hospital visits, and contacts with the nurse or other healthcare providers).

What proportion of home nursing visits are likely to be possible by video link? In three retrospective chart-review studies on the effectiveness of video-visits in palliative home care, some 30–48% of the study home visits could have been conducted through video-visits, which is in agreement with studies in community care generally.[14-16] Criteria for determining if home telehealth was possible included whether the patient was stable and whether they required the delivery of health equipment (e.g. walker, wheelchair), medication administration or hands-on care.[16]

However, a retrospective chart review may not reflect the actual number of visits that can be replaced by video-visits in practice.

In the Alberta study, feedback from nurses and patients indicated that the videophones could have been used to deliver approximately 50% of the visits.[8] However, just because a videophone could have been used does not mean that it would have been used. Readiness factors, the human context of illness, organizational support and work–life or caseload management are all factors that will influence adoption and use.

Conclusion

A number of inextricably linked factors in the provision of palliative home care influence the adoption of home telehealth. The results to date demonstrate some similarities and some differences in the success of video-visiting in different care delivery contexts. The Canadian project found that nurses were less ready than patients, although patients preferred fewer visits overall. The videophones were sometimes found to be effective in palliative home care and when used appropriately could deliver care via video-visits as well as home visits. Some evidence also showed cost-effectiveness if more than five consecutive visits were made and driving distances were great. The American experience in Kansas and Michigan was that patients and caregivers wished to see increased utilization in their own care plan and that nurse–patient communication seemed unaltered. Both studies found providers cautiously enthusiastic about telehospice. A key finding was that long-term experience with telehospice was a significant predictor of provider acceptance.

The factors that were associated with the successful use of home telehealth in the Canadian study were: a care model appropriate for integrating technology (e.g. flexibility in scheduling home visits), support from senior management, adequate initial and ongoing training, frequent enough use of the technology to maintain skills and interest, in-house technical support (e.g. to deliver and set up videophones in the home, as well as to troubleshoot technical problems for nurses and patients), active encouragement of patient and nurse feedback with respect to the intended use and expected outcomes, and local decision-making on programme applications and guidelines for use.

The factors that may impede successful applications include: limited willingness or capacity to consider innovative ways to support patients, making assumptions about appropriate disease criteria and fit, and 'doing business the way we always have'.

How much information is enough to make decisions about using home telehealth? Although many studies have demonstrated that telehealth can be effective in home care, there is no definitive answer in the general context of palliative home care. The decision to use a videophone must include consideration of the patient's characteristics, what care is required, what the nurse is able to deliver, and what the technology can offer patients and caregivers.

Overall, innovation and ongoing evaluation are critical to providing care in the community. In an age of increasing workload, an aging workforce and more acutely ill patients at home, technology-supported care is not only viable and feasible but also desirable. Practitioners and researchers in the telehealth field need to engage each other in the 'action-reflection-action' cycle, so that home telehealth technology becomes a flexible tool to serve a variety of patients and healthcare providers in achieving the common goal of sustainable community healthcare. Hospice palliative care also is undergoing an important evolution, which needs to incorporate the use of technology as well as consider how this will change the ways in which care is delivered.

Further information

Kinsella A. *Telehospice: a resource manual for program development and implementation*. Asheville, NC: Information for Tomorrow, 2004.

References

1 Hospice Foundation of America. *Hospice Foundation of America annual report 2003–2004*. Washington, DC: Hospice Foundation of America, 2006. Available at: www.hospicefoundation.org/aboutUs/annualReport.asp. (last accessed 18 November 2005).
2 Hospice Foundation of America. *What is hospice?* Washington, DC: Hospice Foundation of America, 2006. Available at: www.hospicefoundation.org/hospiceInfo/ (last accessed 18 November 2005).
3 Miccinesi G, Crocett E, Morino P, *et al.* Palliative home care reduces time spent in hospital wards: a population-based study in the Tuscany Region, Italy. *Cancer Causes Control* 2003;**14**:971–7.
4 Coyle N, Khojainova N, Francavilla JM, Gonzales GR. Audio-visual communication and its use in palliative care. *J Pain Symptom Manage* 2002;**23**:171–5.
5 Wong FKY, Liu CF, Szeto Y, *et al.* Health problems encountered by dying patients receiving palliative home care until death. *Cancer Nurs* 2004;**27**:244–51.
6 Kinsella A. Learning home telehealth: new opportunities. *Home Healthc Nurse* 2000;**18**:507–11.
7 Kinsella A. Telehealth in hospice care, or telehospice: a new frontier of telehealth service delivery. *J Palliat Med* 2005;**8**:711–12.
8 Hebert MA, Jansen JJ, Brant R, *et al.* Effectiveness of video-visits in palliative home care: preliminary findings of an RCT in the community. In: *Proceedings of the IASTED International Conference on Telehealth 2005*. Calgary: ACTA Press, 2005:127–30. Available at: www.actapress.com/PaperInfo.aspx?PaperID=21968 (last accessed 9 January 2006).
9 Hebert MA, Paquin MJ, Iversen S. Predicting success: stakeholder readiness for home telecare diabetic support. *J Telemed Telecare* 2002;**8** (Suppl 3):33–6.
10 Utterback K. Supporting a new model of care with telehealth technology. *Telehealth Pract Rep* 2005;**9**(6):3.
11 Hibbert D, Mair FS, May CR, *et al.* Health professionals' responses to the introduction of a home telehealth service. *J Telemed Telecare* 2004;**10**:226–30.
12 Parker Oliver DR, Demiris G. An assessment of the readiness of hospice organizations to accept technological innovation. *J Telemed Telecare* 2004;**10**:170–4.
13 Hebert MA, Paquin MJ, Whitten L. Nursing guideline for video-visits in palliative homecare. *Can Nurse* (submitted).
14 Wootton R, Loane M, Mair F, *et al.* A joint US-UK study of home telenursing. *J Telemed Telecare* 1998;**4** (Suppl 1):83–5.
15 Allen A, Doolittle CG, Boysen CD, *et al.* An analysis of the suitability of home health visits for telemedicine. *J Telemed Telecare* 1999;**5**:90–6.
16 Hebert MA, Paquin MJ, Whitten L, Cai P. Suitability of video-visits for palliative home care: Implications for nursing practice. *J Telemed Telecare* (in press).

17   Whitten P, Doolittle G, Hellmich S. Telehospice: using telecommunication technology for terminally ill patients. *JCMC* 2001;**6**. See jcmc.indiana.edu/vol6/issue4/whitten2.html (last accessed 18 November 2005).

18   Doolittle GC. A cost measurement study for a home-based telehospice service. *J Telemed Telecare* 2000;**6** (Suppl 1):193–5.

▶22

Remote asthma monitoring

Vedran Ostojić

Introduction

Asthma is a chronic inflammatory disease with more or less frequent attacks of wheezing, cough and shortness of breath. Asthma is associated with significant morbidity and mortality, affecting more and more children and adults every year. About five million people in the UK and 15 million people in the US have this disease. The prevalence and severity of asthma have increased over the past 20 years, and asthma is currently the fourth leading cause of limitation of normal daily activities. Asthma can have a significant negative effect on the quality of life. The severity of this condition can vary from mild seasonal attacks of night cough to life-threatening shortness of breath.

Asthma, however, does not have to stop a person living a full and enjoyable life. Although it cannot be cured, asthma can be controlled effectively by long-term use of inhaled, long-acting β_2-agonists and corticosteroids.[1] Properly treated, most patients can live without a single asthmatic attack. For that to be achieved, asthma, like other chronic diseases such as diabetes and high blood pressure, has to be monitored frequently, preferably daily. Morbidity from asthma in both children and adults is related to their adherence to therapy.[2,3] Guidelines are widely available – both electronically and in paper form – and are designed to provide a consistent standard of care for patients with asthma.[4]

Despite proactive asthma care in general practice, only about one-third of people with asthma in the UK attend for their annual review.[5] Adherence to guidelines is very poor and tends to worsen over time. In addition, the awareness of symptoms and perception of their severity are variable and subjective. It is generally agreed that one-time or occasional spirometry severely limits a physician's ability to adequately assess and follow asthma. It is almost impossible to perform these measurements more frequently and under professional supervision, so this has to be done at home. Some pulmonary function tests are particularly suitable for home monitoring, especially peak expiratory flow rate (PEFR) and forced exhaled volume in the first second (FEV_1 – that is, the air volume that can be forcibly exhaled in one second after taking a deep breath). Patients can perform these tests after some training by using small and affordable portable spirometers (Fig. 22.1). Values lower than 80% from the baseline indicate poor control of asthma. Very low values (lower than 50% from the baseline) are an indication for an immediate visit to the physician or admission to a hospital unit.

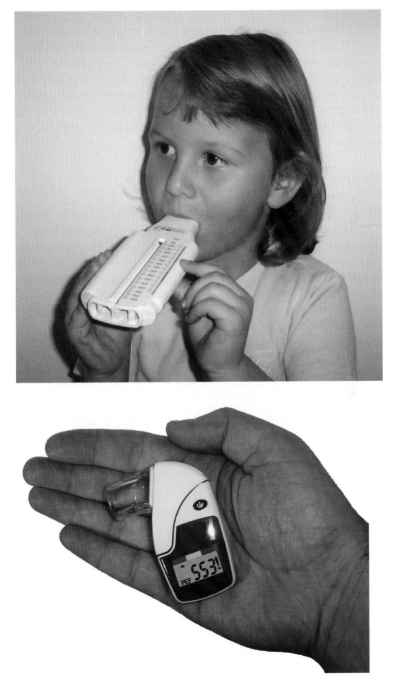

Fig. 22.1. Peak flow meters

Recent data have shown that asthma education programmes, using a self-management plan, are more likely to decrease the utilization of health services. Daily recorded PEFR and FEV_1 values are valuable data that allow a physician to estimate a patient's condition and therapeutic effect. Unfortunately, compliance of patients is very variable, and this is compounded by the difficulties of assessing medication adherence accurately. Bender *et al* investigated child report, mother report, canister weight and electronic measurements of metered-dose inhaler actuation.[6] Electronic adherence monitoring was significantly more accurate than self-reporting or canister weight measures.

Asthma and telemedicine

Telemedicine is attractive to physicians because it gives them the possibility of reaching all patients who need their advice – regardless of distance. Telemedicine is attractive to patients because it gives them a better chance of being reached. Naturally, both groups prefer the face-to face consultation where possible, but sometimes (from many authors' experience, in about 50–80% of cases) consultations can be performed by some form of telemedicine, which is more convenient, cheaper, less time-consuming and equally satisfactory for both parties. Telemedicine may reduce patients' travelling time and time off work, and decrease overall costs.

The treatment of asthma requires extensive patient knowledge, as patients must understand basic asthma information, a self-management plan and metered-dose inhaler technique. Patients may also need to use other specific devices to administer medication and perform simple pulmonary function tests such as PEFR and FEV_1 daily. All this can be very demanding, especially for children and elderly adults. Many web-based systems are available for the general public to improve education in asthma. Systems also exist to provide telemedicine contact with healthcare professionals using videoconferencing and telephone calls.

Table 22.1. Methods of remote asthma monitoring

Method	Example
Real-time	
Communication with patient through messaging	• Email
	• Internet messaging
Communication with patient through conversation	• Telephone
	• Internet
Communication with patient through videoconference	• TV
	• Internet videoconference
Store-and-forward	
Transmission of pulmonary sounds to health professional	• Telephone
	• Internet
Transmission of data on pulmonary function to health professional	• Letter
	• Fax
	• Email
	• Mobile phone text messages
	• Internet

Asthma control includes managing the acute exacerbations, as well as chronic management aimed at reducing the severity and frequency of acute exacerbations and maintaining optimum health and lung function. Health outcomes for children and adults with asthma may be improved through education, adherence to appropriate therapy, regular review and, in the case of young people and adults with asthma, promotion of self-management. Most of these activities can be enhanced or supported by telemedicine.

Several methods of remote asthma monitoring exist. These can be divided into real-time methods of communication, such as the telephone, and store-and-forward methods of communication, such as email (Table 22.1).

Letter and fax

Telemedicine consultations in asthma were probably first conducted by letter. Patients could write to their physicians to describe their signs and symptoms in order to monitor the severity of the disease. Obviously, a patient's view of symptom severity may be subjective. Paper can be used to transmit objective data as well, however, such as the results of pulmonary function tests. This telemedicine method is still used today in the form of the asthma diary, in which patients record their PEFR data and symptoms like night cough, wheezing and shortness of breath. The diary can then be presented directly to the physician during the patient's follow-up visits. The method is simple and cheap, but patient compliance is surprisingly low. Fax transmission of paper documents has not been used widely by patients. The main disadvantages of the 'asthma diary' are poor compliance and the time interval between recording the information and its evaluation by the physician.

Telephone and mobile phone

The first telecommunication device generally available was the telephone, and it is still used widely today. Early developments in telemonitoring with the telephone can be traced back to 1905, when Einthoven transmitted an electrocardiogram from a hospital to his laboratory.[7] Subsequently, the telephone has been used to improve asthma control. Transmission of the results of pulmonary function tests in digital form was made possible by the telephone. To connect a computer to the telephone network requires an electronic device called a modem (a word constructed from MOdulator-DEModulator). This converts the digital information from the computer into audible sounds that can be transmitted and received over the telephone lines. Because of the relatively small number of data needed for transmission of the results of pulmonary function tests, even the early modems were fast enough.

Voice conversation

The first application was to talk directly to the patient. Patients can present their symptoms and any information about their asthma management. The physician can

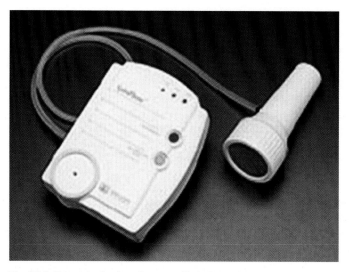

Fig. 22.2. Transtelephonic spirometer (SpiroPhone)

provide useful information as feedback. Many authors have shown the feasibility of telemedicine-over-telephone in reducing the utilization of medical services, improving health status and reducing mortality.[8,9] Some, however, have also expressed concern about the adequacy of telephone interviews compared with face-to-face examinations, because of lack of objective data and dependence on patient feedback.

Respiratory sounds

As well as interviewing the patient, it is also possible to transmit respiratory sounds with an electronic stethoscope. Sound is recorded by a microphone attached to the patient's chest wall, and the remote physician can listen to this recording to assess the severity of the asthma. In order to produce satisfactory sound quality, a few technical enhancements are necessary, including noise suppression, digitization of transmitted sounds and enhanced spectral analysis of received sound. Examples of such devices are telespirometry systems for home monitoring (Fig. 22.2).[10,11]

Audio transmission has been enhanced further with the introduction of mobile phones.[12] The main disadvantages of this method are the need for sophisticated electronic equipment and the difficulty of excluding differential diagnoses.

Internet

The Internet is a ubiquitous communications medium. Several different kinds of telecommunication are possible. Store-and-forward methods include email and the web; real-time methods include instant messaging and videoconferencing.

Email

Email allows rapid delivery of information and easy attachment of text, audio or video files, but it requires access to a suitable computer and is vulnerable to unauthorized access to information. Email is recommended for all kind of textual communication between patient and doctor in settings where real-time interaction is not needed.[13] Email has been used to send video file attachments of patients who have recorded themselves using their inhalers.[14] Patients received feedback from case managers via email, including pointers on inhaler technique. The main disadvantage of email as a communications medium is poor security of the data.

Instant messaging

Instant messaging began as Internet text communication that differed from email because conversations happened in real-time. Modern instant messaging programs allow simultaneous exchange of all kinds of messages – from plain text to videoconferencing. Although this is an interesting way of communicating, there seem to be no reports of its use in patients with asthma. For the general population, there is no obvious benefit compared with the ordinary telephone, except for the lower per-minute cost in international communication.

Web

Many web pages are dedicated to asthma news and education. In addition, several web-based systems for asthma monitoring are available, especially for PEFR, FEV_1 and symptom recording and monitoring (for example, www.myasthma.com and sms.astma.hr). Many authors have found the web to be an excellent tool for delivering patients' pulmonary function results.[11,15] Networking speed was not found to be restrictive because of the non-demanding nature of pulmonary function tests. Even the slowest modem connections are sufficient to transmit all necessary data in a reasonable time (up to 10 minutes). However, higher bandwidth, such as digital (integrated services digital network, ISDN) or broadband lines, is required for videoconsultations.

If secure protocols (HTTPS) and passwords are used for data transmission on the Internet, then security is probably satisfactory. Studies have shown considerable financial benefits from lower hospitalization and medication rates if every asthmatic patient has access to the Internet and the skills to use it. Unfortunately, after an enthusiastic start, some authors have observed a significant decrease in patient compliance with text-based asthma monitoring services.[16]

Videoconferencing

A videoconference enables more direct contact with the physician than is possible by telephone. It enables positive identification of the participants involved and improves confidence and information transfer between patient and doctor. Several examples exist of videoconferencing in the education of patients[17] and supervision of patients while using inhalers or performing pulmonary function tests. Videophones have been used successfully in video communication between patients' homes and a chest clinic to improve treatment. Recently, Internet-based videoconferencing has become popular. It is hard to implement such communication on a large scale, however, because of the difficulties in organizing appropriate times in the busy schedule of physicians.

Text messaging

Many mobile phones offer the short message service (SMS), which allows the sending and receiving of text messages up to 160 characters in length. This can be used for long-term control of patients with asthma. Instead of using a dedicated communication device for sending pulmonary function test results, a universally familiar device is employed. Although many people find Internet communication difficult to use, because it requires basic knowledge of computers, they are often very familiar with their mobile phones and most are capable of sending SMS messages.

Several applications have used SMS transmission successfully in the monitoring of asthma.[18,19] The convenience of sending PEFR results with a mobile phone resulted in better compliance over longer periods. Some services that receive SMS

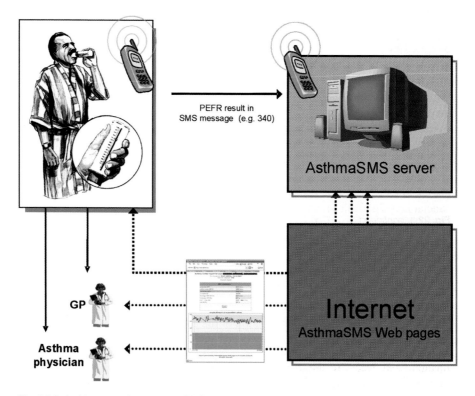

PEFR result in
SMS message (e.g. 340)

AsthmaSMS server

GP

Asthma
physician

Internet
AsthmaSMS Web pages

Fig. 22.3. Architecture of an asthma SMS service

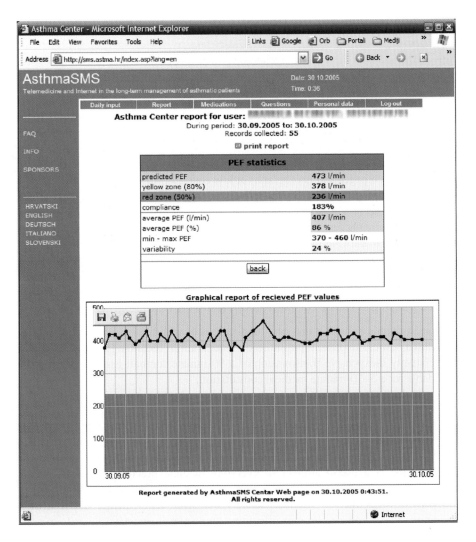

Fig. 22.3. *continued*

messages containing pulmonary function test results provide feedback in the form of graphical and statistical reports (Fig. 22.3). Text messages can be used as feedback from a physician or as a reminder in order to improve asthma control and adherence to medication, especially in schoolchildren with asthma. Text messaging may hold an advantage over the Internet and email, because it is less susceptible to unauthorized access to the message data. The SMS service itself is evolving into a multimedia messaging service (MMS) that is suitable for transmission of text, audio, still images and video.

New mobile communication protocols

New developments in mobile technology will provide further possibilities for telemedicine in asthma. The new mobile communication protocols include:

- EDGE (enhanced data rates for GSM evolution) is a new technology that delivers broadband-like data transmission speeds to mobile devices. This permits high-capacity, Internet-based communication, including colour web browsing, email, visual communication and multimedia messaging. It enables constant 24-hour connectivity to the Internet and transfer of pulmonary function test data, digital images, web pages and photographs at low cost.
- 3GSM (third-generation GSM) delivers advanced mobile services such as the downloading of video and music clips, full multimedia messaging, high-speed colour Internet access and email on the move.
- WiMAX (Worldwide Interoperability for Microwave Access) will bring wireless broadband Internet access to mobile users. WiMAX wireless coverage will allow true wireless mobility, as opposed to the limited coverage ('hot-spots') required by wireless computing at present. It seems that many mobile phone manufacturers are planning to release combined GSM- and WiMAX-capable mobile phones.

It is reasonable to predict that new mobile devices with two-way video capabilities will start a new era in patient–physician communication. Technology that will support the relatively inexpensive transmission of a 90-minute football game will surely be affordable for a 5–10-minute medical consultation.

Conclusion

Telemedicine is a useful adjunct to everyday medical practice, especially in the monitoring of asthma, where it may contribute to better disease control. According to the current experience in asthma management with telemedicine, the following scenarios can be proposed for cost-effective asthma management:

- daily remote monitoring by wireless means (for example, by mobile phone), with automatic transmission of pulmonary function data to a central server (e.g. PEFR, FEV_1 and forced vital capacity, FVC)
- secure, web-based access to statistical and graphical reports for physicians and patients
- frequent telephone or mobile phone consultations – for example, once a month. Videoconsultations by mobile phone may be possible in the future.
- periodic face-to-face follow-up (2–3 times a year, as well as during exacerbations).

Although several feasibility studies of asthma management using telemedicine have proved successful, it is not yet common – except in acute situations where other forms of medical help are not available in a reasonable time. Various barriers exist to its widespread adoption, including privacy and security concerns, and certain medicolegal issues. None of these seem to be irresolvable.

It is important to remember that the intention of telemedicine is not to replace face-to-face consultations but to improve the management of asthma. Intelligent use of telemedicine will improve asthma management and make the quality of life of people with asthma fuller and more enjoyable.

Further information

Global Initiative for Asthma (GINA) website. Available at: www.ginasthma.org (last accessed 2 January 2006).

MyAsthma website. Available at: www.myasthma.com/ (last accessed 2 January 2006).

National Asthma Council of Australia website. Available at: www.nationalasthma.org.au (last accessed 2 January 2006).

Wainwright C, Wootton R. A review of telemedicine and asthma. *Dis Manag Health Outcomes* 2003;**11**:557–63.

References

1   Masoli M, Fabian D, Holt S, Beasley R. *Global burden of asthma. Global Initiative for Asthma (GINA).* Global Initiative for Asthma, 2004. Available at: www.ginasthma.com/download.asp?intId=29 (last accessed 1 January 2006).

2   Schmier JK, Leidy NK. The complexity of treatment adherence in adults with asthma: challenges and opportunities. *J Asthma* 1998;**35**:455–72.

3   Bauman LJ, Wright E, Leickly FE, *et al.* Relationship of adherence to pediatric asthma morbidity among inner-city children. *Pediatrics* 2002;**110**:e6.

4   Global Initiative for Asthma (GINA). *Workshop report. Pocket guide for asthma management and prevention.* Global Initiative for Asthma, 2005. Available at: www.ginasthma.com/download.asp?intId=191 (last accessed 1 January 2006).

5   National Asthma Campaign. Out in the open: a true picture of asthma in the United Kingdom today. *Asthma J* 2001;**6** (Suppl):3–14.

6   Bender B, Wamboldt FS, O'Connor SL, *et al.* Measurement of children's asthma medication adherence by self report, mother report, canister weight, and Doser CT. *Ann Allergy Asthma Immunol* 2000;**85**:416–21.

7   Einthoven W. Le télécardiogramme. *Arch Int Physiol* 1906;**4**:132–64 (in French).

8   Wasson J, Gaudette C, Whaley F, *et al.* Telephone care as a substitute for routine clinic follow up. *JAMA* 1992;**267**:1788–93.

9   Pinnock H, Bawden R, Proctor S, *et al.* Accessibility, acceptability, and effectiveness in primary care of routine telephone review of asthma: pragmatic, randomised controlled trial. *BMJ* 2003;**326**:477–9.

10 Bruderman I, Abboud S. Telespirometry: novel system for home monitoring of asthmatic patients. *Telemed J* 1997;**3**:127–33.

11 Finkelstein J, Hripcsak G, Cabrera M. Telematic system for monitoring of asthma severity in patients' homes. *Medinfo* 1998;**9**:272–6.

12 Anderson K, Qiu Y, Whittaker AR, Lucas M. Breath sounds, asthma, and the mobile phone. *Lancet* 2001;**358**:1343–4.

13 Partridge MR. An assessment of the feasibility of telephone and email consultation in a chest clinic. *Patient Educ Couns* 2004;**54**:11–13.

14 Malone F, Callahan CW, Chan DS, *et al.* Caring for children with asthma through teleconsultation: 'ECHO-Pac, The Electronic Children's Hospital of the Pacific'. *Telemed J E Health* 2004;**10**:138–46.

15 Rasmussen LM, Phanareth K, Nolte H, Backer V. Internet-based monitoring of asthma: a long-term, randomized clinical study of 300 asthmatic subjects. *J Allergy Clin Immunol* 2005;**115**:1137–42.

16   Anhoj J, Nielsen L. Quantitative and qualitative usage data of an Internet-based asthma monitoring tool. *J Med Internet Res* 2004;**6**:e23.

17   Reznik M, Sharif I, Ozuah PO. Use of interactive videoconferencing to deliver asthma education to inner-city immigrants. *J Telemed Telecare* 2004;**10**:118–20.

18   Anhoj J, Moldrup C. Feasibility of collecting diary data from asthma patients through mobile phones and SMS (short message service): response rate analysis and focus group evaluation from a pilot study. *J Med Internet Res* 2004;**6**:e42.

19   Ostojic V, Cvoriscec B, Ostojic SB, *et al*. Improving asthma control through telemedicine: a study of short-message service. *Telemed J E Health* 2005;**11**:28–35.

Section 4: The future

▶ 23

Financial implications of widescale implementation of telecare

David A. Bradley and Simon Brownsell

Introduction

Telehealth services encompass a wide range of provision – these include online access to sources of information and comprehensive telemedicine systems. Home telehealth, sometimes called telecare, is an aspect of telemedicine and e-health generally: the terms are inexact and often used interchangeably. Here 'telecare' refers to the use of telehealth techniques to support people – either ill or well – in their homes.

In relation to telecare services, basic community alarms or personal emergency response systems, as they are sometimes known, provide direct support throughout much of the industrialized world. At the time of writing, more than 1.6 million people use these first-generation telecare systems in the UK alone. Much work on telecare to date, however, has concentrated on the performance of the technologies – often involving trials with relatively small numbers of people. Few studies have attempted to evaluate new telecare systems against more traditional forms of intervention or the associated costs.

As technology develops, second-generation telecare systems are becoming available. These incorporate features such as health monitoring, gas alarms and automatic incident reporting – for example, when a fall occurs. Table 23.1 describes the different generations of telecare systems.

Table 23.1. Evolution of telecare systems

Generation	Capability
First	• Technically simple systems with no embedded intelligence and entirely reliant on user activating calls
Second	• More advanced systems with all features of first-generation system but also providing some level of intelligence either locally or distributed
	• Proactive and intended to detect alert situations and autonomously initiate calls for assistance if required or if user unable to do so
Third	• Encompassing functions of second-generation systems and adding additional support capabilities such as lifestyle monitoring
	• Focus on widespread use of telecommunications
	• Introduce concepts such as virtual neighbourhoods
	• Aim to contribute to improvement in quality of user's life by supporting a range of teleservices
Fourth	• Likely to make use of a range of diagnostic tools based on developing sensor technologies and using advanced information processing

A critical factor in introducing new-generation systems is their cost-effectiveness in relation to other forms of care. Indeed, Whitten *et al* commented that this is one of the most commonly posed questions about assistive technologies and second-generation telecare systems.[1] Furthermore, in 1998, Wootton suggested that cost-effectiveness studies are crucial to the introduction of second-generation telecare systems, as no government will introduce them on a significant scale without firm evidence of this.[2]

Cost elements in telecare

The architecture of a telecare system is illustrated in Fig. 23.1. The home-based elements consist of the sensor(s) used to measure a range of variables associated with the individual, together with the local processing of the resultant information. The infrastructure external to the home supports the transmission of the data and its management, including the responses required. The costs associated with telecare can therefore be considered in relation to the following areas:

- collection and analysis of data in the home (sensors and associated data processing)
- onward transmission of the data (communications infrastructure)
- managing and responding to the data (system-level functions, control centres, skills profiles and training requirements).

Each of these contributes to the overall cost of providing a telecare system.

Sensors and actuators

The sensors and actuators required by first-generation, and to a large extent second-generation, telecare systems are generally straightforward. For example, passive infrared (PIR) sensors and switches, or off-the-shelf items of relatively low cost may be used. In terms of actuators, systems such as door openers are also generally available. Even in those forms of telecare associated with the direct management of clinical conditions such as congestive heart failure (CHF), chronic obstructive pulmonary disease (COPD) and asthma, the sensors required are also readily available. The only difference is the provision of some local intelligence in the user's home to forward data previously gathered in a medical setting.

As the sophistication of systems increases from second-generation to third-generation systems and beyond, additional sensors are required with improved performance, depending on the users' needs. These sensors are likely to be associated

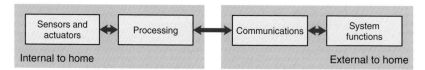

Fig. 23.1. Architecture of a telecare system

with significant development costs and thus will need to be sold in large numbers to enable these costs to be recovered.

Other advanced sensors, including implantable devices for monitoring clinical conditions such as diabetes, are also likely to be associated with substantial development costs. Their underlying technologies, however, may result in them eventually becoming disposable items – in a way that current sensors are not.

Processing and networking

Computer processing power is now comparatively cheap. Where the target user has their own personal computer (PC), it may be possible to install a card in that PC to reduce costs, but careful consideration must be given to liability if the system should fail. In the home, sensors, actuators and system intelligence must be connected by a secure communications network. Here, wireless technologies such as Bluetooth, Wi-Fi and Zigbee reduce costs by eliminating the need for any rewiring.

The system hardware, however, is not likely to represent the major proportion of the cost of a home telecare system. Rather, the cost of software, particularly the software development time required to produce a validated system, is likely to be the major factor. This is particularly the case with third- and fourth-generation systems, for which the aim is to move from responsive systems to predictive and supportive systems that incorporate enhanced client diagnostic functions as well as the self-monitoring and checking of the system itself. Such systems will need to complete a rigorous validation and testing programme, including ensuring compliance with the appropriate national standards for medical devices, which will add significantly to development time and hence costs.

Communications

As indicated by Curry et al,[3] the current (2005) levels of communications traffic associated with telecare can be accommodated by the ordinary telephone network (public switched telephone network, PSTN), as long as most information processing is carried out in the user's home. This, however, tends to assume that no other services require, or are likely to require, similar access to the home telephone line and that no other uses will be developed, such as the creation of virtual communities to support individuals undergoing treatment at home or simply to enhance social interaction.

The evolution of third- and fourth-generation telecare systems is likely to increase the demand for additional telecommunications bandwidth to support the increased functionality. The continuing growth of broadband networks is likely to facilitate the provision of this extra bandwidth, as will the introduction of local intranets by bodies such as housing associations to support communication with tenants, as telecare can be piggybacked onto such networks.

Although an increasing number of households throughout the world are using broadband services, the number of broadband users remains relatively low in comparison with those who use the PSTN.[4] The communications infrastructure is not a significant element with respect to first- and second-generation systems in terms of its contribution to the costs of providing telecare, as most households have access to the telephone network. Additional bandwidth is likely to be required for third- and fourth-generation systems, which will add to system costs.

System functions

Telecare is not just about equipment installation in the individual home or care environment: the network needs to be managed. This management infrastructure typically consists of a control centre to provide an operator response, together with ancillary functions such as technical support. As more people are supported in their own homes, greater numbers of support staff are required to respond to, and provide physical assistance in, the home environment. This shift in staffing profile implies a redistribution of resources from hospitals to the community, which will require significant redesign and restructuring of current service provision.

To support a move to future systems, control centres will have to manage the additional information provided by these systems. There will also be a need to ensure that the requisite information is available to facilitate overall operation of the system, including the growth of home-based services. This brings with it questions of security, access to information and the management of information – as is the case for health-related data stored elsewhere.

Changes at the system level also bring additional training requirements for a wide range of clinical, support and technical staff. Indeed, staff specifically trained to work with the technologies of telecare and provide the assessment of individual need in relation to those technologies are likely to be required. Although it may well be possible to support such staff with a range of tools (including intelligent support systems), the development of these tools and the associated training programmes represents an additional cost at the system level. Identification and provision of an appropriately structured healthcare workforce may in the long term be a determining factor in the success of telecare.

Cost-effectiveness of telecare

Despite the complexities of understanding the true cost-effectiveness of telecare, studies, such as those by Roth et al[5] and Bowes and McColgan,[6] report cost savings associated with the use of specific telehealth services. These reports may not include all possible cost elements, however, so the results may be distorted. In order to allow reliable conclusions to be drawn, telecare services need to progress through four stages:

- development of the technology
- technical performance trial
- limited system trial to learn implementation and delivery lessons
- large-scale trial.

The final stage ideally should be a controlled trial that compares the true costs of the conventional intervention with the new telecare option. Such trials are difficult to conduct, however, and systems often proceed directly to implementation. There is also the problem that by the time all four stages have been conducted, the technology may have developed significantly in terms of more functionality and reduced cost. This perhaps suggests that large-scale, randomized, controlled trials (RCTs) may not be the preferred method for evaluating telecare services.

Little quantitative information exists about the savings that result from using telecare instead of traditional methods. Nevertheless, the levels of evidence described below can inform the debate.

Service level reports

In 2004, the Audit Commission in the UK stated that 'the potential of assistive technology to promote independence and save money across public services is not in doubt'.[7] They also suggested that the NHS could save £63 million in patients with COPD and £118 million in patients with CHF alone by using telecare. A similar indication of the effectiveness of assistive technology in reducing the cost of care comes from the US.[8]

Following the European-funded ASTRID project (a social and technological response to meeting the needs of individuals with dementia and their carers), a countywide assistive technology and telecare service was introduced in Northamptonshire, UK, to support people with dementia and their carers. The 'safe at home project' uses items of equipment such as calendar clocks and medication dispensers to compensate for disabilities caused by dementia. When evaluating the service, the technology seemed to play an important role in enabling people with dementia to maintain independent living for longer. In financial terms, over a 21-month period, the saving per user was estimated as £3690. Across the 233 users, this suggests an overall saving of about £1.5 million.[9]

The Veterans Health Administration in the US is a large-scale user of telecare (see Chapter 9).[10]

Peer-reviewed findings

Some studies have reported cost-effectiveness data, although most of the work relates to telemedicine rather than telecare. Jennett et al provided a comprehensive overview of cost-effectiveness in relation to a number of application areas of interest.[11]

Telephone-based applications can have a significant socio-economic impact. Such applications include patient assessment, patient monitoring and disease management, along with the ability to target people for further professional assessment. Some evidence of socio-economic benefit has been obtained. Home telecare studies have indicated socio-economic benefits such as enhanced quality of life and reduced utilization of services (hospital days or clinic visits).

Evidence suggests that interactive videoconferencing is effective in rural and remote areas. However, economic analysis suggests that cost savings depend on the numbers of patients and distances involved, as well as the perspective of the study. Thus, if only those costs to be met by the healthcare system are included, the telehealth alternative is not always cheaper.

Systematic reviews

Several systematic reviews have been undertaken in the area of telemedicine generally, including telecare. Roine *et al* reported that few studies demonstrated cost benefits from the introduction of a telemedicine service,[12] while Whitten *et al* reviewed 612 articles, of which 55 included actual data on cost benefits.[13] Of these, only 24 met the inclusion criteria for a good-quality review. From this, the authors concluded that no strong evidence shows that telemedicine and telecare are a cost-effective means of delivering healthcare. This inability to provide conclusive evidence from a systematic review has much to do with the lack of robust scientific evidence,[14] as alluded to earlier.

As May *et al* noted,[15] a large body of literature seems supportive of telehealth and telecare, but systematic reviews suggest that a degree of scepticism is reasonable. The field is dominated by reports of small-scale studies that are often short-lived demonstration projects, and there are, as yet, few large-scale clinical trials of telecare systems.

Cost modelling

The complexity of telecare interventions and the relative scarcity of high-quality studies means that one way of obtaining a better understanding of the financial consequences is through modelling. Models allow investigation of the changes that would be associated with the widespread deployment of telecare. One such telecare model compared the current community alarm system for 11 618 users against a replacement second-generation telecare system that costs an average of £700 per installation. Over a 10-year life cycle, an extreme scenario analysis (that is, one that looked at the most pessimistic and optimistic outcomes) suggested that, when compared with the present community alarm system, the worst-case financial saving

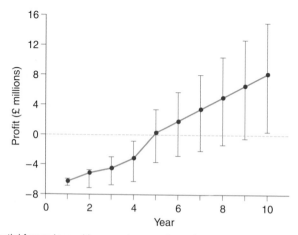

Fig. 23.2. Potential for savings with second-generation telecare system

was of the order of £500 000, while the most optimistic scenario produced savings of about £14 million. The most likely result was savings of some £8 million. The level of sensitivity for the analysis can be seen from Fig. 23.2. Extrapolation of these results to the UK as a whole suggests that if all of the current 1.6 million community alarm users were provided with the second-generation telecare system considered in the model, savings in excess of £1 billion could accrue.[16]

Any model, however, is only as good as its underlying assumptions. The House of Lords Science and Technology Committee have commented that present and prior models do not adequately reflect the impact of telehealth and telecare on the healthcare infrastructure, in part due to the problems of obtaining the information on performance and costs that are required to support robust models.[8]

Discussion

From the above, it is apparent that the cost implications for the large-scale introduction of telecare are unclear. Certainly, reports of cost-effective systems exist, but these are not demonstrated beyond reasonable doubt. As suggested in a recent European report,[17] however, 'although such estimates of cost savings and efficiency gains remain highly speculative due to lack of robust measurement methodologies and the current low rate of uptake of technologies, it is widely accepted that, from an economic point of view, telecare is likely to increase efficiency and productivity in the healthcare industry.' The report goes on to identify key areas as:

- close observation and monitoring of patients, supporting a shift in emphasis from reaction to prevention
- the more efficient use of available resources through the use of online decision support systems, reducing the amount spent on 'unnecessary' or inappropriate care.

Potential for savings

For a telehealth or telecare system to be seen as cost-effective, it must pay for itself by achieving equivalent savings elsewhere in the healthcare system. Studies have identified costs that might be influenced by the presence of an effective telecare system; however, in general, they are difficult to quantify with any degree of accuracy. For instance, at a mundane level, the ability to remotely operate external door locks would eliminate the need for forced entry, saving unspecified repair costs.

A number of factors that also influence cost-effectiveness are not generally capable of being assessed or quantified. It is recognized, therefore, that potential cost benefits exist as a result of an individual feeling more secure and comfortable in their home environment, although establishing a monetary figure for this is difficult, if not impossible.

Where representative figures are available, savings are likely in relation to:

- support services, e.g. day care and helpers
- full-time care, e.g. nursing and care homes

- hospitalization, e.g. bed costs, care and support
- treatment costs, by providing more timely interventions.

The analysis that has been done suggests that relatively modest changes in the care profile, such as delaying entry into full-time care for a period of a few weeks or months, or reducing the average period of hospitalization by one or two days, could result in savings that would cover the cost of the requisite system. It is not surprising, therefore, that much of the focus of interventions to date has been on chronic conditions.

Preventive systems

Loeb has said that 'the general cost-effectiveness of preventing an illness rather than treating it is usually favourable, but the specific cost of the preventive traditionally has to be paid by a party that has not yet incurred the obligation to pay for the illness. Nowhere is this problem more obvious than in the boundaries between hospital, extended care facility and home care for frail but generally healthy patients.'[18] However, although, in general, a preventive approach is likely to be beneficial in terms of resource utilization, and hence cost, this is not always the case. Indeed, situations are likely to exist in which the long-term and cumulative costs of a preventive strategy may outweigh the cost of treatment (in financial terms at least).

Such decisions will remain a matter of clinical judgement; however, future generations of telecare can be seen to have a major preventive role. This balance between prevention and treatment has not necessarily been taken into account in relation to previous decisions about healthcare provision. To quote the conclusions of the House of Lords Committee on Science and Technology report referred to earlier: 'The initiation of studies of the cost-effectiveness of spending resources on prevention rather than treatment must be an important consideration…'.[8]

Urban–rural split

In Scotland, significant problems result from the sparsely distributed rural population and the requirement to meet their expectations for healthcare provision.[19] Telehealth may be important in supporting independent living – especially when distance is a problem.

Telecare has an important role in enabling individuals to remain at home and increasing their feelings of independence and dignity, especially in rural environments such as parts of Australia, Canada and the US. In the UK, the extension of broadband networks into rural areas should facilitate the introduction of telecare services. In addition to supporting individuals in maintaining their independence, such a strategy is likely to benefit the community as a whole by ensuring or maintaining its overall viability.

Economies of scale

Clearly a relationship exists between the cost of a telecare system and the number of systems being installed and operated. In many cases, particularly in first- and second-generation systems, the basic sensors for the systems are relatively low-cost items. The overall installation costs, however, are often 10 or more times higher than the cost of the sensors. The main reason for this is the cost of the associated software and infrastructure necessary to provide the system-level support and decision-making. Software development and validation costs remain relatively high, particularly in a safety critical environment such as healthcare. These costs must be spread over a large number of installations if they are not to dominate the cost of telecare. This means that the financial viability of telecare services is a question of scale.

This has been recognized by the UK government. The statement of evidence presented to the House of Lords Science and Technology Committee included, for example, 'We [the Department of Health] are big purchasers...we have people...who have an expertise in understanding the market place...I have got them working on how we can best drive down the price of technologies.'[8]

Conclusion

Telecare is characterized by an absence of direct evidence for its cost-effectiveness, the need for a significant capital investment and the fact that any savings are likely to accrue to others in the healthcare system – not those making the investment. This means that an element of financial risk undoubtedly exists when telecare is embraced. Anyone who is considering the introduction of a telecare service is thus faced with a series of decisions, supported by relatively little evidence in critical areas such as cost-effectiveness. However, this does not mean that telecare should be neglected or abandoned. In pockets of telecare work, positive, and significant, financial returns are being reported. Numerous intangible benefits also are associated with telecare, and patient satisfaction is often reported as high. What is required is greater attention to generating the evidence as the field matures. Cost-effectiveness work from structured and well-controlled trials must be used to prioritize telecare applications that provide the greatest returns – both financially and for the user.

Further reading

Audit Commission. *Implementing telecare. Strategic analysis and guidelines for policy makers, commissioners and providers*. London: Audit Commission, 2004. Available at: www.audit-commission.gov.uk/Products/NATIONAL-REPORT/ BDBE0111-764C-44a4-8A66-1CB25D6974A4/Telecare.pdf (last accessed 15 November 2005).

Brownsell S, Bradley D. *Assistive technology and telecare: forging solutions for independent living*. Bristol: Policy Press, 2003.

Department of Trade and Industry. *Technology and delivery of care for older people – a mission to Japan*. London: Department of Trade and Industry, 2004. Available at: www.oti.globalwatchonline.com/online_pdfs/36238MR.pdf?pubpdfdload=05%2F 535 (last accessed 10 December 2005).

References

1   Whitten P, Kingsley C, Grigsby J. Results of a meta-analysis of cost-benefit research: is this a question worth asking? *J Telemed Telecare* 2000;**6** (Suppl 1):4–6.
2   Wootton R. Telemedicine in the National Health Service. *J R Soc Med* 1998;**91**:614–21.
3   Curry RG, Trejo Tinoco M, Wardle D. *Telecare: using information and communication technology to support independent living by older, disabled and vulnerable people. Report for UK Department of Health.* London: Department of Health, 2003. Available at: www.icesdoh.org.uk/downloads/ICT-Older-People-July-2003.pdf (last accessed 8 December 2005).
4   Ofcom. *Digital television, internet and broadband update – April 2004* Document 11. London: Ofcom, 2004. Available at: www.ofcom.org.uk/research/telecoms/reports/bbresearch/int_bband_updt/may2004/#content (last accessed 8 December 2005).
5   Roth A, Gadot R, Kalter E. Tele-cardiology for patients with chronic heart failure: the 'SHL' experience in Israel and Germany. *Stud Health Technol Inform* 2005;**114**:235–7.
6   Bowes A, McColgan G. *Smart technology at home: users' and carers' perspectives.* Stirling: University of Stirling, 2005. Available at: www.dass.stir.ac.uk/curr-proj/documents/Interimreport.pdf (last accessed 10 December 2005).
7   Audit Commission. *Independence and well-being 4: assistive technology.* London: Audit Commission, 2004. Available at: www.audit-commission.gov.uk/reports/NATIONAL-REPORT.asp?CategoryID=&ProdID=BB070AC2-A23A-4478-BD69-4C19BE942722 (last accessed 8 December 2005).
8   House of Lords Committee on Science and Technology. *Ageing: scientific aspects.* London: Stationery Office, 2005. Available at: www.parliament.the-stationery-office.co.uk/pa/ld200506/ldselect/ldsctech/20/20.htm (last accessed 8 December 2005).
9   Woolham J. *Safe at home.* London: Hawker Publications, 2005.
10   Department of Veterans Affairs. *General telehealth in VA.* Washington, DC: Department of Veterans Affairs, 2006. Available at: www.va.gov/occ/THinVA.asp (last accessed 8 December 2005).
11   Jennett PA, Affleck Hall L, Hailey D, *et al.* The socio-economic impact of telehealth: a systematic review. *J Telemed Telecare* 2003;**9**:311–20.
12   Roine R, Ohinmaa A, Hailey D. Assessing telemedicine: a systematic review of the literature. *CMAJ* 2001;**165**:765–71.
13   Whitten PS, Mair FS, Haycox A, *et al.* Systematic review of cost effectiveness studies of telemedicine interventions. *BMJ* 2002;**324**:1434–7.
14   Magnusson L, Hanson E, Borg M. A literature review study of information and communication technology as a support for frail older people living at home and their family carers. *Technol Disabil* 2004;**16**:223–35.
15   May C, Williams T, Mort M, *et al. What factors promote or inhibit the effective evaluation of telehealthcare interventions? Final report.* Newcastle: University of Newcastle, 2002.
16   Brownsell S, Bradley D. *Assistive technology and telecare: forging solutions for independent living.* Bristol: Policy Press, 2003.
17   Constantelou A, Zambarloukos S. *Civilising technologies in healthcare provision: experiences and prospects for Europe.* Milan: Project STAR c/o Databank Consulting, 2005. Available at: www.databank.it/star/list_issue/h_5.html (last accessed 9 December 2005).
18   Loeb GE. *Telecare: enabling the virtual housecall.* Milwaukee, WI: Marquette University, 1999. Available at: www.eng.mu.edu/wintersj/HCTWorkshop/HCT-pos_GL-telecare.htm (last accessed 15 November 2005).
19   NHS Scotland. *Building a health service fit for the future.* Edinburgh: Scottish Executive, 2005.

▶ 24

Conclusion

Richard Wootton, Susan L. Dimmick and Joseph C. Kvedar

Introduction

This book shows that technology makes it possible to deliver high-quality healthcare to the home. Doctors can once again make home visits – albeit virtually – but they can also engage their patients in a healthcare partnership that brings benefits for both. Patients can take more responsibility for monitoring their symptoms and transmitting their physiological data, so that doctors and nurses can deliver better targeted, 'just-in-time' healthcare.

If home telehealth is to be adopted widely, however, it will need to be seen by healthcare planners as a cost-effective alternative to conventional practice. The problem is not that the studies to date have provided strong evidence against efficacy but rather that their methods preclude definitive statements. Many have used sample sizes that limit statistical power and others have been performed in settings that may not be generalizable to real clinical settings. Most studies have been based on convenience samples of patients rather than the populations that might benefit most from improved access to health services, such as those who are indigent and/or have complex chronic diseases.[1]

This pattern is not unique to home telehealth – or even telemedicine generally. Frequently, when new technologies are introduced into practice, they are introduced without a clear idea of which patients will benefit most, the balance of benefits and harms, and the value for money that technologies offer.[2] Frequently, such introductions do not stand the test of time.

Technology adoption in medicine

Health service and technology assessment is part of the general move towards evidence-based medicine. Health technology assessment can be used to promote access to safe, efficacious and cost-effective technologies and – at least in principle – to discourage access to undesirable ones. Of course, home telehealth is not strictly a technology. It is more than this – it is a technique. Nonetheless, home telehealth will need to jump the hurdle of formal health technology assessment if it is to be adopted on a wide scale.

Adoption of technology into the mainstream of healthcare practice involves more than simply assessing the cost-effectiveness of a particular new development. There are actually three stages (Fig. 24.1). These are:

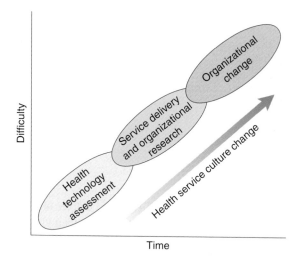

Fig. 24.1. Health technology assessment is only the first step in the change in organizational culture required for adoption of new techniques into mainstream healthcare service delivery

- Health technology assessment – the cost-effectiveness of a particular intervention may be examined, e.g. telemonitoring in patients with congestive heart failure.
- Service delivery and organizational research – if a likely-looking intervention can be identified, then service delivery and organizational research will be required to answer questions such as: what is the appropriate setting for the intervention, e.g. primary or secondary care?
- Organizational change – having identified a cost-effective intervention and decided how best to make use of it, the last stage is to bring about the necessary change in practice.

In many ways, the last step to widespread adoption – bringing about organizational change – is the most difficult in healthcare, where organizations tend to be large and to have huge inertia. It may be recalled that the *Titanic* (Fig. 24.2) was an 'organizational unit' that had great difficulty in changing direction when faced with an unexpected problem …

Current problems

As this book shows, telehealth is already an option deserving of serious consideration for delivering healthcare services to the home. In addition to the delivery of clinical care, the educational aspects of telemedicine can provide important health information to patients, families and healthcare practitioners. Despite this significant and emerging role, a number of problems and unresolved issues remain. Principal among these is the lack of evidence from research or programme evaluation to support the quality of clinical care provided by home telehealth compared to in-home, traditional contact.

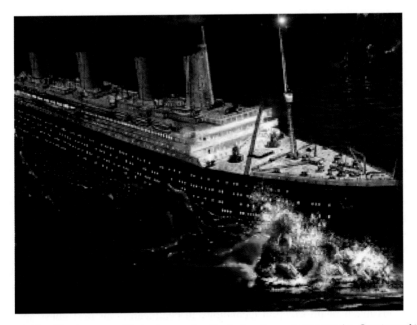

Fig. 24.2. The *Titanic* was unable to change direction in time to avert catastrophe. Courtesy of the Titanic Nautical Resource Center (www.titanic-nautical.com/Legal.html)

Innovation, demand and investment in telehealth will be impeded as long as formal evidence of its clinical efficacy and cost benefit is unavailable or not accepted widely.[3] Nonetheless, some evidence exists (see Chapter 6).

In the US, and perhaps to a lesser extent elsewhere, important issues of reimbursement need to be solved. This may require more effective coordination of planning, policy-making and allocation of resources among government, academic and private organizations than has occurred so far. Table 24.1 shows the central issues identified in home telehealth.[4]

Fear of change might also be added to this list. As Chapter 4 shows, the behavioural issues are perhaps the least of the obstacles to be overcome.

Table 24.1. Central issues in home telehealth[4]

Category	Potential barrier
Technical	• Lack of technical knowledge
	• Fear of technology
Economic	• Lack of third-party reimbursement
	• Financial obstacles for home-health agency
Organizational	• Lack of organizational support
	• Inadequate workflow processes
Behavioural	• Resistance from healthcare staff
	• Resistance from patients and caregivers

Many home telehealth programmes currently operate as research programmes or part of new initiative grants. The cost-effectiveness and economic sustainability of home telehealth programmes independent from research or other grants need to be studied carefully. Certain medicolegal aspects of the delivery of healthcare at a distance remain unresolved issues.

Place of telehealth in home care

What then is the place of telehealth in home care? The editors of this book are not blind advocates for the use of home telehealth (nor for telemedicine in general), and in particular, we do not suggest that telehealth will completely replace physical outreach services or that patients will never need to be transferred to hospitals in the future. Rather, we have tried to present the current and potential applications of home telehealth in a disinterested way, identifying the benefits but at the same time highlighting the limitations and unresolved issues. As the book shows, telemedicine seems to have great potential in the home healthcare field, and its many applications deserve careful investigation. Hopefully, it will not fall victim to the hyperbole that surrounds much of information technology in healthcare. Our best guess about the place of telehealth in future home care is that it will form a valuable part of the disease management process. When used intelligently, home telehealth will supplement conventional delivery techniques – not replace them.

The future

The successful use of home telehealth allows clinical services to be redesigned. Nurses can reduce their travelling time and consequently manage a bigger caseload. Furthermore, telehealth allows providers to apply their expertise across the country – or even between countries. This permits 'time-shifting', thus allowing more flexibility in employing staff to deliver out-of-hours services at more convenient times. We have already seen the provision of out-of-hours radiology services in the US, which are delivered by board-certified radiologists based in Australia (Box 24.1). Similar developments can be expected to occur in home telehealth as more widespread adoption occurs.

Telemedicine can also provide educational benefits for patients, families and health professionals alike. Incremental education over time affords both patients and caregivers the opportunity to have care concepts reinforced.

Future research into home telehealth should include evaluation of its utility and cost-effectiveness compared to traditional services and care provided in person. It also should include evaluation of the effectiveness of education and information provided to consumers and health professionals. Continued expansion of home telehealth services combined with rigorous research and evaluation will determine the definitive place of telemedicine in the armamentarium of home healthcare.

Box 24.1. NightHawk Radiology Services

NightHawk Radiology Services is based in Sydney, Australia, and provides teleradiology services to hospitals and radiology groups in the US. The company mainly supplies radiology coverage to emergency departments during evening and night hours in the US – this corresponds to daytime and evening work hours in Australia. This time difference is attractive for recruiting and retaining highly qualified radiologists to provide out-of-hours services.

NightHawk Radiology Services provides rapid preliminary radiological interpretations at the time of the patient visit to the emergency department. Official (primary) interpretations are provided by local radiologists at the hospital the following day. A key to the company's success has been in employing well-qualified radiologists. All are certified by the American Board of Radiology, and many also have fellowship subspeciality training. The radiologists are fully licensed in all American states and have credentials in all hospitals for which they provide their radiology services.

Summary

The experience reported in this book shows that no single 'correct answer' exists to what is fundamentally a multidisciplinary problem – often several different solutions are possible. Home telehealth, although at an early stage, seems to be an exciting technique that deserves serious consideration. An index of 'civilization' is the way that society treats its elderly and its sick;[5] on this measure, many countries might be considered to have failed. Perhaps home telehealth can be used in the future to improve the way that elderly and infirm people are looked after.

References

1   Brantley D, Laney-Cummings K, Spivack R. *Innovation, demand and investment in telehealth.* Washington, DC: US Department of Commerce, 2004. Available at: www.technology.gov/reports/ TechPolicy/Telehealth/2004Report.pdf (last accessed 15 November 2005).
2   Stevens A, Milne R, Lilford R, Gabbay J. Keeping pace with new technologies: systems needed to identify and evaluate them. *BMJ* 1999;**319**:1291.
3   Hersh WR, Wallace JA, Patterson PK, *et al. Telemedicine for the Medicare population: pediatric, obstetric, and clinician-indirect home interventions.* Rockville, MD: Agency for Healthcare Research and Quality, 2001. Available at: www.ahrq.gov/clinic/tp/telemedsuptp.htm (last accessed 23 December 2005).
4   Essey M, ed. *Home telehealth reference 2005.* Pittsburgh, PA: Quality insights of Pennsylvania, 2005. Available at: www.tmf.org/homehealth/telehealth/ (last accessed 8 January 2006).
5   Carter J. *The measure of a society is found in how they treat their weakest and most helpless citizens.* Available at: quotationnation.com/quote_20211.htm (last accessed 16 January 2006).

Index